Vitamin and Carrier Functions of Polyprenoids

World Review of Nutrition and Dietetics

Vol. 31

Series Editor
Geoffrey H. Bourne, St. Georges University School of Medicine,
Grenada, West Indies

S. Karger · Basel · München · Paris · London · New York · Sydney

Symposium on Vitamin and Carrier Functions of Polyprenoids, Bangalore, December 8–11, 1976

Vitamin and Carrier Functions of Polyprenoids

Volume Editors
H.R. Cama and P.S. Sastry, Bangalore

47 figures and 55 tables, 1978

S. Karger · Basel · München · Paris · London · New York · Sydney

World Review of Nutrition and Dietetics

Vol. 26: Human and Veterinary Nutrition. G.H. Bourne, Atlanta, Ga. (ed.)
XII + 274 p., 22 fig., 21 tab., 1977. ISBN 3–8055–2392–0
Vol. 27: Some Aspects of Human Nutrition. G.H. Bourne, Atlanta, Ga. (ed.)
X + 178 p., 17 fig., 81 tab., 1977. ISBN 3–8055–2393–9
Vol. 28: Some Aspects of Human and Veterinary Nutrition. G.H. Bourne, Atlanta, Ga. (ed.)
XII + 260 p., 21 fig., 37 tab., 1978. ISBN 3–8055–2672–5
Vol. 29: Toxicology and Nutrition. R. Truhaut, Paris, and R. Ferrando, Alfort (eds.)
X + 190 p., 27 fig., 41 tab., 1978. ISBN 3–8055–2697–0
Vol. 30: Human and Veterinary Nutrition, Biochemical Aspects of Nutrients.
G.H. Bourne, Grenada, West Indies (ed.)
X + 236 p., 22 fig., 20 tab., 1978. ISBN 3–8055–2789–6

Cataloging in Publication
Symposium on Vitamin and Carrier Functions of Polyprenoids, Bangalore, 1976
Vitamin and carrier functions of polyprenoids: Symposium on Vitamin and
Carrier Functions of Polyprenoids, Bangalore, December 8–11, 1976/
volume editors, H.R. Cama and P.S. Sastry.–Basel; New York: Karger, 1978
(World review of nutrition and dietetics; v. 31)
Sponsored by the Indian National Science Academy and other agencies.
1. Vitamin A–physiology–congresses 2. Vitamin D–physiology–congresses
3. Vitamin E–physiology–congresses
I. Cama, H.R., ed. II. Sastry, P.S., ed. III. Indian National Science Academy
IV. Title V. Series
W1 W0898 v.31 QU 165 S989v 1976
ISBN 3–8055–2801–9

ISBN 3–8055–2801–9

Advisory Board

Contents

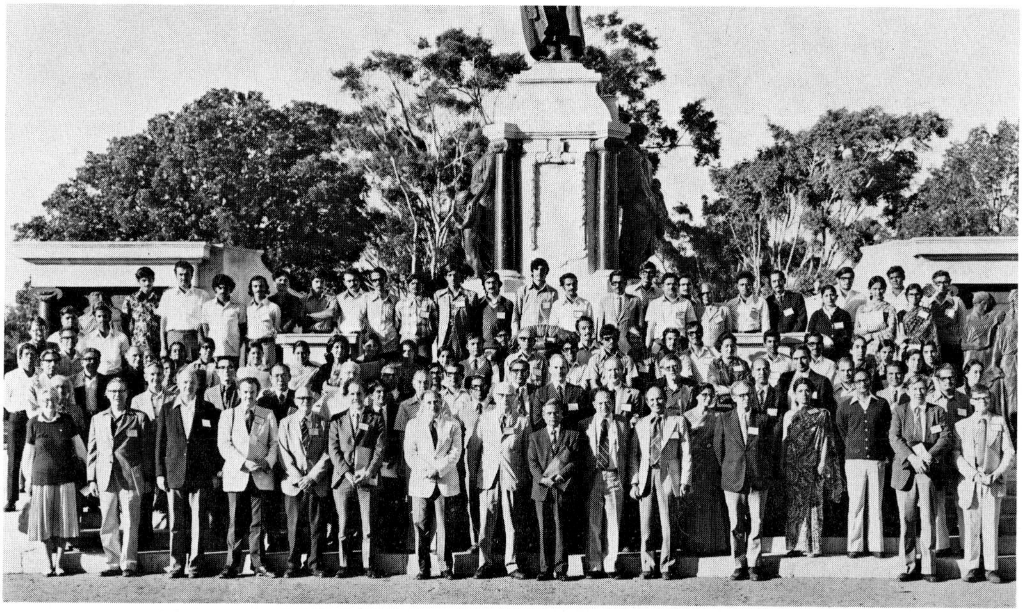

Participants of the Symposium held at the
Department of Biochemistry of the Indian Institute of Science, Bangalore, India

Professor R.A. Morton, F.R.S.
Born – 1899 : Died – 1977

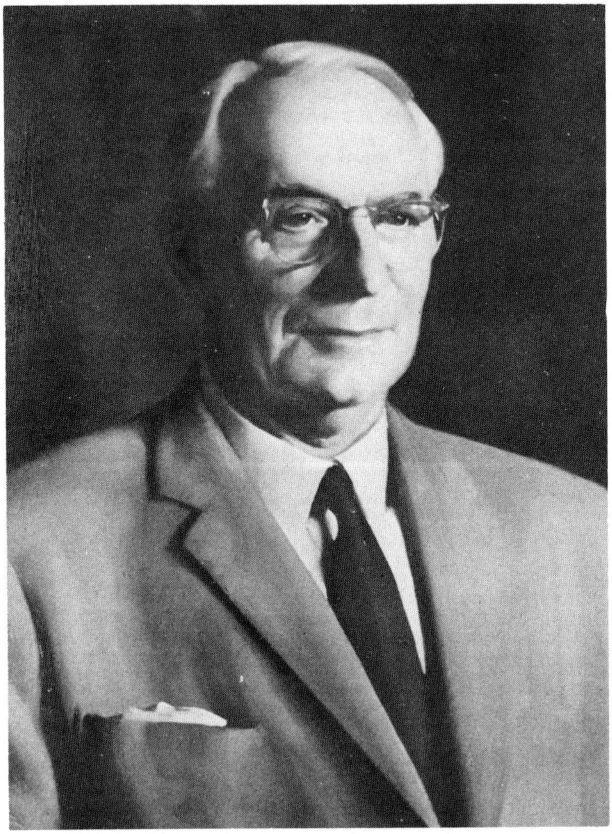

Professor *Richard Allan Morton*, F.R.S., obtained his Ph.D. in 1923, and D.Sc. in 1928, from the University of Liverpool. He was elected in 1944 to the Johnstone Chair of Biochemistry at the University of Liverpool, which position he filled with great distinction for about 22 years. He was elected Fellow of the Royal Society in 1950. His research interests were in spectroscopy, biochemistry of vitamins, food additives and general biochemistry and his work on several aspects of carotenoids, vitamins A_1 and A_2, visual pigments and ubiquinones has been outstanding. He was the author of several publications, reviews and books on 'Absorption spectra of vitamins and hormones', 'Biochemistry of quinones', and his two recent volumes on 'Biochemical spectroscopy' are of immense benefit to the biochemical community. With great qualities of head and heart, he enjoyed the respect of biochemists and scientists all over the world.

A number of national and international symposia were organized in his honour. His last international commitment was to participate and preside over the International Symposium on 'Vitamin and carrier functions of polyprenoids' held at the Indian Institute of Science, Bangalore, during December 8–11, 1976. He was in excellent health and enjoyed the scientific meeting and 'get-together' of scientists. It is sad to record that within two months of the International Symposium at Bangalore, Professor Morton died suddenly at his home after a short illness. The privilege of honouring him for the last time has fallen on me, who was associated with him for over 5 years at the University of Liverpool. May His Soul Rest in Eternal Peace.

H.R. Cama
Convener of the Symposium

Preface

The fat-soluble vitamins, A, D, E and K have been known for a long time and their deficiency syndromes have been well characterized. However, in spite of the many advances made in this field, their mode of action in molecular terms still remains obscure. A good deal of research is being carried out all over the world on polyprenoids, especially the fat-soluble vitamins, and it is gratifying that this is also an active area of sustained research in many laboratories in India. The symposium on 'Vitamin and carrier functions of polyprenoids' was planned to bring together scientists from abroad with those from India and provide a forum for exchange of views and ideas so that this important area would receive renewed impetus and thrust.

We are very happy that about forty scientists, in roughly equal numbers both from abroad and from India, participated in the symposium, and that a number of young research workers from various Indian universities and research institutions also attended. Inevitably, the majority of papers were on vitamin A, but other areas were also fairly well represented. In particular, the characterization and role of binding-proteins in vitamin A transport and metabolism received a great deal of attention. The recent developments on the role of vitamin K in the carboxylation of preprothrombin were brought sharply into focus. Another refreshing aspect of the symposium was the discussion on social relevance of the current researches, particularly on carotenoids and vitamin A in clinical nutrition. The excellent work being carried out in different parts of the world in combating blindness due especially to want of nutritional factors in the vulnerable group of the population, was highlighted. The publication of the deliberations of the symposium should be of considerable help in our appreciation of the metabolic role of fat-soluble vitamins and other polyprenoids.

Many scientific organizations in India and abroad supported this symposium. For their sponsorship and financial assistance, we are grateful to the following: Indian National Science Academy, University Grants Commission,

Indian Council of Medical Research, Council of Scientific and Industrial Research, Department of Atomic Energy, Department of Science and Technology, Indian Institute of Science, Ministry of Defence, Society of Biological Chemists (India), Royal Institute of Chemistry (Deccan Section) and the Chemical Society. We wish to thank science foundations and societies abroad for making travel grants available to enable several scientists to come and participate in this symposium. We must record our sincere appreciation of the excellent assistance given to us in the organization of the symposium by the authorities of our Institute and by many of our colleagues, in particular, Professors *N. Appaji Rao* and *T. Ramasarma.*

Bangalore, India, May 1977

H.R. Cama
P.S. Sastry

Wld Rev. Nutr. Diet., vol. 31, pp. 1–9 (Karger, Basel 1978)

Retinaldehyde-Protein Pigments

R.A. Morton
University of Liverpool, Liverpool

I wish to thank the organizers of this symposium for the honour they confer on me by inviting me to preside over the conference.

We are meeting in 1976, almost exactly 100 years since Franz Boll presented a classical paper to the Berlin Academy (23 November, 1876). He described how a freshly excised frog retina was pink in colour and became 'bleached' on exposure to light. The colour, associated with retinal rods was due to a pigment designated *sehrot* found in the retinas of many species. Boll's work was brilliantly extended by F.W. Kuhne (1877, 1878) and his designation *sehpurpur* was translated as 'visual purple'. Kuhne probably made as much progress as was then possible. The next advances came with the development of spectrophotometry about 20 years later. Soon after World War I, Hecht, using new methods, made further progress.

Then came the isolation of vitamin A_1 and the discovery of vitamin A_2, visual purple became rhodopsin and new related pigment porphyropsin was discovered by *Wald*, who described retinene$_1$ and retinene$_2$ as decomposition products. The retinenes were then shown to be the aldehydes derived from retinol and 3-dehydroretinol (vitamin A_2).

The biochemistry department in this institute has, for many years, sustained the interest in vitamins A, their chemistry and physiology, and many advances have come from here. Many of your visitors, too, have struggled to elucidate aspects of the modes of action of this and other fat-soluble vitamins. We all share the hope that the confluence of experiences, of ideas and techniques will be effective. The more unexpected the outcome the better we shall be pleased.

There is now a vast body of knowledge about visual pigments due to contributions by workers from many disciplines (for a survey, see *Morton* (25)), and the photochemistry of rhodopsin itself is complex. There is now general agreement that retinaldehyde forms a Schiff-base with a lipoprotein opsin, probably with an ϵ-amino group of a lysine moiety, and that the base becomes protonated

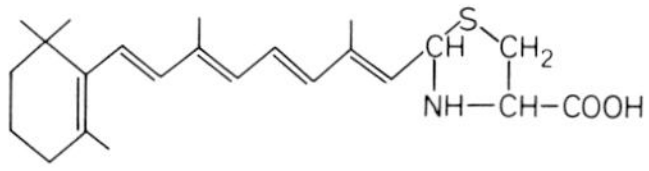

Fig. 1. Retinal and cysteine yielding a thiazolidine carboxylic acid.

with a displacement of λ-max into the visible region. Further displacements are characteristic of the various opsins and are often attributed to interactions between the protonated retinylidene derivatives and certain amino acid residues. There is, however, no full explanation of such effects apart from the postulate of conformation changes.

Wald's group (38) found that all-*trans* retinyl esters could be isomerised to 11-*cis* retinyl esters, or all-*trans* retinol to 11-*cis* retinol, which was changed to 11-*cis* retinal (via an alcohol dehydrogenase), which united with opsin to form rhodopsin. Under the action of light the rhodopsin (after the intermediate stages) yielded all-*trans* retinal which was then converted to all-*trans* retinol. Porphyropsin, occurring with rhodopsin in the eyes of many fish species, was shown to be based on 11-*cis*-3-dehydroretinal (14).

In the fly *Calliphora, Burkhardt*'s pioneer work (3) using intracellular micro-electrodes, revealed three types of cells, with sensitivity peaks at 470, 490 and 520 nm, together with a second peak at about 345 nm in each type of cell. At that stage it seemed that each pigment had both a visible peak and the 345 nm peak. This suggestion has been contested and the issue is important.

A considerable body of elegant physiological work has added much information in this multi-disciplinary area (1, 6, 15, 16). In the higher *Diptera* the ommatidia show, in cross-section, seven distinct rhabdomeres (six (1–6) grouped outside a central one made up of two smaller retinula cells 7 and 8). The six outer retinula cells are effective in dim light and the central ones in bright light. *Horridge and Mimura* (15) showed by polarization studies that the two peaks of the spectral sensitivity curves of *Calliphora* corresponded to two visual pigments. The peak sensitivity to polarized light for the 345 nm pigment is at an angle to that for the 490 nm pigment. The pigments are separated in proximal and distal parts of the rhabdomere with a twist between the two parts. *Horridge et al.* (16) found that in the drone fly *Eristalis tenex* most of the photoreceptors had double peaks (350 and 450 nm) as well as occasional cells with one peak (at 350, 450 or 520 nm) but *Bishop* (1) had observed cells with only one type of visual pigment. It is, however, agreed that the species has an ultraviolet-sensitive receptor substance distinct from the pigments of the visible region (fig. 1).

Goldsmith (11) had already discussed the problem of accounting for a peak at 345–350 nm occurring in a derivative of retinaldehyde. *Peskin and Love* (32) has found that retinaldehyde and cysteine combined to give a thiazolidine carboxylic acid with λ-max *ca.* 335 nm and displaying no displacement on acidification. It is reasonable to explore the idea that a cysteine terminal residue in a polypeptide chain of an opsin can form a holoprotein with *h*-max *ca.* 345 nm. The hypothesis is consistent with retaining retinaldehyde as the prosthetic group, but it allows little for effects on protein conformation. The difficulty, from a chemistry standpoint, is to devise a structure related to that of retinaldehyde which accounts for a considerable shift of the retinaldehyde peak in the direction of shorter wavelengths but retains the photochemical lability necessary for a light receptor.

Gogola et al. (9), using 2% aqueous digitonin, extracted a visual pigment of the ultraviolet receptor of the neuropteran *Ascalaphus macaronius Scop.* The solution absorbed maximally at 345 nm. When the pigment is irradiated with ultraviolet light at pH 5.2 the photoproduct shows λ-max 483 nm. If the pH is changed to 9.3, the 483 nm pigment is converted to a stable form with λ-max 375 nm. When the ultraviolet pigment is denatured, the liberated prosthetic group is retinal. The ultraviolet pigment incorporating a Schiff-base must have a shorter conjugated double bond system than that of rhodopsin. The problem has not been solved, but I offer a suggestion for scrutiny.

It will be remembered that vitamin A (retinol) is readily dehydrated to give anhydrovitamin A, and that when this is fed to rats it is converted to rehydrovitamin A (*retro*-retinol). Vitamin A_2 yields a 4-alkoxy anhydroretinol and apparently a rehydrovitamin A_2 occurs naturally. Once it is admitted that *retro*-retinol can exist in nature, *retro*-retinol, an aldehyde lacking α,β-unsaturation, becomes the simplest candidate for a retinylidene Schiff-base not readily susceptible to bathochromic shifts. It could in principle exhibit a resonance form with an exocyclic double bond (28).

Oesterhelt and Christoffel (27) used bacterioopsin in testing retinaldehyde analogues. *Sumper et al.* (34) had grown halobacteria in the presence of 1 m*M* nicotine and found that, although there was no change in generation time, there was no biosynthesis of retinal and no formation of purple pigment. *Oesterhelt and Schuhmann* (29), by removing the prosthetic group with hydroxylamine, also obtained the membrane apoprotein before successfully reconstituting the pigment. *Oesterhelt and Christoffel* (27) recorded that the aldehyde group was indispensable for regenerating bacteriorhodopsin, but the C_{25} and C_{30} analogues of retinal failed to work. The positions of the methyl groups were necessarily those of retinol and retinal, and bacterioopsin would only form pigments with the 9-*cis* and 11-*cis* of retinal isomers. 3-Dehydroretinal and bacterioopsin combined to give a functional chromoprotein (blue in colour). Pigments were also formed with 4-hydroxyretinal and 5,6-epoxyretinal, but they were not effective in proton pumping.

Laser light has been used in the study of ultra-fast physical and chemical changes by spectroscopic methods (4) and very intense pulses lasting a few picoseconds (10^{-12} s). *Kaufman et al.* (17) found that the rate of formation of the first intermediate in the photo-cycle of bacteriorhodopsin is approximately $10^{11}\,s^{-1}$. A transient absorption peak occurs near 580 nm and has been tentatively ascribed to an excited singlet state. Bacteriorhodopsin has all-*trans* retinal, and the possibility arises that the primary process does not allow enough time for the 11-*cis* ⟶ all-*trans* rearrangement. *Busch et al.* (5) using a 530 nm laser found that prelumirhodopsin (i.e., bathorhodopsin) with *h*-max 560 nm was formed from bovine rhodopsin in 6 ps and had a life-time of 30 ns.

Montal (24) has argued that the classical rhodopsin photo-chemical change from 11-*cis* retinal to all-*trans* (21, 35) changes the protein conformation leading to conductance changes in the retinal photoreceptor cell membrane (13). *Montal* has presented a case that rhodopsin acts as a light-activated ion translocator. Accepting that Ca^{2+} is the transmitter, *Montal*'s model proposes a channel closed in the dark with Ca^{2+}-dependent ATPase pumping Ca^{2+} into the rod discs. On bleaching, the channel opens and allows Ca^{2+} to diffuse down to its concentration gradient. The efflux of Ca^{2+} would close the channel. This, with the photo-regeneration of rhodopsin and functioning of the pump, would restore the membrane to the dark adapted state.

The current state of knowledge still leaves much to be elucidated about the visual pigments that mediate daylight vision. Dim light vision involving rhodopsins is not of course more important than bright light colour vision, but its historical significance in the development of ideas is crucial. Retinochrome is, perhaps, a special aspect of the larger problem but, again, its role together with the unusual properties of squid rhodopsin constitute a significant widening of ideas. Bacteriorhodopsin, considered as a part of the overall set of problems, is an almost unique biological adaptation, but its action as a photochemical proton pump – a new and special case of photophosphorylation – brings it into a central, incompletely understood, area of biochemistry. The existence of an ultraviolet photoreceptor in insect eyes reminds us that size is a factor of great importance. The membranes in the small and delicate eyes of insects transmit radiations which would fail to pass through similar tissues of larger creatures. The biological advantages of an insect ultraviolet receptor can be appreciated even if the detailed chemistry eludes us at present.

The C_{50} carotenoids of halobacteria constitute separate, but real, challenges (18).

We may now scrutinise current ideas on the original problem. When the decomposition of rhodopsins is studied at different temperatures and at different pH values, a very complex situation emerges. The initial effect, at the temperature of liquid helium, depends on the wave-length of the filtered light used to effect a change. Thus, wave-lengths greater than 540 nm (i.e., 540–575 nm absorbed) convert rhodopsin to hypsorhodopsin, so named because λ-max undergoes a hypochromic shift from 500 to 430 nm. Hypsorhodopsin exposed to radiation of wave-length 406 nm forms a compound bathorhodopsin (λ-max 543 nm), so called because of the bathochromic shift. Irradiation with light of wave-length 437 nm converts rhodopsin (reversibly) to bathorhodopsin. It may be that bathorhodopsin is the significant initial product leaving hypsorhodopsin as an alternative under special conditions of irradiation. Lumirhodopsin, metarhodopsin I and metarhodopsin II appear at higher temperatures. According to *Yoshizawa* (37) the prosthetic group retinal changes from 11-*cis* to all-*trans* at the initial stage and the final step is perhaps the decomposition of metarhodopsin II to give the protein opsin and all-*trans* retinal. The latter undergoes isomerization to 11-*cis* retinal which forms a Schiff-base with opsin to regenerate rhodopsin.

It is of course possible that at physiologic temperatures the whole sequence proceeds, but with very great speed. It may, however, be prudent to inquire whether some of the earliest steps do, in fact, occur at body temperature.

If bathorhodpsin is considered to be the initial product, the obvious need is to find a structural explanation of the 500–543 nm displacement. The significance of such a shift gains importance from the fact that it also occurs with squid rhodopsin and that iodopsin has a 560–640 nm shift and porphyropsin 523–592 nm.

Oseroff and Callender (31) used resonance Raman spectroscopy to study retinal rod disc membranes at –190°C. The pigment, under laser irradiation, set up a photostationary state containing rhodopsin, isorhodopsin (13-*cis*) and bathorhodopsin. *In situ* rhodopsin contains 11-*cis* retinal and opsin joined by a protonated Schiff-base which can be deuterated so that a stretching vibration is displaced (1655–1630 cm^{-1}). Bathorhodopsin shows three good peaks at 856, 877 and 920 cm^{-1} absent from all-*trans* retinylidene solutions.

Fransen et al. (8), doubting that the 11-*cis*-all-*trans* step occurred at the initial stage, postulated a different explanation for the resonance Raman spectra and invoked a *retro*-structure with an exomethylene double bond at C_{18} (fig. 2).

They attributed a 1539 cm^{-1} peak to the ene-amine structure shown in a protonated Schiff-base and the 877 cm^{-1} peak to a wagging vibration of a 1,1-dialkyl substituted ethene. Terpenes like sabinene, nopinine and camphene with an exomethylene bond show strong peaks at 920, 877 and 856 cm^{-1}. Cholecalciferol, which also has an exomethylene group, also has peaks at 930, 894, 880 and 863 cm^{-1}.

If the *retro*-retinal structure were an intermediate in the rhodopsin photolysis, at some stage in the thermal processes following the formation of bathorhodopsin, a hydrogen atom would have to be reattached at C_{18} so as to obtain all-*trans* retinal. *Fransen et al.* (8) observed some (5–7%) incorporation of deuterium in retinal extracted from rhodopsin regenerated from D_2O-incubated opsin-11-*cis* retinal mixtures. It was felt that all the evidence pointed to hydrogen exchange between chromophore and apoprotein during photolysis.

Kropf (20) was not satisfied by the proton transfer hypothesis for the initial

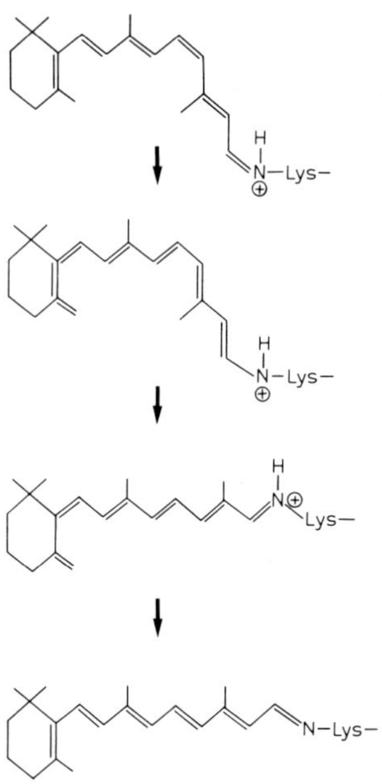

Fig. 2. (a) Probable structure of prosthetic group of native rhodopson (11-*cis*); (b) postulated structure of bathorhodopsin showing resonance Raman peaks at 856, 877 and 920 cm^{-1}. Peaks at 856, 877 and 920 cm^{-1} are shown by terpenes with an exomethylene double bond (sabinene, nopinene and camphene) and also by calciferol; (c) transient thermally produced product; (d) all-*trans* Schiff-base. Lys- stands for a lysyl group in a protein.

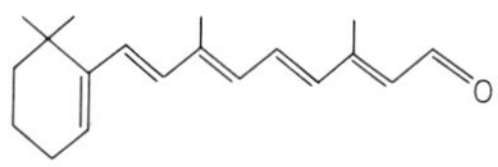

Fig. 3. Desmethyl retinal.

photochemical step in vision. He said that the 920, 877, 856 cm^{-1} peaks were matched in the spectra of crystalline 11-*cis* retinal. He prepared 5-desmethyl-retinal and obtained the all-*trans*, 9-*cis*, 11-*cis* and 13-*cis* isomers. Of these only the 11-*cis* and 9-*cis* forms combined with opsin from ox retinas, and they did so at 1% of the normal rate for retinal. The 5-desmethyl-retinals yielded rhodopsin analogues with λ-max 480 nm and a bathorhodopsin analogue with λ-max 525 nm (fig. 3).

The results showed that a batho-intermediate can be formed from a retinal analogue lacking an allylic methyl group in the molecule. Without such a group, *Kropf* said it was impossible to transfer a hydrogen atom or ion from a group on the ionone ring to opsin. The structure proposed for bathorhodopsin was, therefore, in his view to be rejected; but the infrared peaks cannot be dismissed easily.

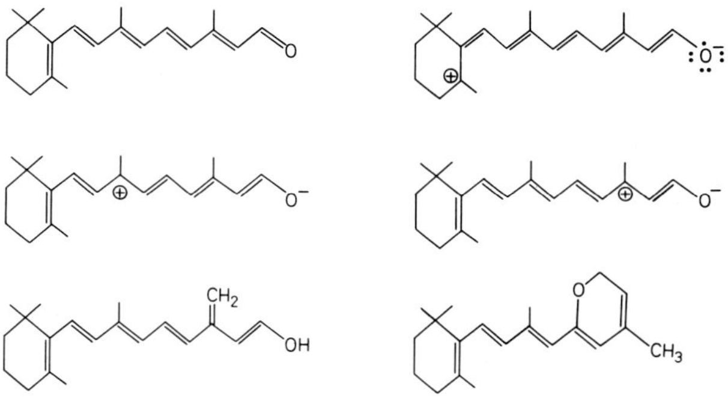

Fig. 4. (a), (b), (c) and (d) – Resonance forms of retinal; (e) and (f) – possible photoenolic forms.

Mathies and Stryer (23) studied the spectra of retinal, in an intense electric field. They examined all-*trans* retinal, its protonated base with n-butylamine and Cl-salt of the protonated Schiff-base. They recorded that retinal has a highly dipolar vertically excited singlet state, and found this consistent with an electrostatic mechanism for generating large spectral displacements. They regarded the plausible structures as (a) and (b) in resonance (fig. 4).

Emrich and Reich (7) using isolated bovine rod outer segments studied the metarhodopsin I-II equilibrium, using absorption changes measured by rapid flash photometry and found that H^+ uptake accompanied the transition. The equilibrium was pH-dependent in parallel with the proton uptake. Metarhodopsin-II conformation is stabilized by the protonation of an amino group which cannot be re-enfolded into the hydrophobic core as it is too polar. The binding group is not in the chromophoric region of rhodopsin. This fits well with the cascade of dark reactions in which metarhodopsin-I (λ-max 480 nm) yields metarhodopsin-II (λ-max 380 nm) and 11-*cis* retinal is replaced by all-*trans* retinal. The reaction time MI ⟶ MII fits the latency period for excitation and it is suggested that the conformation change triggers visual excitation.

Shichi and Somers (33) argued that the regeneration of rhodopsin from opsin and all-*trans* retinal involves separate reactions, first the isomerization all-*trans* ⟶ 11-*cis* and, second, the binding of 11-*cis* to opsin. Phospholipid is required for the isomerization, but phosphatidyl choline has no effect while phosphatidyl serine is inhibitory. Phosphatidyl ethanolamine forms a complex with all-*trans* retinal and the protonated Schiff-base (with λ-max 455 nm, $^{\epsilon}$max 43,600) effects a non-enzymic isomerization. Bleached rod outer segments form a complex (λ-max 458) with all-*trans* retinal in the dark and in light the aldehyde becomes 11-*cis*. The most effective radiation is in the region 450–460 nm. Isomerization activity in partially delipidated rod outer segments is restored by adding phosphatidyl ethanolamine. Some 30% of the latter associated with rod outer segments is involved in complex formation with all-*trans* retinal. The retinal remains in the complex after isomerization. Schichi and Somers consider that this is not inconsistent with an ϵ-amino group of lysine uniting with 11-*cis* retinal to form rhodopsin. Numerous other studies on retinals are relevant to further discussion (23) but not on this occasion.

It may be that the new ideas will be found compatible with the electrophysiological studies on the early receptor potential. But it is worthwhile to note again that the *Rentzepis* school find that the first spectroscopic change to bathorhodopsin occurs with a light flash of 6 ps and the decay time is 30 ns. Now the speed of light means that in 33 ps, the distance travelled is only 1 cm. As *Rentzepis* suggests and *Wald* agrees, the time allowed for the initial response is embarrassingly short. *Cis-trans* isomerization does of course occur, but it may not be the first, or possibly the most significant, step.

References

1 *Bishop, L.G.:* J. comp. Physol. *91:* 267 (1974).
2 *Brody, S.S.:* Z. Naturforsch *28c:* 157 (1973).
3 *Burkhardt, D.:* Symp. Soc. exp. Biol. *16:* 86 (1962).
4 *Busch, G.E. and Rentzepis, P.M.:* Science, N.Y. *194:* 276 (1976).
5 *Busch, G.E.; Applebury, M.L.; Lamola, A., and Rentzepis, P.M.:* Proc. natn. Acad. Sci. USA *69:* 2802 (1972).
6 *Eckert, M.:* Kybernitik *9:* 145 (1971); ibid. *14:* 1 (1973).
7 *Emrich and Reich, R.:* Z. Naturforsch *29c:* 577 (1974).
8 *Fransen, M.R.; Luyten, W.C.M.M.; van Thujil, J., Lugternburg, J.; Jansen, P.A.A.; van Breugel, P.J.G.M., and Daeman, F.J.M.:* Nature, Lond. *260:* 726 (1976).
9 *Gogola, M.; Hamdorf, K., and Schwemeor, J.:* Z. vergl. Physiol. *70:* 410 (1970).
10 *Goldsmith, T.H.:* Proc. natn. Acad. Sci. USA *44:* 123 (1958).
11 *Goldsmith, T.H.:* Handbook of sensory physiology; in *Dartnall* Photochemistry of vision; vol. VII/1, p. 683 (Springer, Berlin 1972).
12 *Grumbach, K.H. and Lichtenthaler, H.K.:* Z. Naturforsch. *28c:* 439 (1973).
13 *Hagins, W.A.:* Ann. Rev. Biophys. Bioeng. *1:* 131 (1972).
14 *Hara, T. and Hara, R.:* Handbook of sensory physiology; in *Dartnall* Photochemistry of vision; vol. VII/1, p. 720 (Springer, Berlin 1972).
15 *Horridge, G.A. and Mimura, K.:* Proc. R. Soc. Lond. *B190:* 211 (1975a).
16 *Horridge, G.A.; Mimura, K., and Tsukahara, Y.:* Proc. R. Soc. Lond. *B190:* 225 (1975b).
17 *Kaufman, J.J.; Rentzepis, P.M.; Stoeckenius, W., and Lewis, A.:* Biochem. biophys. Res. Commun. *68:* 1109 (1976).
18 *Kelly, M., Norgord, S., and Liaaen-Jensen, S.:* Acta chem. scand. *24:* 2169 (1970).
19 *Kleudgen, H.K. and Lichtenthaler, H.K.:* Z. Naturforsch *29c:* 142 (1974).
20 *Kropf, A.:* Nature, Lond. *264:* 92 (1976).
21 *Kropf, A.; Brown, P.K., and Hubbard, R.:* Nature, Lond. *183:* 146 (1959).
22 *Lichtenthaler, H.K. and Grumbach, K.H.:* Z. Naturforsch. *29c:* 532 (1974).
23 *Mathies, R. and Stryer, L.:* Proc. natn. Acad. Sci. USA *73:* 2169 (1976).
24 *Montal, M.:* Biochem. Soc. Trans. *4:* 560 (1976).

25 *Morton, R.A.:* Biochemical spectroscopy; in *Hilger* vol. 2; p. 543 (London 1975).
26 *Oesterhelt, D.:* Angew. Chem. *15:* 17 (1976).
27 *Oesterhelt, D. and Christoffel, V.:* Biochem. Soc. Trans. *4:* 556 (1976).
28 *Oesterhelt, D.; Hartmann, R.; Fischer, U.; Michel, H., and Schrekenbach, Th.:* Proc. FEBS 10th Meet. *40:* 239 (1975).
29 *Oesterhelt, D. and Schuhmann, L.:* FEBS Lett. *44:* 262 (1974).
30 *Oroshnik, W.; Brown, P.K.; Hubbard, R., and Wald, G.:* Proc. natn. Acad. Sci. USA *42:* 578 (1956).
31 *Oseroff, A.R. and Callender, R.H.:* Biochemistry *13:* 4243 (1974).
32 *Peskin, J.C. and Love, B.B.:* Biochim. biophys. Acta *78:* 751 (1963).
33 *Schichi, H. and Somers, R.L.:* J. biol. Chem. *249:* 6750 (1974).
34 *Sumper, M.; Reitmeier, H., and Oesterhelt, D.:* Angew. Chem. *15:* 187 (1976).
35 *Wald, G.:* Angew. Chem. *80:* 857 (1968).
36 *Yekowaski, N. and Brody, S.S.:* Z. Naturforsch. *29c:* 327 (1974).
37 *Yeshizawa, T.:* Handbook of sensory physiology; in *Dartnell* Photochemistry of vision; vol. VII/1, p. 146 (Springer, Berlin 1972).
38 *Yoshizani, T. and Wald, G.:* Nature, Lond. *201:* 340 (1964).

Dr. *R.A. Morton*, †, Emeritus Professor of Biochemistry, University of Liverpool, *Liverpool* (England)

Wld Rev. Nutr. Diet., vol. 31, pp. 10–15 (Karger, Basel 1978)

Isoprene Units:
Their Role in the Structure and Function of Terpenes, Carotenoids and Other Fat Soluble Vitamins

Ivan M. Sharman

Dunn Nutritional Laboratory, University of Cambridge and Medical Research Council, Cambridge

Isoprene – the polyene obtained by passing the vapour of dipentene over red hot platinum – is a secondary unsaturated hydrocarbon with a five-membered carbon chain. As its name suggests the chain is branched. It was first isolated by Willstatter and Mieg in 1907 and has since been shown to have the molecular formula C_5H_8 and the structural formula:

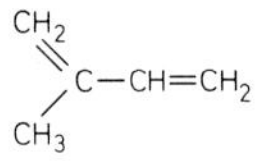

Fig. 1. Formula of isoprene.

Isoprene is a liquid of boiling point 34°C. When heated to 300°C under pressure it yields dipentene. Under certain conditions isoprene polymerises to caoutchouc, the hydrocarbon constituent of rubber.

The basic carbon skeleton of isoprene appears either singly, or repeated, in a large number of compounds which are both of chemical and biological importance, though, as will be seen later, the double bonds may undergo extensive rearrangement. Such compounds are known as polyprenoids, and occur extensively in plant and animal material. Thus this type of structure appears frequently in volatile oils of plants, the so-called essential oils, valued from early times because they carried the *Quinta essentia,* the delicious fragrance of the plants. Because of the occurrence of this type of compound in oil of turpentine the name 'terpenes' was given to them. As a result of the work of Perkin, Semmler, and others around the beginning of the century, the chemical nature of the terpenes became elucidated.

Terpenes

Terpenes are cyclic hydrocarbons of the general formula $(C_5H_8)_n$ and occur widely distributed in nature. They are the chief constituents of the essential oils obtained by distilling with steam the sap and tissues of certain plants, particularly those of the coniferous and citrus families. Essential oils or ethereal oils, prepared in this way, are used in the production of perfumes and in pharmacology.

Hydrocarbons of this type are generally subdivided into hemiterpenes C_5H_8 (of which isoprene itself is an example), terpenes $C_{10}H_{16}$, sesquiterpenes $C_{15}H_{24}$, diterpenes $C_{20}H_{32}$, triterpenes $C_{30}H_{48}$ and tetraterpenes $C_{40}H_{64}$. The various classes are readily distinguished by the marked differences in boiling points, the boiling points rising with increasing molecular weight.

The terpenes are all unsaturated hydrocarbons containing either one or two ethylene bonds in the molecule, according to which they are again divided into monocyclic and dicyclic terpenes. The majority of monocylcic terpenes are derived from *p*-cymene and have the following carbon skeleton:

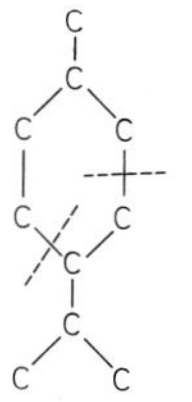

Fig. 2. Carbon skeleton of *p*-cymene.

The dotted lines indicate how the molecule may be regarded as made up of 2 isoprene units. Limonene, the chief constituent of the oil of orange rind, is a typical monocyclic terpene and has the formula:

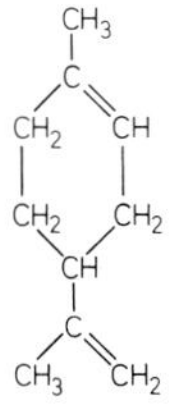

Fig. 3. Formula of limonene.

It also occurs along with pinene in oil of lemons. Small amounts, 11–17 mg/100 g, are present in commercial marmalades. However, there is no evidence that the compound has any nutritional value.

Many other monoterpenes and monoterpenoids, as their oxygen-containing derivatives are called, have been isolated from the essential oils. Examples are geraniol, menthol, and camphor; also about 150 sesquiterpenoids are known; half of these have already had complete structural formulae assigned to them. They can all be regarded as made up from 3 isoprene units; an example is the alcohol farnesol $C_{15}H_{25}OH$.

Diterpenoids

Diterpenoids are often present in high boiling fractions of essential oils and in the residues of the distillation of oleoresins, such as colophony obtained from pine trees. Related are a number of bitter substances, the plant hormone gibberellic acid, and the diterpene alkaloids. Most of these compounds have one or more ring systems. Phytol is the only naturally occurring representative of the acyclic series. Its occurrence in green plants as part of the chlorophyll molecule makes it one of the most widespread of the diterpenes.

The number of monocyclic structures in this group is also small. It includes α-camphorene, a constituent of camphor oil, and retinol. This is important for the present symposium as it is a vitamin.

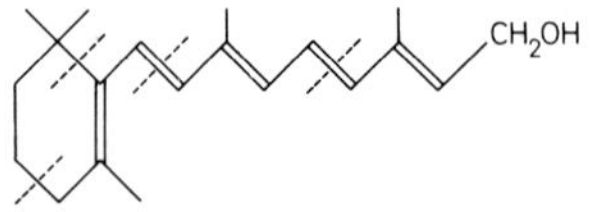

Fig. 4. Formula of retinol.

Vitamin A_2 has an extra double bond, is present in position 3, and is therefore known as 3-dehydro-retinol.

A congener of retinol, kitol (from Greek *kitos* = whale) has been prepared from whale-liver oil. Elementary analysis of the compound corresponded to $C_{20}H_{30}O$ and molecular weight determinations were in agreement with $C_{40}H_{60}O_2$. The compound is biologically inactive but it can be broken down to retinol by heating to over 200°C. Its structure, based mainly on NMR spectral data, has been reported by *Burger et al.* (1). This shows the molecule to have 3 rings and 4 asymmetric carbon atoms. This formula has been confirmed by *Giannotti et al.* (2) using mass spectroscopy and other methods.

Retinol is conveyed in the blood by attachment to a protein, named by de Witt Goodman, retinol binding protein (RBP). In an unusual case of self-imposed vitamin A deficiency the levels of carotenoids and retinol in the blood were measured. A young man, aged 20, who had been suffering epileptic fits from the age of 12 read an article in 'The New Scientist' entitled 'What too much vitamin A does to cells'. It mentioned the influence of the vitamin on membrane permeability. It is not clear how the patient was led by the article to believe that vitamin A was responsible for his epileptic condition, but he forthwith resolved to cut out all sources of the vitamin from his diet. This he did so effectively that his vitamin A blood levels fell to the lowest ever recorded in Great Britain, e.g., 7.8 and 4.1 μg retinol/100 ml plasma. Details of this case have already been published (5). On other occasions when blood specimens were taken the analysis was extended to include measurements of RBP carried out by Dr. Goodman. The results showed that when blood levels of retinol were very low the levels of RBP were also low. When the subject had ingested vitamin A and his blood levels of the vitamin were near normal, the RBP levels were found to have increased. These results are in keeping with the suggestion that the key action of retinol may be to catalyse the synthesis of RBP.

Triterpenoids

The formulae of triperpenes contain 30 carbon atoms and theoretically structures based on 6 isoprene units. Many compounds where this applies only to a part of the structure have been called triterpenoids. The steroids could strictly be included in this group of compounds but in practice are usually regarded as a separate class. Triterpenes are found in many plants in the free state and in combination with sugars and with acids as esters. The saponins are a widely distributed group.

An acyclic triterpene occurring extensively in animals is the compound squalene $C_{30}H_{50}$. It was originally isolated from a shark liver oil and later found to occur in other fish oils. It is also present in human earwax and hair oil. Squalene has been shown by Bloch to be a progenitor of cholesterol and is, therefore, of widespread occurrence.

Examples of triterpenoids are cholesterol and the triterpene alcohol lanosterol.

Tetraterpenoids

This group of compounds includes what are perhaps the most interesting and certainly the most colourful of the terpenoids. Most of the known members are found among the yellow and red pigments obtained from plants and animals. These carotenoid and xanthophyll pigments contain 8 isoprene units. The two halves of the molecule are arranged in such a way that the carbon skeletons can be constructed from 2 phytol chains in mirror-like fashion.

As a result of the new separation methods, e.g., thin layer chromatography, the number of individual carotenoids has increased from about 80 in 1948 (4) to the present total of over 300 (3). Furthermore, the great advances that have been made in methods for determining structure, such as spectroscopic measurements and mass spectra, have enabled the configuration of most of these compounds to be elucidated.

β-Carotene, the yellow colouring matter of the carrot is, of course, the best known of these compounds. In the combining together of the 8 isoprene units to form the molecule of β-carotene, 8 hydrogen atoms have to be discarded, and the double bonds have to be extensively rearranged. In regard to the spacing of the methyl groups in the central chain, 5 carbon atoms intervene between the 1st and 2nd, and 3rd and 4th methyl groups, but the 2nd and 3rd methyl groups are divided by 6 carbon atoms. This is due to the reversal of the asymmetric isoprene molecule which is orientated inwards from each ionone ring.

β-Carotene contains 2 β-ionone rings and is the most active isomer. Other forms are α-carotene, which contains one β-ionone ring and one α-ionone ring, and γ-carotene which contains one intact β-ionone ring and one opened β-ionone ring.

Other carotenoids of interest are the acyclic compounds, lycopene, phytofluene, ζ-carotene, and neurosporene.

Terpenoid quinones

The vitamin discovered by Dam in 1935 to prevent bleeding in chickens, was named by him vitamin K (Koagulations-vitamin). Another form of the vitamin discovered by Doisy is known as vitamin K_2. It possesses a C_{35} 7 isoprene-unit side chain. A lower isoprenolog with a C_{30} side chain has also been found in putrified fish meal, the source of the original K_2. Vitamin K_1 has long been established as 2-methyl-3-phytyl-1,4-napthoquinone. Both compounds are important biologically as the antihaemorrhagic vitamin. However, their biological activity does not depend on the presence of the long phytyl side chain as evidenced by the fact that menadione, which contains no side chain, is equally active. This compound, however, does not occur naturally.

Another class of terpenoids with more than 8 isoprene units is exemplified in the ubiquinones. As their name implies, these compounds are very widespread in nature occurring especially in liver and intestinal tissue. These substituted benzoquinones have a poly-terpenoid side chain of 25–50 carbon atoms. Several forms have been synthesized. The importance of this group in electron transport is wellknown. Coenzyme Q, one of the ubiquinones, has been shown to be essential in the reduction of cytochrome-*c* by succinate.

Terpenoid chromanes

Another group of biologically important compounds are based on the nucleus which is best known in vitamin E, α-tocopherol. This compound, necessary for the fertility of rats and other animals, also has antioxidant properties which are believed to be responsible for its physiological activity. Seven tocopherols, each a derivative of the parent substance tocol, 2-methyl, -2-(trimethyltridecyl)-6-hydroxychromane, have been found in nature.

The seven possible compounds arise from the fact that one, two, or three methyl groups can be substituted for hydrogen atoms in various positions in the tocol molecule. They are all antioxidants. The trimethyl tocol, α-tocopherol, is the most active. The dimethyl compounds are less active, and the monomethyl compounds still less active than α-tocopherol.

If the tocopherols are regarded as derived from a substituted phenol by ring closure, thereby forming the heterocyclic oxygen-containing ring, the chain length is that of 4 isoprene units.

Another series of compounds with vitamin E activity are the tocotrienols; these have double bonds in the phytyl side chain. These compounds occur in various plant products and their biological role is now being given much attention.

References

1 *Burger, B.V.; Garbers, C.F.; Pachler, K.; Bonnett, R., and Weedon, B.C.L.:* Chem. Commun. 588 (1965).

2 *Giannotti, C.; Das, B.C., and Lederer, E.:* Chem. Commun. 28 (1966).

3 *Isler, O.:* Carotenoids (Birkhauser, Basel 1971).

4 *Karrer, P. and Jucker, E.:* Carotenoids (Elsevier, New York 1950).

5 *Sharman, I.M.:* Am. J. clin. Nutr. *22:* 1134 (1969).

Dr. *I.M. Sharman,* Dunn Nutritional Laboratory, University of Cambridge and Medical Research Council, Milton Road, *Cambridge CB4 1XJ* (England)

Wld Rev. Nutr. Diet., vol. 31, pp. 16–20 (Karger, Basel 1978)

Mannosylretinyl Phosphate: Transfer of Mannose to Protein

S. Masushige, Gloria Chi Rosso and G. Wolf

Department of Nutrition and Food Science, Massachusetts Institute of Technology, Cambridge, Mass.

It is our hypothesis that one of the possible functions of vitamin A is to act as a lipid intermediate in the transfer of sugar moieties from nucleotide sugars to the growing oligosaccharide chains of glycoproteins. The synthesis, both *in vitro* and *in vivo,* of such lipid intermediates as mannosyl and galactosylretinyl phosphate has been amply documented, both in our laboratory and by others (1, 5, 6). The requisite precursor, retinyl phosphate, was shown to be present in the intestinal mucosa (2).

It was necessary to show that the sugar moiety was transferable to a protein acceptor. The characterization of this transfer reaction, from mannosylretinyl phosphate (MRP) to protein, forms the substance of this report.

We prepared ^{14}C-MRP from chemically synthesized retinyl phosphate and GDP-^{14}C-mannose by the liver microsome system and separated the MRP from dolichylmannosyl phosphate (DMP) by differential solvent extraction (6). DMP has been shown to serve as a substrate in mannosyl transfer reactions (4).

When incubating rat liver microsomes, acting as enzyme source and endogenous acceptor, with labeled MRP and DMP separately (fig. 1) we could get about 18% transfer of mannose to protein from MRP and 8% from DMP. Of course, the true meaning of these percentages is not clear, since we do not as yet know the pools of endogenous MRP and DMP in these preparations and hence their specific activities. That this represents true transfer to protein of mannose from MRP is clear. That this is not due to reversal of the reaction, from MRP to GDP-mannose and hence via newly-formed DMP to protein, was shown by the independence of the transfer reaction of Mn^{++} (table I) and the fact that addition of an excess of non-radioactive GDP-mannose had no effect on the reaction (fig. 2). It was interesting to note that during the transfer reaction with MRP, no radioactivity could be extracted into chloroform:methanol:water (10:10:3), suggesting that no oligosaccharide-lipid appeared to be formed as intermediate, whereas fully one-half of the radioactivity transferred from DMP could be recovered in this extract.

Table I. Effect of *Mn*$^{++}$ ion on ^{14}C-mannose transfer from ^{14}C-MRP to protein

Experiment	Substrate MRP, cpm	Addition of Mn^{++} (10 mM)	Protein cpm
A	2,800	–	442
		+	599
B	22,000	–	1,580
		+	1,650

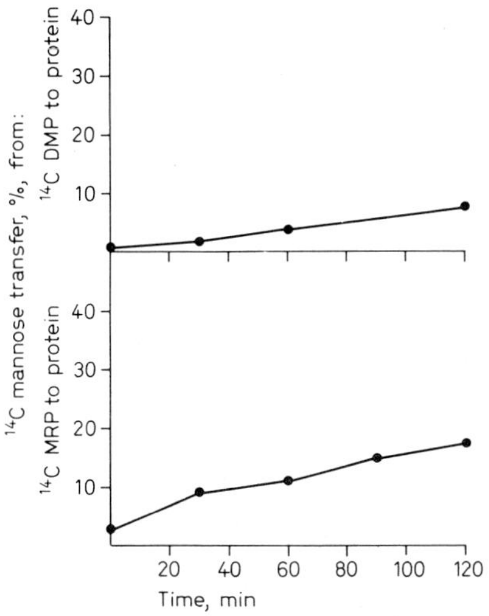

Fig. 1. Time-course of transfer of mannose from mannosylretinyl phosphate (MRP) to total protein in microsomes, compared to transfer from dolichylmannosyl phosphate (DMP).

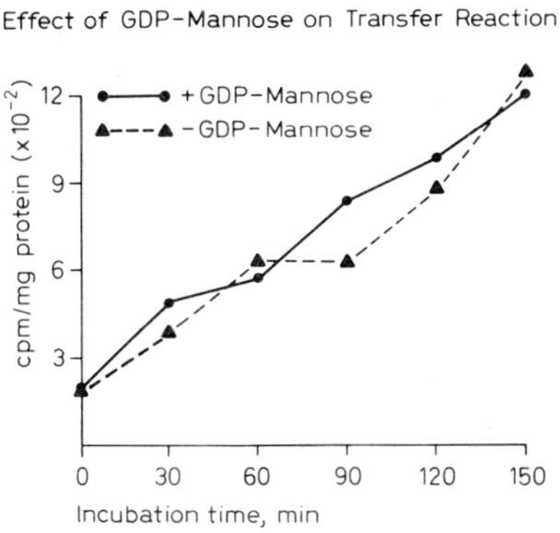

Fig. 2. Effect of addition of a 10-fold molar excess of non-radioactive GDP-mannose on transfer of ^{14}C-mannose from ^{14}C-mannosylretinyl phosphate to protein in microsomes.

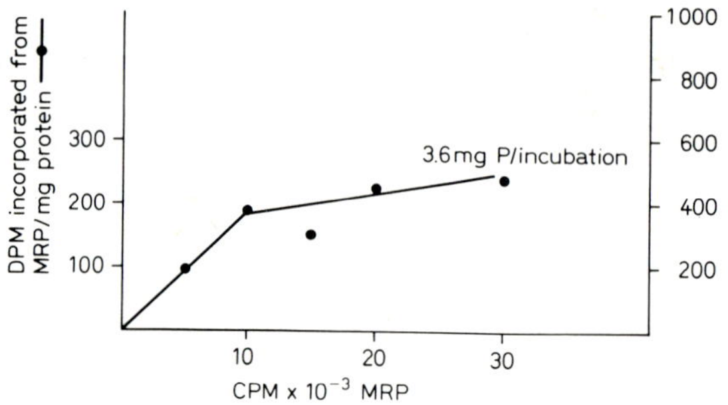

Fig. 3. Effect of concentration of ^{14}C-mannosylretinyl phosphate on transfer of ^{14}C-mannose to protein in microsomes.

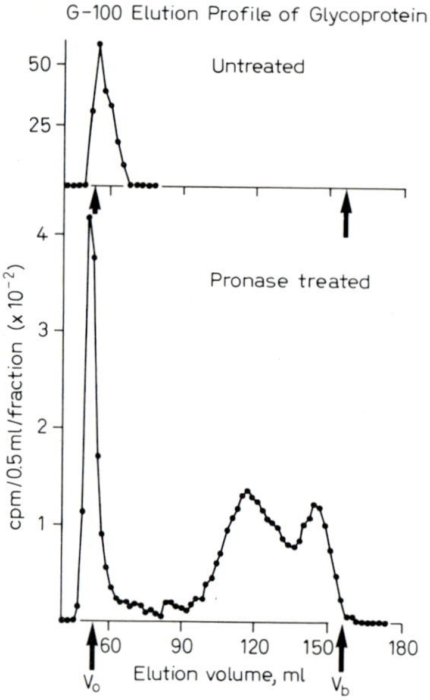

Fig. 4. Gel filtration chromatography of labeled glycoprotein from microsomes. Microsomes treated with SDS-mercaptoethanol to dissolve labeled glycoprotein following incubation with ^{14}C-mannosylretinyl phosphate, and chromatography of the extract on Sephadex G-100, before and after treatment with proteolytic enzyme (pronase).

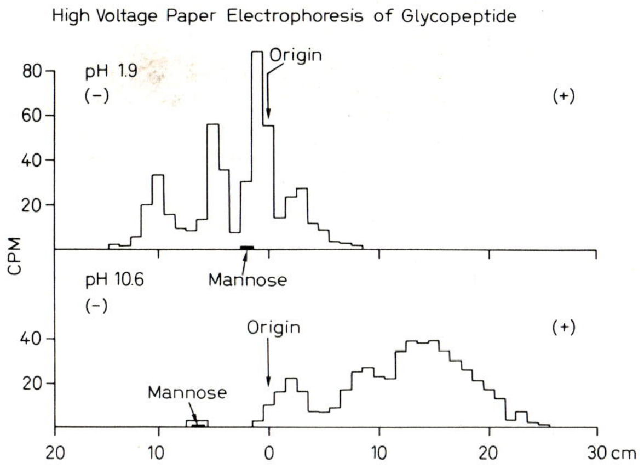

Fig. 5. High-voltage paper electrophoretic separation of the ^{14}C-glycopeptides obtained by pronase digestion of the ^{14}C-glycoprotein (Fig. 4) labeled from ^{14}C-mannosylretinyl phosphate at low and high pH.

The reaction showed pH dependence with a maximum at pH 7.2, and also increased with the amount of MRP incubated (fig. 3). To show that the product was truly a protein, we extracted it (90%) from the microsomes at the end of the reaction by solubilizing with SDS-mercaptoethanol, and showed that after preliminary purification on Sephadex G-25, it could be found in the void-volume of Sephadex G-100. If it was then treated with protease, glycopeptides were found to be eluted after the void volume of G-100 (fig. 4) and these glycopeptides were shown to be zwitterionic by high-voltage electrophoresis (fig. 5).

Finally, using highly-purified jack-bean α-mannosidase, we were able to remove 50% of the mannose added by MRP from these glycopeptides.

These results suggest that vitamin A can function in the transfer of sugar moieties from nucleotide sugars, in the form of a retinylsugar phosphate, to what appears to be large molecular weight glycoprotein acceptors present in liver microsomes. The possibility exists, and is currently under investigation in our laboratory, that the serum glycoprotein α_1-macroblobulin, which is most probably made in the liver and contains mannose residues, may receive mannose via mannosylretinyl phosphate, since we have good evidence that this serum glycoprotein is vitamin A-sensitive (3). However, we found a non-enzymatic reaction also occurs in which mannose from MRP becomes attached to protein. We are currently attempting to distinguish between the enzymatic and non-enzymatic products.

References

1 *Barr, R.M. and De Luca, L.:* Biochem. biophys. Res. Commun. *60:* 355 (1974).
2 *Frot-Coutaz, J.P.; Silverman-Jones, C.S., and De Luca, L.:* J. Lipid Res. *17:* 220 (1976).
3 *Kiorpes, T.C.; Molica, S.J., and Wolf, G.:* J. Nutr. *106:* 1659 (1976).
4 *Lennarz, W.J.:* Science N.Y. *188:* 986 (1975).
5 *Peterson, P.A.; Rask, L.; Helting, T.; Ostberg, L., and Fernstedt:* J. biol. Chem. *251:* 4986 (1976).
6 *Rosso, G.C.; De Luca, L.; Warren, C., and Wolf, G.:* J. Lipid Res. *16:* 235 (1975).

Dr. *G. Wolf,* Department of Nutrition and Food Science, Massachusetts Institute of Technology, *Cambridge MA 02139* (USA)

Wld Rev. Nutr. Diet., vol. 31, pp. 21–26 (Karger, Basel 1978)

Control of Retinol Transport in Plasma

J. Glover, R.C. Kershaw and Suzanne Large
Department of Biochemistry, University of Liverpool, Liverpool

The main vitamin A reserves of an animal are stored in the esterified form within lipid droplets in the parenchymal cells of the liver. The retinol is then gradually released into the plasma for transport to target tissues in the alcohol form bound to a specific carrier, retinol-binding protein (RBP) which has one binding site for the vitamin (9). It is necessary for several reasons for the distribution of retinol to be tightly controlled. Firstly, the molecule is amphipathic and is capable of causing disruption of membranes (2); secondly, metabolism of excess retinol can lead to the formation of retinoic acid known to be toxic in moderate excess (20).

Within the plasma, RBP (22,000 daltons) associates with thyroxine-binding prealbumin (54,000 daltons) forming a 1:1 complex which is considered of physiological value in preventing undue loss of the vitamin and its carrier from the circulation by reducing the filtration rate through the kidney (18). However, although some RBP does pass through into the glomerular filtrate, it is readily reabsorbed by the proximal tubules and there utilised and metabolised while the surplus retinol is possibly returned to the bloodstream (4, 17).

The uptake of the vitamin by the various target tissues (e.g., the eye or the intestine) appears to be mediated by RBP acceptor proteins on the cell membranes (8, 17) and by intracellular binding protein for retinol (1). These proteins could also form critical control factors in individual tissues.

Retinol is multifunctional in the animal in that the metabolite, retinoic acid, can satisfy the normal growth requirement of epithelial tissues but retinol itself is a necessary precursor of retinal, the cofactor for the various photoreceptors in the eye. Retinol is also needed to maintain key reproductive tissues (20). It is reasonable to assume that the latter may at particular stages of development require a different level of supply of retinol compared to other tissues so that the plasma concentration of RBP may fluctuate in accordance with the needs of the animal. It is, thus, of interest to know how the level is controlled.

Distribution of Retinol in Liver Cells and Possible Control Step

Initially, the distribution of retinol was studied between the various organelles within the liver cells of sheep and of man (4). In normal sheep, a large proportion of retinol (90% approx.) was found to be esterified and localised mainly in lipid globules while the remaining free retinol was dispersed in the endoplasmic reticulum and cytosol. The equilibrium between the two fractions is maintained by esterase. Some of the alcohol will be associated with liposomes and the lipid fraction of membranes, and some with retinol-binding cell protein (1), but only one tenth of the free retinol present is attached to retinol-binding (plasma) protein, ready for secretion into the bloodstream. Retinol has a high affinity for apo-RBP $Ka = 5.6 \times 10^6 M^{-1}$ (7) and, in normal animals with adequate vitamin reserves, the apo-RBP will be fully saturated as it is formed. The supply of apo-RBP is, however, dependent to some extent on the amino acid pool maintained by the diet. With large excess of free retinol in the cells over that bound to RBP, it is more likely that the availability of the latter will be a major factor in controlling the rate of secretion of holo-RBP into the plasma rather than the action of esterase. This is supported by experiments with rats maintained on a low protein diet of poor quality (13) and by many observations on protein-energy-malnourished (PEM) pre-school children who have a plasma concentration of RBP of the order of 10 μg/ml compared to about 25 to 30 μg/ml plasma in normal healthy children.

Again, marked changes in plasma concentrations of RBP have been observed in subjects with diseases of the liver or kidney affecting either the normal synthesis or metabolism of the protein (15, 19). The principal aim of the present study is, however, to obtain information on the normal hormonal control of the plasma level in healthy subjects.

Changes in Plasma RBP Concentration of Retinol-Deficient Rats after Administration of the Vitamin

The administration of retinol to the vitamin A-deficient rat on a good protein diet causes a rapid release of the RBP which has accumulated in the liver during the previous period of deficiency (13, 14). The plasma level attains a peak about 3 h after dosing and then declines sharply over the next few hours as the various target tissues take up their quota of the vitamin and the organism attempts to restore a balance between protein biosynthesis and metabolism. The variation in the mean plasma concentrations of a group of 4 male rats were followed daily for a period of 10 days, employing the procedure described earlier (6). The concentration was found to oscillate slowly between maxima and minima. Again, the mean coefficient of variance for daily values determined in 3

Table I. Effect of lighting conditions on the plasma concentration of retinol-binding protein in the male rat

Rat No.	Period	Plasma RBP concentration, μg/ml			
		dark (D) mean ± SEM	light (L) mean ± SEM	difference (L–D)	signif-icance P
1	10 days	34.5 ± 1.2	35.5 ± 1.4	1.0	N.S.
2	10 days	31.7 ± 1.5	36.3 ± 1.2	4.6	∠ 0.05
3	10 days	33.1 ± 1.4	36.9 ± 1.4	3.8	∠ 0.1
4	10 days	35.6 ± 1.7	41.3 ± 1.5	5.7	∠ 0.025
5	10 days	28.8 ± 1.4	33.0 ± 1.3	4.2	∠ 0.05
6	10 days	28.5 ± 1.2	34.0 ± 1.5	3.5	∠ 0.025
	Average	32.0 ± 1.2	36.2 ± 1.2	4.2	∠ 0.025

male rats over 7 days and 6 rats over 10 days was 20%, compared to 3% for 6 replicate analyses on a single sample, indicating that the fluctuations were real and did not arise from experimental error. These fluctuations in plasma RBP concentration had no correlation with the food intake, and body weights remained constant. Thus, the changes in plasma concentration in these male rats arise from a hormone-controlled rhythm such as one might expect to see in the female over the oestrus cycle.

The relatively rapid switches in RBP concentration indicated that there might be an underlying circadian-type rhythm, but over a period of a week or 10 days. Consequently, plasma samples were taken from a further group of 3 male rats on a 14 h day/10 h night cycle at 2 h intervals, over a period of 2 days and RBP values were obtained on the samples. The RBP concentration was higher following the light period, and lower towards the end of the dark period. Furthermore, the mean daily plasma RBP concentrations of a group of rats under continuous lighting for 2 weeks were then compared with the mean values for the same animals kept for 2 weeks in the dark. The results are shown in table I. In a number of the rats, values for the light period were significantly higher than those for the dark period; in a few others there was no significant difference. Although it looks as if the lighting variable has an indirect effect on the plasma RBP concentration in the rat, further work needs to be done before this can be regarded as proved.

Seasonal Changes in Plasma RBP Concentration of Sheep

The holo-RBP concentrations in plasma of groups of ewes and wethers (castrated rams) were determined monthly throughout the year (3). It was found that the concentrations in both groups of animals passed through minimal levels (20–30 μg/ml) in the summer when the day length was longest, but in late August and early September rose to peak values (80–100 μg/ml) i.e., about 3-fold higher than the minimum level. The maximum occurred just after the September equinox and levels remained elevated over the breeding season except for a dip in the values in mid-October. During November and December, the concentration declined steadily and returned to the January level of 40 μg/ml for the rams and 30 μg/ml for the ewes. The RBP values for the rams remained slightly higher than those for the ewes throughout the annual cycle. RBP levels in the male are also known to be normally higher than in the female in the case of the rat and human.

These cyclic changes in RBP values in both sexes appears to be associated with the development of the gonads which is known to be triggered in the sheep by the shortening of the day length after mid-summer via the pineal-hypothalamo-hypophyseal hormone axis. So RBP must clearly be affected by the same system. It is unlikely that the gonadal steroid hormones are involved since the same changes also occurred in the castrated males.

These earlier observations have now been confirmed in birds which become sexually active in spring (5). The holo-RBP concentration in Japanese quail rises steeply in January and reaches an initial peak value towards the end of March, dips a little in April, but rises to a second peak in early May before declining steadily to minimal levels in June/July, in the case of the male birds, and July/August for females. The two-peak feature of the elevated RBP levels in the Japanese quail over the spring resembles the pattern in the correspondingly high values for sheep in the autumn. It is interesting to note that in the quiescent period of the annual cycle, the male plasma levels lie within the range 140 to 170 μg/ml and are much higher than the female values within the range 80 to 100 μg/ml, whereas in the spring the mean female level (in the range 250–280 μg/ml) overtakes that of the male (190–250 μg/ml). This is slightly different from the situation in sheep; the very high levels may be necessary for the egg-laying which makes a high demand on the vitamin.

It is clear that the 2 to 3-fold increase in plasma RBP takes place at a time when the gonads are growing rapidly in both species. A similar increase in plasma RBP occurs in young rats (10) and in young children at puberty (16). These findings, coupled with the previous observations of *Thompson et al.* (20) who demonstrated that reproductive tissues have a specific requirement for retinol as opposed to retinoic acid, emphasise the role retinol must play in the rapid growth and functioning of gonadal tissues.

It is of interest to know the hormonal mechanism by which RBP is mobilised from the liver, and to this end information would be useful on the temporal sequence of the RBP changes in relation to other known hormonal changes during the development of gonadal tissue. A considerable amount of work has been done on the hormonal changes in the polyoestrous rat over the pubertal development period, which in some ways resembles the changes occurring in the seasonally sexually active species.

Plasma levels of holo-RBP were measured in a sequence of 8 groups of 4 weanling male rats of similar mean weight as they grew from 21 days to 70 days. The accelerated growth phase for the gonads occurs between days 13 and 22 after weaning, just as the plasma RBP doubles in value from about 25–55 μg/ml. This is similar to the 2 to 3-fold rise seen in sheep and Japanese quail. Similar observations were made in female rats, but their plasma levels were, in general, slightly lower and the growth of gonadal tissue smaller. This and other work on changes over the oestrus cycle will be reported separately.

The above well-sustained changes in holo-RBP concentration do not seem to show any direct correlation with the plasma changes in luteinizing hormone and follicle-stimulating hormone during the rats' sexual maturation as reported by other workers (12, 13).

The findings of the latter are themselves somewhat variable so it is difficult to gauge the physiological significance of the temporal sequence of changes in gonadotrophin levels with those of RBP. Nevertheless, it seems that gonadal tissue must grow to a certain stage of development with the participation of retinol before FSH and LH can really carry out their full function. The nature of the hormone, however, which triggers the increasing RBP and the simultaneous rapid growth of the gonads remains to be determined. There is little doubt that the additional cyclic changes in RBP in the seasonal breeding animals are associated with gonadal development and regression, whereas the tonic or basal levels are required for general turnover and maintenance of all the body tissues once growth has settled down. Consequently, any scheme on the mechanism of the sexual maturation of the animal must take retinol supply into account. Again, the nature of any feedback control system on RBP levels in plasma has still to be elucidated.

Acknowledgement

We wish to thank the World Health Organisation (Grant No. N3/181/51) and the Agricultural Research Council (Grant No. AG 26/117) for their financial support.

References

1 *Bashor, M.M. and Chytil, F.:* Biochim. biophys. Acta *411:* 87 (1975).
2 *Dingle, J.T.:* Biochem. J. *79:* 509 (1961).
3 *Glover, J.; Jay, C.; Kershaw, R.C., and Reilly, P.E.B.:* Br. J. Nutr. *36:* 137 (1976).

4 *Glover, J.; Jay, C., and White, G.H.:* Vitams Horm. (New York) *32:* 251 (1974).
5 *Glover, J. and Large, S.:* Proc. Nutr. Soc. *36:* 85A (1977).
6 *Glover, J.; Moxley, L.; Muhilal, H., and Weston, S.:* Clinica chim. Acta *50:* 371 (1974).
7 *Glover, J. and Muhilal, H.:* Biochem. Soc. Trans. *3:* 744 (1975).
8 *Heller, J.:* J. biol. Chem. *250:* 3613 (1975).
9 *Kanai, M.; Raz, A., and Goodman, DeW.S.:* J. clin. Invest. *47:* 2025 (1968).
10 *Kershaw, R.C.; Large, S., and Glover, J.:* Unpublished results.
11 *McKennon, P.C.B.; Mattock, J.M., and Ter Haar, M.B.:* J. Endocr. *70:* 361 (1976).
12 *Mijachi, Y.; Nieschlag, E., and Lipsett, M.B.:* Endocrinology *92:* 1 (1973).
13 *Muhilal, H., and Glover, J.:* Br. J. Nutr. *32:* 549 (1974).
14 *Muto, Y.; Smith, J.E.; Milch, P.O., and Goodman, DeW.S.:* J. biol. Chem. *247:* 2542 (1972).
15 *Peterson, P.A., and Berggard, I.:* J. biol. Chem. *246:* 25 (1971).
16 *Peterson, P.A.; Nilsson, S.F.; Ostberg, L., and Vahlquist, A.:* Vitams Horm. (New York) *32:* 181 (1974).
17 *Peterson, P.A.; Rask, L.; Ostberg, L.; Andresson, L.; Kamwendo, F., and Pertoft, H.:* J. biol. Chem. *248:* 4009 (1973).
18 *Raz, A; Shiratori, T., and Goodman, DeW.S.:* J. biol. Chem. *245:* 1903 (1970).
19 *Smith, F.R. and Goodman, DeW.S.:* J. clin. Invest. *50:* 2426 (1971).
20 *Thompson, J.N.; Howell, J. McC., and Pitt, G.A.J.:* Proc. R. Soc. B. *115:* 510 (1964).
21 *Thompson, J.N. and Pitt, G.A.J.:* Nature *188:* 672 (1970).

Dr. *J. Glover,* Department of Biochemistry, University of Liverpool, P.O. Box 147, *Liverpool L69 3BX* (England)

Wld Rev. Nutr. Diet., vol. 31, pp. 27–30 (Karger, Basel 1978)

Cellular Retinol and Retinoic Acid-Binding Proteins

Frank Chytil

Departments of Biochemistry & Medicine, Vanderbilt University School of Medicine, Nashville, Tenn.

Although the molecular mechanism of retinol and retinoic acid action in tissues other than the eye still remains to be elucidated, it has become evident in recent years that a cell which is under the influence of retinol deals with at least three distinct systems, which show a considerable specificity towards the vitamin A-like compounds. The first system is that responsible for the transport of retinol to target cells, represented by serum or plasma retinol-binding protein, traditionally abbreviated RBP (9, 18). To clearly distinguish this protein from those binding proteins found inside the cells, we propose to name it SRBP (serum RBP). The second system, recently located on the plasma membranes of some epithelial cells, interacts specifically with SRBP and shows characteristics of a membrane receptor for SRBP (8). It is presumably involved in 'admission' of retinol into the target cell, leaving SRBP outside. Lastly, the third system is represented by at least two intracellular binding proteins, one of which specifically binds retinol, and it has been proposed (12) that it be called cellular retinol-binding protein (CRBP). The other (13) protein specifically binds retinoic acid and should be named cellular retinoic acid-binding protein (CRABP). To call these intracellular binding proteins 'receptors' by analogy with the steroid receptors is, we believe, premature. Though considerable effort has been given to characterize these proteins, our knowledge of the mode of action of these proteins is still meager and the 'receptor' title is, therefore, not justified and might be confused with the above receptor for SRBP.

Here an attempt is made to review the progress achieved in the field of these cellular binding proteins in our laboratory. Other laboratories have also been interested in this problem (6, 19, 20, 21, 23, 24).

Cellular Retinol-Binding Protein (CRBP)

An intracellular binding protein for retinol was discovered by *Bashor* who, working in our laboratory, applied the technique of sucrose gradient centrifug-

Table 1. Characteristics of rat serum retinol-binding protein (SRBP) and cellular retinol-binding protein (CRBP) from rat testis

Characteristic	SRBP	CRBP
Molecular weight	20,000 (10)	14,000 (13)
Binding of retinoic acid or retinal	yes (7)	no (1, 13)
Fluorescence excitation spectrum (maximum, nm)	334 (10)	350 (13)
Antigenic towards antiserum against (SRBP)	yes (11)	no (2)
Level in testis in vitamin A deficiency	depressed (11)	no change (17)

References to literature in parentheses.

ation (5–20%) to detect a protein showing a sedimentation of 2 S and binding (15–^{3}H) retinol (1). The binding protein was shown to be saturable, reversible as nonradioactive retinol reduced binding (1, 2). The binding was specific as radioactive retinol, or retinoic acid in an excess over ^{3}H retinol did not reduce binding. This binding was not observed in serum. This protein is widely distributed in organs of adult animals, only could not be detected in serum and muscle CRBP (1). The size of this protein was determined by gel filtration to be about 14,000 daltons (13). Subsequently this protein was purified 1000-fold. It has been clearly established that it represents a protein different from the SRBP as summarized in table I and documented by differences in size, fluorescence spectra and antigenicity.

Furthermore, the binding specificity of CRBP towards various vitamin A active compounds was studied (12). It was also shown that this protein carries retinol *in vivo* (17). When rats are depleted of retinol, testicular CRBP no longer carries retinol but its level is not altered (17). In pair-fed rats only about 40% of the total CRBP is saturated by retinol (17). The reason for this phenomenon is not known.

Cellular Retinoic Acid-Binding Protein (CRABP)

The specificity of CRBP for retinol is striking and all evidence accumulated pointed away from the possibility that this protein could mediate action of retinoic acid, known to be able to support growth but not vision (5) or reproduction (22). *Ong,* in this laboratory, while purifying CRBP, discovered a second protein specific for retinoic acid (13), called cellular retinoic-acid-binding protein (CRABP) when high speed supernatants from homogenates of some tissues are incubated with ^{3}H retinoic acid and submitted to sucrose gradient centrifugation under conditions identical to those used for detection of CRBP, again a peak of radioactivity in the 2 S region can be observed. This binding is also saturable and specific as not retinol or retinal, but only retinoic acid compete for binding of radioactive retinoic acid. The organ distribution of this protein is different from that of CRBP (13). Some organs, for instance testes or uterus, contain both CRBP and CRABP. It was, therefore, suggested that in order to maintain the reproductive function both retinal and retinoic acid are necessary (3).

That we are indeed dealing with two separate proteins was ascertained by separation of these proteins by column chromatography (13). Further study was devoted to the binding specificity of CRABP towards ring analogues of retinoic acid and a striking correlation of the binding affinity with growth-promoting ability of these analogues was observed (4). Whether this protein carries retinoic acid *in vivo*, as well as the extent of saturation by this ligand, remains to be shown. The levels of this protein in testes of vitamin A-depleted rats appears to be unchanged (17).

CRBP and CRABP during Perinatal Development

These proteins are present in the tissues of the fetal rat. As mentioned above, CRBP is still present in most tissues of the adult rat. On the other hand, CRABP was not detected in some tissue, including lung, liver, intestine and kidney. During prenatal development of rat lung the level of CRBP remains relatively constant, while the level of CRABP peaks at 10 days postnatally, then declines. It is not detectable in lungs from 21 day-old animals. In liver, however, CRABP is not detectable later than 5 days, postnatally, while CRBP rises sharply near birth, declining only after 21 days. From these experiments it can be concluded that the alterations in the levels of these two binding proteins suggest different and changing requirements for retinol and retinoic acid in organ development and differentiation (16).

CRBP and CRABP in Cancer

Vitamin A appears to have an inhibitory effect on the development of some tumors (for review see 15). Earlier testing has shown that some experimental tumors did not contain CRBP (2). The screening was then expanded for both proteins and more tumors. It was found that some tumors contain both binding proteins, some only CRABP and in some none of these proteins has been detected (15). It is interesting to note, that a correlation between the responsiveness to vitamin A treatment and presence of CRABP does exist (15). The binding specificity of tumor CRABP (mouse skin papillomas) towards ring analogues of retinoic acid has been found not to be significantly different from that of testes (4). We have found also that CRABP is present in human breast and lung carcinomas, while it was not detectable in adjacent normal tissue (14).

Acknowledgements

This work was supported by grants from United States Public Health Service. The support and generous gift of vitamin A derivatives from the Hoffmann-La Roche Company is appreciated.

The author is indebted to the National Science Foundtion (USA) for a travel grant.

References

1 *Bashor, M.M.; Toft, D.O., and Chytil, F.:* Proc. natn. Acad. Sci. USA *70:* 3483 (1973).
2 *Bashor, M.M. and Chytil, F.:* Biochim. biophys. Acta *411:* 87 (1975).
3 *Chytil, F.; Page, D.L., and Ong, D.E.:* Int. J. Vitam. nutr. Res. *45:* 293 (1975).
4 *Chytil, F. and Ong, D.E.:* Nature *260:* 49 (1976).
5 *Dowling, J.E. and Wald, G.:* Proc. natn. Acad. Sci. USA *46:* 587 (1960).
6 *Futterman, S.; Saari, J.C., and Swanson, D.E.:* Expl Eye Res. *22:* 419 (1976).
7 *Glover, J.; Jay, C., and White, G.M.:* Vitams Horm. *32:* 215 (1974).
8 *Heller, J.:* J. biol. Chem. *250:* 3613 (1975).
9 *Kanai, M.; Raz, A., and Goodman, D.S.:* J. clin. Invest. *47:* 2025 (1968).
10 *Muto, Y. and Goodman, D.S.:* J. biol. Chem. *247:* 2533 (1972).
11 *Muto, Y.; Smith, J.E.; Milch, P.O., and Goodman, D.S.:* J. biol. Chem. *247:* 2542 (1972).
12 *Ong, D.E. and Chytil, F.:* Nature *74:* 255 (1975).
13 *Ong, D.E. and Chytil, F.:* J. biol. Chem. *250:* 6113 (1975).
14 *Ong, D.E.; Page, D.L., and Chytil, F.:* Science N.Y. *190:* 60 (1975).
15 *Ong, D.E. and Chytil, F.:* Cancer Lett. *2:* 25 (1976).
16 *Ong, D.E. and Chytil, F.:* Proc. natn. Acad. Sci. USA *73:* 3976 (1976).
17 *Ong, D.E.; Tsai, C.H., and Chytil, F.:* J. Nutr. *105:* 204 (1976).
18 *Peterson, P.A.:* J. biol. Chem. *246:* 34 (1971).
19 *Saari, J.C. and Futterman, S.:* Expl Eye Res. *22:* 425 (1976).
20 *Sani, B.P. and Hill, D.L.:* Biochem. biophys. Res. Commun. *61:* 1276 (1974).
21 *Sani, B.P. and Hill, D.L.:* Cancer Res. *36:* 409 (1976).
22 *Thompson, J.N.; Howell, J.McC., and Pitt, G.A.J.:* Proc. R. Soc. B *159:* 510 (1964).
23 *Wiggert, B.O. and Chader, G.J.:* Expl Eye Res. *21:* 143 (1975).
24 *Wiggert, B.O.; Bergsma, D.R., and Chader, G.J.:* Expl Eye Res. *22:* 411 (1976).

Dr. *F. Chytil,* Departments of Biochemistry & Medicine, Vanderbilt University School of Medicine, *Nashville, TN 37232* (USA)

Wld Rev. Nutr. Diet., vol. 31, pp. 31–36 (Karger, Basel 1978)

Retinol-Binding Protein in Tubular Proteinuria of Patients with Itai-Itai Disease[1]

Masamitsu Kanai, Takao Iwanaga, Noboru Hagino and Yasutoshi Muto

Central Clinical Laboratories, Shinshu University Hospital, Asahi, Matsumoto City; Hagino Hospital, Fuchu, Toyama Prefecture, and Department of Nutrition, School of Health Sciences, Faculty of Medicine, University of Tokyo, Tokyo

Retinol circulates in human plasma bound to a specific carrier protein, retinol-binding protein (RBP) which interacts strongly with plasma prealbumin to form the RBP-prealbumin complex (3). It is found that patients with tubular proteinuria excrete large amounts of RBP (4, 5, 8) and β_2-microglobulin (1, 7) associated with other well-defined low molecular weight proteins (6). In this report, RBP and β_2-microglobulin were isolated and four immunologically identical RBP subfractions were separated from the urinary protein fractions of patients with Itai-Itai (ouch-òuch) disease, a chronic cadmium poisoning (2). This disease usually attacks elderly, multiparaous women, who live in a specific localized area around the central basin of the Jinzu river, in the upper reaches of which Kamioka mine is located. Clearance values of serum albumin, prealbumin, RBP and β_2-microglobulin of the patients were compared with the average values in normal persons. The major increase of the RBP and β_2-microglobulin clearance favours grossly impaired tubular reabsorption of the low molecular weight proteins in the kidney. A differentiation of patterns of proteinuria was also studied by measuring urinary excretion of albumin, RBP and β_2-microglobulin.

Purification of Urinary RBP

DEAE-Sephadex A-50 column chromatography of lyophilized urinary protein from the patients with Itai-Itai disease eluted with linear gradient from 0–0.6 M NaCl resulted in resolution of urinary proteins into several peaks. Materials with fluorescence were eluted in three positions. It was found that the first two peaks, emerging with albumin, constitute the main urinary free un-

[1] This work was partially supported by the US-Japan Co-operative Research Program Grant 5R037 from the Japan Society for Promotion of Science.

complexed forms of RBP, and the third peak represents RBP-prealbumin complex. They were separately pooled and subjected to gel chromatography on Sephadex G-100 columns. Free RBP was isolated in the low molecular weight protein fraction that emerged after albumin. The RBP-prealbumin complex was dissociated by preparative polyacrylamide disc electrophoresis and separately purified by gel filtration, as reported earlier (3).

For further purification of RBP and separation of RBP species, sulfopropyl Sephadex C-50 column chromatography was carried out. Several peaks were eluted with a linear gradient of sodium acetate buffer. Electrophoretic analyses were performed on aliquots of the fractions. From this data, it was found that apo-2 and holo-2 RBP can be obtained from the first, and apo-1 and holo-1 RBP from the second fluorescent peak of the DEAE-column fractions.

A major portion of urinary RBP in the patients with Itai-Itai disease, occurring in free forms as apo- and holo-RBP, should originate from the two forms of free RBP in plasma (9, 11, 13). *Rask et al.* (11) reported structural differences of the two forms of RBP; however, the microheterogeneity of RBP found in the present study remains to be solved.

Polyacrylamide disc electrophoretic pattern of urinary protein from patients with Itai-Itai disease revealed the presence of four heterogeneous RBP species in post-albumin and α-globulin zone with β_2-microglobulin and transferrin. These protein fractions constitute a characteristic electrophoretic pattern of the disease. By use of immunoelectrophoretic technique, more than ten plasma protein subfractions were identified, including α_1-acid glycoprotein, α_1-antitrypsin, α_2-heat stable glycoprotein, haptoglobin, IgG and IgA.

Biochemical Abnormalities and Renal Function Study (Itai-Itai Disease)

Results of the study of biochemical constituents in sera and renal function of 18 patients with the disease revealed elevated level of serum creatinine and reduction of endogenous creatinine clearance in all of the cases. In about half of them, retention of urea and elevation of alkaline phosphatase level in serum were observed. Serum levels of total protein, albumin and prealbumin were within normal range with few exceptions. RBP level had a tendency to be high in the cases of moderate nitrogen retention. One patient had definite anemia, hypoproteinemia and azotemia which was severe.

Differentiation of Proteinuric Patterns

Differentiation of patterns of proteinuria in renal disorders of varying etiologies was studied by measuring urinary excretion of total protein, albumin

Table I. Differentiation of four types of proteinuria

No. of subjects	Type of proteinuria	mg/24 h Total protein	Albumin	RBP	Albumin/ total protein	Albumin/ RBP
26	Normal	10–37 (22)	3.6–17.6 (8.6)	0.06–0.23 (0.11)	0.14–0.77 (0.41)	28–188 (84)
16	Glomerular	187–8610 (2290)	120–4700 (1390)	0.1–3.51 (0.82)	0.28–0.87 (0.63)	735–10300 (2830)
19	Tubular	180–1020 (590)	34–108 (58)	20–126 (65)	0.04–0.19 (0.11)	0.4–4.6 (1.1)
9	Mixed	365–6550 (2400)	190–2950 (1174)	2.4–143 (32)	0.31–0.78 (0.49)	5–179 (80)

[1] Mean in parenthesis.

and RBP (table I). Ratio of albumin to total protein, and that of albumin to RBP, indicate characteristic features in normal, glomerular and tubular proteinuria. In addition to the three types of patterns, a mixed glomerular tubular type was classified which can be differentiated from the normal type by an increased excretion of proteins in the former type. Also, an average daily excretion of prealbumin markedly increased in Itai-Itai disease, ranging from 3.4–22 mg, in contrast to an average normal excretion of 0.05 mg. In the present study, the glomerular pattern was found in cases of chronic glomerulonephritis, nephrotic syndrome and diabetic nephropathy; the tubular pattern mainly in the cases of Itai-Itai disease; the mixed pattern in renal insufficiency with diabetic nephropathy, multiple myeloma and other etiologies, which suggests the presence of a threshold mechanism for the tubular reabsorption of RBP (free RBP fractions) similar to other low molecular weight proteins.

A nomogram was constructed to differentiate types of proteinuria (fig. 1). The urinary excretion of albumin was plotted on a double logarithmic scale against that of RBP of the same persons. The distribution separated four different zones of normal (N), glomerular (G), tubular (T) and mixed glomerular-tubular (M) types of proteinuria. Serial determinations of the patterns of proteinuria in the same patient were found to be useful for following the course of the disease and involvement of the site of lesion in the kidney. The differentiation of proteinuric patterns as described above with measurement of albumin and β_2-microglobulin was reported earlier by *Peterson et al.* (7).

Recently, evidence for a serum threshold for the tubular reabsorption of β_2-microglobulin was shown by *Wibell et al.* (14). The present study also suggests the presence of a similar threshold mechanism for RBP. Low molecular weight proteinuria together with albuminuria (12), called nephron loss protein-

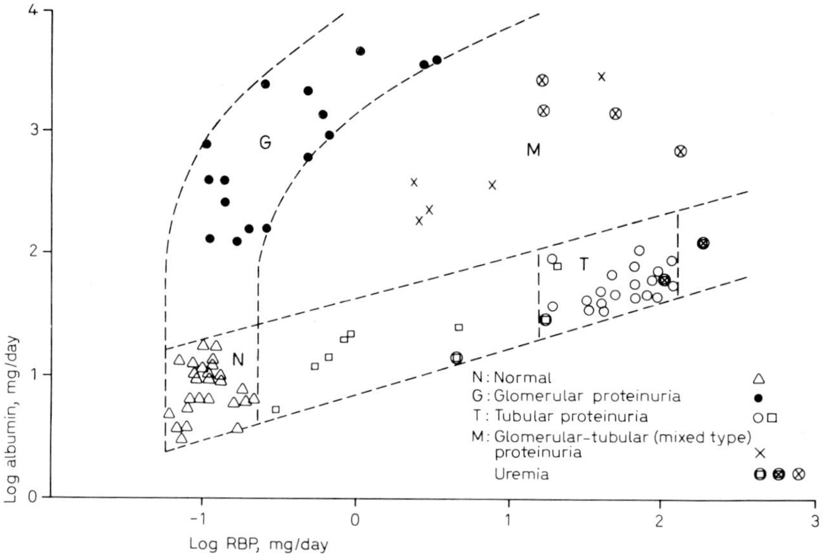

Fig. 1. A nomogram for the differentiation of proteinuria.

uria (14), corresponds to the mixed glomerular tubular type of proteinuria in the present study, commonly found in renal insufficiency with varying etiologies. In the absence of renal insufficiency, below a serum threshold, the excretion of RBP and albumin can be used for the early detection of tubular proteinuria and differentiation of proteinuric patterns.

Renal Clearance Study of Proteins in Patients with Itai-Itai Disease

To elucidate a pathophysiological mechanism for the increased excretion of various proteins, clearance values of serum albumin, RBP and prealbumin of 12 patients with the disease were calculated in terms of μl/min, corrected for their body surface and compared with the average values in normal persons shown in parenthesis: albumin clearance 1.2 (0.14); prealbumin clearance 26 (0.1); RBP clearance 1260 (2.0) (table II). A major increase of the RBP clearance compared with that of the albumin clearance favours the grossly impaired reabsorption in renal tubules in the patients. However, a more complicated mechanism would be involved for more pronounced increase of prealbumin clearance than that of albumin clearance. An interrelationship in plasma levels of RBP and prealbumin was reported in various pathologic conditions which affect the retinol transport system (13) and in experimental studies of vitamin A deficiency in rats (10). The

Table II. Serum and urine levels of three proteins and creatinine in patients with Itai-Itai disease compared with those of normal persons

		Albumin	Prealbumin	RBP	Creatinine
Serum, mg/litre	P[1]	44×10^3 (29–51) $\times 10^3$	278 (146–360)	46 (35–95)	22 (11–52)
	N	43×10^3	250	40	8
Urine, mg/day	P	64 (34–108)	8.2 (4.2–15.3)	65 (20–125)	
	N	8.6	0.05	0.11	
Clearance, µl/min	P	1.23 (0.6–1.85)	26 (13–60)	1260 (380–1950)	27×10^3 (8–58) $\times 10^3$
	N	0.14	0.1	2.0	67×10^3

[1] Mean and ranges of 12 patients.

marked increase in prealbumin clearance in the disease together with that of RBP would suggest a metabolic interrelationship in the kidney for the excretion of the two proteins.

In a separate study with 12 patients, the mean clearance value of β_2-microglobulin was 9.0 (range, 3–22.4) ml/min and that of creatinine was 20.8 (range, 8.3–40.5) ml/min. Thus, clearance of β_2-microglobulin amounts to 42% (range, 22–25%) of that of creatinine. In contrast to β_2-microglobulin, existing in the same uncomplexed form in serum and urine, a major portion of serum RBP (over 90% of total RBP) exists as a complex with prealbumin, with a small fraction of uncomplexed form (9, 13), which largely explains the difference in clearance values of the two proteins.

Relationship of RBP and Prealbumin in Blood and Urine

In blood, an average of 40–50% of prealbumin circulates in the form of a complex with RBP. Besides RBP-prealbumin complex, a small portion of RBP is in free form. In urine, RBP excretion occurred in three forms, a larger portion as free RBP in the form of apo- and holo-RBP, and a smaller portion as RBP-prealbumin complex. These findings suggest that circulating free RBP is easily filtered through glomerular membrane and excreted in large amounts in urine because of grossly impaired tubular reabsorption of the protein. However, the mechanism for the increased excretion of RBP-prealbumin complex remains to be solved.

References

1 *Berggård, I. and Bearn, A.G.:* J. biol. Chem. *243:* 4095 (1968).
2 *Friberg, L.; Piscator, M.; Nordberg, G.F., and Kjellström, T.:* Cadmium in the environment (CRC Press, 1974).
3 *Kanai, M.; Raz, A., and Goodman, D.S.:* J. clin. Invest. *47:* 2025 (1968).
4 *Kanai, M.; Nomoto, S.; Sasaoka, S., and Muto, Y.:* Jap. Conf. Biochem. Lipids (Jap) *3:* 115 (1971).
5 *Kanai, M.; Sasaoka, S., and Naiki, M.:* Proc. Symp. Chem. Physiol. Pathol. (Jap) *12:* 319 and 325 (1972).
6 *Laterre, E.C. and Manuel, Y.:* In *Manuel, Revillard and Betuel* Proteins in normal and pathological urine, p. 172 (Karger, Basel 1970).
7 *Peterson, P.A.; Evrin, P.E., and Berggård, I.:* J. clin. Invest. *48:* 1189 (1969).
8 *Peterson, P.A. and Berggård, I.:* J. biol. Chem. *246:* 25 (1971).
9 *Peterson, P.A.:* Eur. J. clin. Invest. *1:* 437 (1971).
10 *Peterson, P.A.; Nilsson, S.F.; Ostberg, L.; Rask, L., and Vahlquist, A.:* Vitams Horm. *32:* p. 181 (Academic Press, 1974).
11 *Rask, L.; Vahlquist, A., and Peterson, P.A.:* J. biol. Chem. *246:* 6638 (1971).
12 *Ravnskov, U.:* Scand. J. Urol. Nephrol. *8:* 37 and 45 (1974).
13 *Smith, F.R. and Goodman, D.S.:* J. clin. Invest. *50:* 2426 (1971).
14 *Wibell, L.; Evrin, P.E., and Berggård, I.:* Nephron *10:* 320 (1973).

Dr. *M. Kanai,* Central Clinical Laboratories, Shinshu University Hospital, *Asahi, Matsumoto City* (Japan)

Wld Rev. Nutr. Diet., vol. 31, pp. 37–41

Xerophthalmia

G. Venkataswami, J. Glover, M. Cobby and A. Pirie

Nutrition Rehabilitation Centre, Government Erskine Hospital, Madurai; Department of Biochemistry, University of Liverpool, Liverpool, and Nuffield Laboratory of Ophthalmology, Oxford University, Oxford

Blindness, either partial or complete, and usually irreversible, is the frequent outsome of xerophthalmia. In many developing countries xerophthalmia is the most common single cause of blindness in infants and pre-school children (14).

Vitamin A deficiency leads to pathological changes in the retina, the conjunctiva and the cornea. Night-blindness is an early sign of retinol deficiency, but is often not recognised by parents as an important warning sign. If vitamin A is not given to the child at this stage, the conjunctiva becomes dry and wrinkled and a whitish elevated area, a Bitot spot, may develop. Conjunctival xerosis precedes xerosis of the cornea, which loses its lustre and has the appearance of ground-glass. This change is confined to the corneal epithelium. All these signs are fully reversible if vitamin A is given. Further changes, involving ulceration of the corneal stroma and perforation of the cornea, are not fully reversible but leave the cornea with varying degrees and sizes of opacity which may or may not affect vision. The final stage is a rapid sloughing of large areas of the cornea, with collapse of the eyeball and, sometimes, extrusion of the lens. Such an eye is totally and permanently blind. The biochemical basis of night-blindness is understood but the basis for the changes in the cornea is still unclear. The xerosis of conjunctival and corneal epithelium resembles that of epithelia in other parts of the body in vitamin A deficiency, but we have yet to learn the biochemical changes that cause this metaplasia of the cells.

Both mild and severe xerophthalmia, due basically to vitamin A deficiency but complicated by infection and malnutrition, are still widespread. It has only relatively recently been eradicated from Europe. More recently it has disappeared from Singapore due to increased wealth, increased child care and a government ban on all imports of dried skim or tinned milk not fortified with vitamin A. Sri Lanka has also conquered xerophthalmia, with greater prosperity, through increased health education in schools, and child care.

Children who develop corneal xerophthalmia seem, in some ways, to be a different group from the far larger group of children who show conjunctival signs of Bitot spot and conjunctival xerosis. In India, for example, the peak age for a Bitot spot is 5–7 years (*P. Chandra* – unpublished) but the peak age for corneal xerophthalmia is 2–3 years and the younger the child the more likely he is to have the severe form (2). Such children are almost always, or have recently been, suffering from diarrhoea and/or other infections known to reduce absorption of vitamin A.

Active corneal xerophthalmia is rarely found in prevalence surveys. *WHO* (14) suggests that a prevalence of 1:10,000 in children under 5 years of age is sufficient to indicate a public health problem, while a prevalence of 2% conjunctival signs is needed before action should be taken. If we consider that xerophthalmia progresses through conjunctival xerosis to corneal xerosis, ulceration and destruction, then we must consider that almost all children with conjunctival xerosis get over it without treatment. If this were not so, there would be too many blind or half-blind children to count.

With the help and cooperation of the Government of Tamilnadu and the Royal Commonwealth Society for the Blind (UK), a nutrition centre was set up at the Government Erskine Hospital, Madurai, to treat children with clinical xerophthalmia who could not be accommodated in the wards (12). This centre started with the philosophy that educating the parent on this subject was equally important. A diet was devised which was adequate in protein (all from vegetable sources), calories and β-carotene, using local foods at a cost the poor could afford. The parent accompanying the child helped in buying and cooking the food and the main meals were much the same for parent and child. A garden, in which the parents helped, grew many of the vegetables. General medical care was given on admission together with vitamin A as directed. About half of those with conjunctival xerophthalmia or with corneal xerosis were recorded as having received 100,000 IU water-miscible vitamin A by injection as out-patients. Almost all those with severe corneal xerophthalmia received one or more doses by injection and orally. Dosage was decided on by the medical staff before admission of the child to the nutrition centre.

Two hundred and ninety-one children were followed up. Analyses showed that some 'catch up' growth was evident, the improvement being the same whether vitamin A was given or not. No conjunctival case deteriorated, and of the forty children with corneal xerosis those not given vitamin A cleared as well as those who were given it (12). It seemed, therefore, either that the diet itself, rich in protein and β-carotene, was sufficient or that some factor was inhibiting the expression of vitamin A benefit. Protein deficiency needing to be corrected before holo-retinol-binding protein (RBP) could circulate, appeared an obvious factor. This has been studied by estimating prealbumin and RBP in serum on admission of the child and at various times thereafter, using the radial immunodiffusion technique (7) with plates supplied by Hoechst, W. Germany (13).

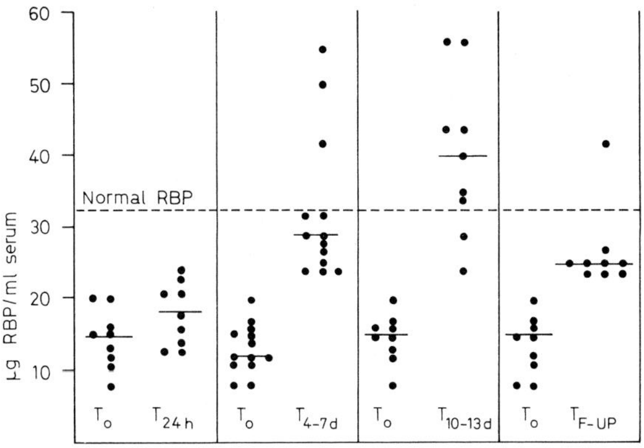

Fig. 1. Increase in serum retinol binding protein at various times after start of treatment and after return home (follow-up). Within each sub-section, values are given for children on admission (T_0) and for these same children after the specified time interval (13).

On admission, children with conjunctival xerophthalmia had median RBP of 22.1 µg/ml serum and those with corneal xerophthalmia, 13.5 µg/ml, $p < 0.001$. The normal level is about 32 µg/ml serum.

We next assessed the effect of dosage with vitamin A given at the same time as *ad lib* food. In rats deficient solely in vitamin A, even a small dose of retinol palmitate, raises the serum RBP, within an hour or so, from a very low level to well above normal and this returns to the normal level within 24 h (8). Vitamin A-deficient children who are also severely malnourished do not respond with a similar rise in RBP on vitamin A administration (4, 9, 10). This suggests that there is a functional defect in release of vitamin from the liver due to lack of hepatic store of RBP. This must be rectified through new synthesis of RBP from food proteins before holo-RBP can be released and circulated. *Venkatachalam et al.* (11) found that serum vitamin A levels increased when protein alone was given to nursing mothers and *Arroyave* (1) confirmed this in malnourished children. Recently, *Ingenbleek et al.* (6) found that both RBP and vitamin A increase in serum of malnourished children given food containing only traces of vitamin A but plenty of protein.

Children at Madurai given 100,000 IU of water-miscible vitamin A by injection on arrival, together with food *ad lib* showed an increase in RBP from a median level of 15 µg/ml to one of 18 µg/ml serum at 24 h. RBP did not reach normal until about 7 days later (fig. 1). Prealbumin, which *Ingenbleek et al.* (5) consider a good indicator of serum protein status was 107.6±7.03 µg/ml serum in those children with conjunctival xerophthalmia and 76.2±4.36 µg/ml serum in those children with corneal xerophthalmia. This is about one third the normal. Prealbumin recovered rather more slowly than RBP.

Table I. Retinol-binding protein in serum of severely malnourished children with X2, X3A, xerophthalmia, before and after dosage with vitamin A and on an improved diet

Age	Nutrition/ diagnosis	Retinol-binding protein, μg/ml								
		at outset			24 h after dose plus diet			5–10 days after dosing plus diet		
		total Madurai	total apo	holo	total Madurai	total apo	holo	total Madurai	total apo	holo
2.5[1]	IV[2]/MK[3], X3A[4]	20	17	14	25	28	30	56	53	48
5	IV/M, X3A	9	7	0	15	18	19	29	24	23
2	III[2]/M, X2[4]	23	–	–	23	27	25	38	29	18
2	III/M, X3A	20	9	0	24	20	19	41	53	58
2.5	III/M, X3A	–	–	–	31	23	23	49	41	31
2.5	IV/M, X2	15	11	0	21	22	21	29	37	33
2	IV/MK, X3A	11	12	0	15	18	20	55	–	56
6	Normal	35	36	29	38	38	38	–	–	–

[1] This child received vitamin A before reaching the nutrition centre.
[2] Nutrition grade IV ia 50% and grade III is 60% normal weight for age.
[3] M = marasmus, K = kwashiorkor.
[4] X2 = corneal xerosis, X3A = corneal xerosis with ulceration.

Some blood samples were analysed for total and holo-RBP in Liverpool by the method of *Glover et al.* (3). In general, the total RBP (apo- and holo-) corresponded with the values found in Madurai. No holo-RBP was found in four samples taken on admission, but 24 h after dosage with vitamin A and food *ad lib,* nearly all the RBP in serum was combined with retinol, the level ranging from 19–23 μg/ml in six children. Five to ten days later holo-RBP was normal or above normal in five out of seven children. All these children were severely malnourished, judging by their wt/age and all showed corneal xerosis or ulceration (table I) (13).

It seems reasonable to conclude that such children need protein in their food from which to synthesize RBP and prealbumin before they can fully utilize vitamin A and restore retinol transport. This is probably one factor explaining our earlier results (12) which showed that children with conjunctival or corneal xerosis progressed equally well with or without vitamin A dosage. A high protein diet which included β-carotene from green vegetables was sufficient. This is no indication that vitamin A should not be given, but protein-rich food needs to be given at the same time. There are many parts of the world where vitamin A preparations are not available and in such places the usefulness of dark green leafy vegetables, carrots and yellow or red fruits should be stressed. Diets can be devised which are within the parents' means and can prevent xerophthalmia and cure it in the early stages.

References

1 *Arroyave, G.:* Am. J. clin. Nutr. *22:* 1119 (1969).
2 *Doesschate ten, J.:* Thesis Uni. of Jakarta, Indonesia (1968).
3 *Glover, J.; Moxly, L.; Muhilal, H., and Weston, S.M.:* Clinica chim. Acta *50:* 371 (1974).
4 *Goodman, D.S.:* Vitams Horm. *32:* 167 (1974).
5 *Ingenbleek, Y.; De Visscher, M., and De Naeyer, P.:* Lancet *ii:* 106 (1972).
6 *Ingenbleek, Y.; van den Schriek, H.G.; de Naeyer, P., and De Visscher, M.:* Metabolism *24:* 633 (1975).
7 *Mancini, G.; Carbonara, A.O., and Heremans, T.F.:* Immunochem. *2:* 235 (1965).
8 *Muto, Y.; Smith, J.E.; Milch, P.O., and Goodman, D.S.:* J. biol. Chem. *247:* 2542 (1972).
9 *Smith, F.R.; Goodman, D.S.; Zaklama, M.S.; Gabr, M.K.; El Maraghy, S., and Patwardhan, V.S.:* Am. J. clin. Nutr. *26:* 973 (1973).
10 *Smith, F.R.; Suskind, R.; Thanangkul, O.; Leitzmann, C.; Goodman, D.S., and Olson, R.E.:* Am. J. clin. Nutr. *28:* 732 (1975).
11 *Venkatachalam, P.S.; Belavady, B., and Gopalan, C.:* J. Pediat. *61:* 262 (1972).
12 *Venkataswamy, G.; Krishnamurthy, K.A.; Chandra, P.; Kabir, S.A., and Pirie, A.:* Lancet *i:* 1120 (1976).
13 *Venkataswamy, G.; Glover, J.; Cobby, M., and Pirie, A.:* Am. J. clin. Nutr. *30:* 1968 (1977).
14 *WHO* Technical Report Series 390 (1976).

Dr. *Antoinette Pirie,* University of Oxford, Nuffield Laboratory of Ophthalmology, Walton Street, *Oxford OX2 6AW* (England)

Wld Rev. Nutr. Diet., vol. 31, pp. 42–44 (Karger, Basel 1978)

Transport of Retinol to Ocular Tissues

An Overview[1]

Joram Heller

Jules Stein Eye Institute, UCLA School of Medicine, Los Angeles, Calif.

It has been known for about 40 years that retinol (vitamin A) is essential for vision. The participation of retinol in vision is in the form of its aldehyde derivative, retinal, acting as the chromophoric group of all known visual pigments. As a matter of fact, this direct participation of retinol in vision is the only function of vitamin A that is understood in molecular terms. Since retinol is a vitamin and has to be supplied in the diet, it is clear that it has somehow to reach the ocular tissue following its absorption from the intestine.

In 1968 Goodman and his colleagues discovered that retinol circulates in blood as a tight complex with a small protein, the so-called (serum) retinol-binding protein of RBP. Recently, I have been interested in elucidating the mechanism of retinol transfer from its complex with RBP to its site of action in the photoreceptors. The present article is a short personal overview of work done in my laboratory.

Cell Surface Receptors for Serum Retinol-Binding Protein

In view of the great stability of the retinol-RBP complex, we postulated that the target organ(s) possess specific cell surface receptor for RBP and that the interaction between this receptor and the binding protein facilitates the transfer of retinol. Indeed, when the protein moiety of retinol-RBP was labeled, it was found that isolated pigment epithelial cells from bovine eyes have high affinity, low capacity binding sites for serum RBP (3). The binding of RBP is specific and is shown only by the pigment epithelial cells and not by photoreceptors. It should be recalled that the pigment epithelium is a monolayer of cells interposed

[1] This study was supported by grants EY 00704 and EY 00331 from the National Eye Institute, NIH.

between the rich choroidal blood supply and between the neuroretina (including the photo-receptors). The pigment epithelium is the site of the so-called blood retinal barrier, a barrier that prevents proteins and other molecules from freely diffusing into the retina. Each pigment epithelial cell has an average of about 5.10^4 receptors. The binding of RBP to the receptor is rapid (complete in about 1 min), temperature dependent and reversible. Debinding studies have shown that even after long incubation periods it is possible to displace all the bound RBP from the cell and it is thus clear that the protein moiety of RBP does not penetrate the pigment epithelial cells. Also, apo-RBP was bound to the receptor less firmly than retinol-RBP. This finding suggests a possible mechanism of physiological debinding whereby, once retinol was delivered to the interior of the cell, the apo-RBP still bound at the receptor will be displaced by a molecule of retinol-RBP since the latter has, presumably, a higher binding constant than the apo form.

Autoradiography of isolated pigment epithelial cells (5) and *in vivo* injection of (^{125}I)-labeled retinol-RBP (1) shows that the specific RBP receptor is localized to the choroidal surface of the cell, i.e., the surface facing the systemic blood supply. Autoradiography confirmed the binding studies that show the absence of internalization of RBP by the pigment epithelium, even 1 h following an *in vivo* injection of RBP. Autoradiography also failed to demonstrate RBP receptors on the photoreceptors.

Transport of Retinol into Pigment Epithelial Cells

Isolated intact bovine pigment epithelial cells are capable of accumulating retinol when incubated with retinol-RBP complex. The fact that retinol has to be supplied as a complex with the specific binding protein is critical; neither free retinol, nor retinol-bovine serum albumin complex can support uptake by pigment epithelial cells (2). Double labeling of the retinol-RBP complex demonstrated that only retinol was taken up by the cells, while the protein moiety was not internalized and could be displaced from the cell surface by excess unlabeled RBP. In other words, the process of retinol uptake by pigment epithelial cells involves the dissociation of the ligand from the protein. The uptake of retinol was fairly rapid, non-saturable and temperature-dependent process. Pigment epithelial cells are also capable of uptake of retinoic acid when presented with retinoic acid-RBP complex. The internalized retinoic acid is apparently reduced to retinol-like material. *In vivo* experiments indicate, though, that the product of retinoic acid reduction is not retinol itself, since retinoic acid is not incorporated into rhodopsin after an injection of labeled retinoic acid-RBP complex. Retinol, on the other hand, is rapidly and efficiently incorporated into rhodopsin under similar conditions (unpublished results).

Intracellular Binding of Retinol in Ocular Tissue

When labeled retinol is added to cytosol preparations from either pigment epithelial cells or photoreceptors, the retinol binds to a high molecular weight lipoglycoprotein (4). After uptake of retinol by intact, isolated pigment epithelial cells, retinol is found bound to the same lipoglycoprotein (2). The intracellular binding proteins from photoreceptor and pigment epithelial cells are similar, but not identical. The molecules are complex, with several protein subunits of varying molecular weight; they contain cholesterol and phosphatidylcholine and covalently linked carbohydrates. The molecular weight of these molecules is at least 1.5×10^6 as determined by gel filtration chromatography. Work is currently in progress to determine the role of these lipoglycoproteins in retinol (or retinal) transport between the pigment epithelium and the photoreceptors.

References

1. *Bok, D. and Heller, J.:* Expl Eye Res. *22:* 395 (1976).
2 *Chen, C.C. and Heller,* J. biol. Chem. *252:* 5216 (1977).
3 *Heller, J.:* J. biol. Chem. *250:* 3613 (1975).
4 *Heller, J.:* J. biol. Chem. *251:* 2952 (1976).
5 *Heller, J. and Bok, D.:* Am. J. Ophthal. *81:* 93 (1976).

Dr. *J. Heller,* Jules Stein Eye Institute, UCLA School of Medicine, *Los Angeles, CA 90024* (USA)

Wld Rev. Nutr. Diet., vol. 31, pp. 45–51

Comparative Studies on Vitamin A Transport in Plasma of the Mammalian and Non-Mammalian Vertebrates

Yasutoshi Muto

Department of Nutrition, School of Health Sciences, Faculty of Medicine, University of Tokyo, Hongo, Tokyo

A comparative study on plasma vitamin A transport started with the isolation and partial characterization of its specific protein, retinol-binding protein (RBP), initially from human plasma (8) and later from rat (12). Purified RBP from both sources exhibited very similar physico-chemical properties: a single binding site for one molecule of retinol with α-mobility on electrophoresis and a molecular weight close to 20,000. Despite these similarities, no cross-immunoreactivity was observed between the two proteins (12). A further comparative immunological study, using radioimmunoassays specifically developed for both human and rat RBP, revealed a high degree of immunological specificity within a given order of the vertebrates, including 5 mammalian orders and the classes *Aves, Amphibia* and *Pisces* (13).

It has also been established that RBP circulates in plasma as a tight complex with prealbumin (PA) on 1:1 molar basis, which has a molecular weight of about 55,000 (10, 21). In general, the association of RBP with PA increases the stability of the retinol-RBP complex (3, 4) and is assumed to prevent the ready filtration of RBP through the renal glomerulus. Since then a similar transport system for retinol in plasma has been confirmed and/or newly demonstrated in many mammalian species including man (16), rat (18), monkey (24), pig (20), steer (6) and dog (13, 19). However, no convincing information has yet been made available as to whether or not this transport system of vitamin A in plasma is widely applicable to all vertebrate species.

This paper deals mainly with the recent studies being conducted in our laboratory on the comparative biochemistry of plasma vitamin A transport, i.e., isolation and characterization of rabbit, chicken and piscine RBP, and the phylogenetic relationship of RBP molecule in the vertebrates.

Molecular Form of Vitamin A-Containing Protein and its Binding Affinity for Human PA in Native Plasma

When fresh plasma from man, rat, dog (adult), cow, swine and chicken were immediately applied to a column of Sephadex G-200, retinol-containing proteins were eluted in volumes consistent with a molecular weight of approximately 70,000–80,000 (i.e., complexed RBP), as previously reported (13). In the present study (22) it was also observed that major fractions of plasma retinol from rabbit (*Oryctolagus cuniculus*), snapping turtle (*Trionyx sinensis japonicus*) and bullfrogs (*Rana catesbeiana*) were associated with proteins having a molecular weight of about 75,000. In sharp contrast, it was noted that vitamin A in plasma from tadpoles (larvae of bullfrogs) as well as three fishes; carp (*Cyprinus carpio*), blue sharks (*Pronace glauca*) and young yellowtails (*Seriola quinqueradiata*), were transported exclusively by proteins with a distinctly smaller molecular size of less than 20,000.

When fresh plasma from man, rat, chicken, turtle and bullfrog were applied to a column of human PA-coupled Sepharose, all retinol-containing proteins were initially adsorbed to the column, and then eluted as peak 2 under a low ionic strength. In contrast, retinol-containing proteins from tadpoles and the three fishes were found to be eluted as peak 1 without any strong binding to human PA. In addition, isoelectric points of protein-bound retinol in plasma of the three fishes were found to be 4.1 to 4.3 by isoelectric focusing in polyacrylamide gel, being distinctly lower than those of rabbit (5.1), chicken (4.9) and turtle (5.1).

These findings strongly suggest that a distinctly different transport system of vitamin A in plasma is available in larvae of bullfrogs and fish, both of which belong to the non-mammalian and non-terrestrial vertebrates. Further studies will obviously be needed in a variety of other mammalian and non-mammalian vertebrate species to elucidate the relationship of RBP molecule.

Rabbit RBP Isolated from Tubular Proteinuria due to Experimental Chronic Cadmium Poisoning

Rabbit RBP is now a well-characterized mammalian RBP. However, it was obtained from the urine of a rabbit chronically poisoned with cadmium (14). When the rabbit was exposed to Cd at a dose of 0.8–1.5 mg/kg of body weight by subcutaneous injections 5 times per week and given a saline solution instead of tap water, large amounts of protein were excreted in the urine from day 80 to 118. The electrophretic patterns of the urinary protein showed two fluorescent bands specific for protein-bound retinol in the α-region (i.e., RBP) as well as β-globulins with smaller molecular weights. Histological study of the kidneys

(Cd; 121 μg/g) from this rabbit revealed damage localized in the proximal tubules, showing atrophy and degeneration of the epithelium (tubular proteinuria).

Rabbit RBP was purified to a homogeneous component by physical and immunological criteria from the pooled urine by a sequence of procedures which included gel filtration on Sephadex G-100, chromatography on DEAE- and SP-Sephadex and preparative isoelectric focusing in gel. The properties of rabbit RBP resembled those of human RBP in many ways: a molecular weight of about 20,000, α-mobility on electrophoresis, ultraviolet and fluorescence spectra and amino acid compositions (4 residues of tryptophan).

The RBP species, identical with regard to both molecular size and immunoreactivity, were further separated into four fractions by means of gel electrophoresis which yielded two holo- (H_2 and H_1) and two apo-RBP (A_2 and A_1) species (15). The urinary excretion ratio of these fractions ($H_2:H_1:A_2:A_1$) was found to be 70:6:21:3. No distinct difference of amino acid composition between holo- and apo-RBP was observed. Using the separated molecular species of rabbit RBP as well as of human RBP, their interactions with human PA were examined: purified rabbit holo-RBP exhibited almost the same binding ability to human PA as did human RBP. In addition, retinol within RBP molecule enhanced the affinity for PA, presumably through the change of tertiary structure, although the presence of retinol was not essential for the protein-protein interaction.

These findings are consistent with urinary excretion of RBP observed in patients with Itai-Itai disease (chronic entero-osteo-nephropathy cadmium) in a limited district of Japan (9) and with tubular proteinuria due to chronic Cd intoxication in Sweden (17).

Since the rabbit urinary RBP has a binding site for human PA and complete immunological identity with serum RBP (14), it is conceivable that a major fraction of holo-RBP; H_2 is derived from a metabolically active pool of plasma RBP in chronic Cd poisoning, mainly due to selectively impaired tubular reabsorption of the protein.

Chicken RBP in Plasma and Developing Embryo

We attempted to isolate and characterize chicken RBP in order to find out the vitamin A transport system in non-mammalian vertebrates and to study RBP metabolism in developing chick embryo. Chicken RBP-PA complex was isolated from plasma (2 litres) by a sequence of procedures which included three different kinds of DEAE-Sephadex chromatography and gel filtration on Sephadex G-100 (1). The molecular weight of the 1:1 molar complex was estimated to be 76,000 by gel filtration, and the sedimentation coefficient was found to be

5.2 S. RBP and PA were then dissociated from the purified complex by means of CM-Sephadex chromatography. Chicken RBP was isolated by a combination of human PA affinity chromatography and preparative gel electrophoresis. The RBP was homogeneous by physical and immunological criteria and resembled other mammalian RBP in molecular weight close to 20,000 by gel filtration, SDS-gel electrophoresis and sedimentation equilibrium analysis (2.0 S), α-mobility on electrophoresis, ultraviolet and fluorescence spectra and amino acid composition. On the other hand, the molecular weight of PA was determined to be 54,000 by gel filtration and sedimentation equilibrium analysis (3.9 S) and 13,000 by SDS-gel electrophoresis. It was also shown that the four subunits of PA (each with a molecular weight of 13,000) are identical by peptide mapping experiments (1). Chicken RBP and PA were immunologically distinct from those of human, rat and rabbit.

These findings have been generally confirmed and supported by other investigators (7, 11) and give strong evidence that vitamin A is transported as an RBP-PA system in chicken plasma, similar to other mammalian species.

Using monospecific anti-sera against chicken RBP and PA (2) both immunoreactive RBP and PA were detected in chick embryo (particularly in brain and eye) at higher concentrations than those in serum, exhibiting a peak at day 6 (well ahead of rhodopsin formation). More recently we have detected immunoreactive RBP in the ependymal cells as well as inside the matrix cells of the embryonic brain by immunohistochemical examinations, using anti-chicken RBP conjugated with horseradish peroxidase (*Hirosawa and Muto* – unpublished observations). Furthermore, embryonic RBP was found to contain vitamin A (holo-RBP) with a molecular weight of about 20,000 and molar ratio of PA to RBP in the embryo was about 1.1 at day 6. Since both RBP and PA could be detected in the egg-yolk (7), it is suggested that the embryonic RBP and PA arise exogenously, although synthesis (and secretion) of the proteins in the liver remains to be explored.

Piscine RBP Isolated from Young Yellowtails

Isolation of retinol-containing protein from plasma (250 ml) of 31 young yellowtails (cultivated for 20 months), as a representative piscine RBP, was attempted as described previously. Piscine RBP was purified (1,000-fold) to a homogeneous component by a sequence of procedures which included gel filtration on Sephadex G-100, chromatography on SP-Sephadex, preparative isoelectric focusing in polyacrylamide gel and finally semipreparative gel electrophoresis (22). This RBP showed physicochemical properties distinctly different from mammalian and chicken RBP. It showed a smaller molecular weight of approximately 16,000, lower isoelectric point of 4.3, a pre-albumin mobility on gel electrophoresis and complete lack of specific binding affinity for human PA. However, piscine RBP displayed similar characteristics in several ways, including the presence of one binding site on RBP for one molecule of retinol (i.e., the formation of a 1:1 molar retinol-RBP complex) and the presence of a high content of tryptophan (4 residues) in the molecule. It was also observed that (^{14}C)-retinol previously bound to piscine RBP was not completely displaced by 170-fold molar excess of retinoic acid (58%) whereas it was completely replaced by 3-dehydroretinol (100%), which dominates in the plasma of freshwater fish.

These findings strongly suggest that piscine RBP is a prototype of the specific vitamin A-transporting protein in plasma, being modified later in evolution to acquire a binding site for PA on the molecule during phylogenetic development of the vertebrates.

Vitamin A Transport in Plasma of Cyclostomes: Lampreys (Entosphenus Japonicus)

A study was conducted to explore a vitamin A transport system in plasma of the lowest class of the vertebrates: cyclostomes (22). When fresh plasma from lampreys was applied to Sephadex G-200, retinol-containing protein was eluted in the void volume of the column, suggesting that a macromolecular protein was responsible for vitamin A transport. It was also revealed that most of vitamin A (80%) was recovered in the lipoproteins of hydrated density less than 1.21, and was found to exist as an ester by TLC analysis.

These findings correspond well with the extraordinarily high content of vitamin A ester in the gut and flesh of lampreys which have been recommended in Japan for centuries as an efficacious diet for the curing of night-blindness. In order to prove that this vitamin A transport system in the lamprey is representative of all cyclostomes, further study will be required, particularly in the hagfishes which are more primitive, and entirely marine without metamorphosis.

Vitamin A Transport Systems in Plasma of Vertebrates

The evidence now available from this and previous reports indicates that at least four different transport systems for vitamin A and its derivatives are available in plasma of the vertebrates, as follows: (i) retinol-RBP circulating as a tight complex with PA (the presence of binding site for PA); classes higher than *Amphibia* (post-metamorphic stage); (ii) monomeric retinol-RBP (without binding site for PA); classes lower than *Amphibia* (pre-metamorphic stage); (iii) retinylester (and carotenoids) associated with lipoproteins; and (iv) retinoic acid circulating with albumin (23). The last two are likely to represent non-

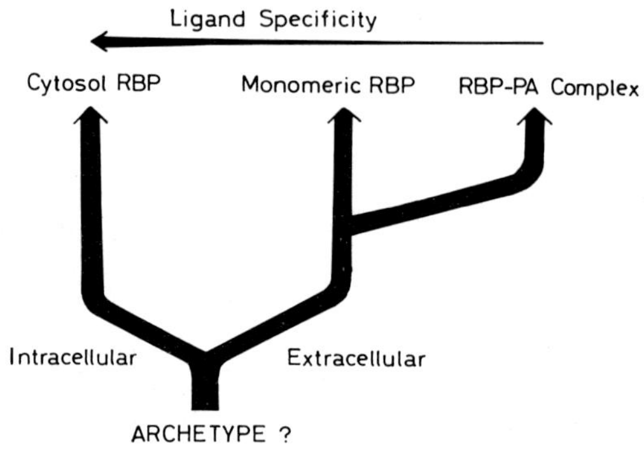

Fig. 1. Possible phylogenetic development of RBP.

specific or collateral systems which may function in abnormal or exceptional states to carry the vitamin to peripheral tissues in a manner that is not finely regulated. In contrast, RBP plays a physiological role in specifically delivering vitamin A to appropriate sites in target tissues; this delivery process may involve specific receptor site(s) for RBP on the cell surface of target tissues (5). Hence, comparative study on phylogenetic development of specific transport protein; RBP, in relation to the cell surface receptor(s) for the protein warrants further investigation. Further efforts are needed to gain an insight into the 'archetype' of vitamin A-binding proteins from which extracellular (or plasma) and/or intracellular (or cytosol) binding proteins have phylogenetically originated (see fig. 1).

Acknowledgement

I am grateful to my colleagues who have participated in the studies summarized in this review. The work from our laboratory reported here was supported in part by US-Japan Co-operative Research Program grant 5R037 from the Japan Society for Promotion of Science, and by grants 057053 and 157068 from the Ministry of Education.

References

1 *Abe, T.; Muto, Y., and Hosoya, N.:* J. Lipid Res. *16:* 200 (1975).
2 *Abe, T.; Muto, Y., and Hosoya, N.:* Life Sci. *17:* 1579 (1975).
3 *Goodman, D.S. and Leslie, R.B.:* Biochim. biophys. Acta *260:* 670 (1972).
4 *Goodman, D.S. and Raz, A.:* J. Lipid Res. *13:* 338 (1972).
5 *Heller, J.:* J. biol. Chem. *250:* 3613 (1975).
6 *Heller, J.:* J. biol. Chem. *250:* 6549 (1975).
7 *Heller, J.:* Devl Biol. *51:* 1 (1976).

8 *Kanai, M.; Raz, A., and Goodman, D.S.:* J. clin. Invest. *47:* 2025 (1968).
9 *Kanai, M.; Nomoto, S.; Sasaoka, S., and Naiki, M.:* Proc. Jap. Conf. biochem. Lipids *13:* 115 (1971).
10 *Kanda, Y.; Goodman, D.S.; Canfield, R.E., and Morgan, F.J.:* J. biol. Chem. *249:* 6796 (1974).
11 *Mokady, S. and Tal, M.:* Biochim. biophys. Acta *336:* 361 (1974).
12 *Muto, Y. and Goodman, D.S.:* J. biol. Chem. *247:* 2533 (1972).
13 *Muto, Y.; Smith, F.R., and Goodman, D.S.:* J. Lipid Res. *14:* 525 (1973).
14 *Muto, Y.; Nakanishi, M., and Shidoji, Y.:* J. Biochem. *79:* 775 (1976).
15 *Nakanishi, M. and Muto, Y.:* J. Nutr. Sci. Vitaminol. *22:* 271 (1976).
16 *Peterson, P.A.:* J. biol. Chem. *246:* 34 (1971).
17 *Peterson, P.A. and Berggard, I.:* J. biol. Chem. *246:* 25 (1971).
18 *Peterson, P.A.; Rask, L.; Ostberg, L.; Andersson, L.; Kamwendo, F., and Pertoft, H.:* J. biol. Chem. *248:* 4009 (1973).
19 *Poulik, M.D.; Farrah, D.; Malek, G.H.; Shinnick, C.J., and Smithies, O.:* Biochim. biophys. Acta *412:* 326 (1975).
20 *Rask, L.:* Eur. J. Biochem. *44:* 1 (1974).
21 *Raz, A. and Goodman, D.S.:* J. biol. Chem. *244:* 3230 (1969).
22 *Shidoji, Y. and Muto, Y.:* J. Lipid Res. *18:* 679 (1977).
23 *Smith, J.E.; Milch, P.O.; Muto, Y., and Goodman, D.S.:* Biochem. J. *132:* 821 (1973).
24 *Vahlquist, A. and Peterson, P.A.:* Biochemistry *11:* 4526 (1972).

Dr. *Y. Muto,* Department of Nutrition, School of Health Sciences, Faculty of Medicine, University of Tokyo, *Hongo, Tokyo* (Japan)

Wld Rev. Nutr. Diet., vol. 31, pp. 52–58 (Karger, Basel 1978)

Vitamin A Transporting System in Plasma

Physico-Chemical Studies on Retinol-Binding Protein (RBP), Prealbumin (PA) and RBP-PA Complex from Goat and Chicken

K. Sreekrishna, M. Krishna Bhat, S.K. Podder and H.R. Cama

Department of Biochemistry, Indian Institute of Science, Bangalore

Vitamin A is stored in liver and transported in the plasma to various target cells as a 1:1 complex with a specific carrier protein 'retinol-binding protein' (RBP, mol wt ≅ 20,000) (9). RBP, isolated from the plasma of a variety of animal species has similar physico-chemical properties (7, 10, 20, 23, 24, 28, 31), although immunologically it is species specific (23). It is generally present as 'complexed RBP' (mol wt ≅ 75,000) and the associated protein is characterized as prealbumin (PA, mol wt ≅ 50,000–60,000) in the sera of primates, rodents and aves (1, 10, 24). Information is lacking regarding the occurrence and nature of PA or any other equivalent RBP binding protein in other animal species. PA is also one of the three proteins for plasma transport of thyroxine (26). Human PA has been studied in detail both with respect to its structure and its interaction with RBP and thyroxine (10, 25), while such studies have been recently initiated with chicken prealbumin (17, 18). There exists a certain degree of heterogeneity in the prealbumin which is characteristic of the animal species (19, 32), for example, rat plasma has two prealbumins, PA_1 and PA_2, of which only PA_2 binds to RBP (22).

The formation of both retinol-RBP and retinol-RBP-PA is of great physiological significance in the plasma transport of vitamin A (9). Studies with human RBP have indicated qualitatively that retinol is tightly bound to its carrier and associated PA stabilizes further retinol-RBP complex (9). However, to understand the molecular mechanism of interaction of retinol-protein complex with target cells during the delivery of retinol, the evaluation of thermodynamic and kinetic parameters of the formation of the complex from its components, is warranted. Quantitative determination of such a parameter for retinol-protein interaction poses problems particularly due to the water-insoluble and labile nature of retinol. Only very recently was such a study initiated (6, 11, 21).

The present work has connection with: (i) nature of retinol transport system in ruminants, (ii) evaluation of binding affinity for retinol-protein interaction and (iii) heterogeneity of chicken prealbumin.

Nature of Protein-Bound Retinol (PBR) Present in Ruminant Plasma

The sera obtained from cow, sheep, goat and buffalo were analysed for the nature of protein-bound retinol by DEAE-Sephadex A-50 and Sephadex G-100 column chromatography. PBR was monitored either by measuring absorbance at 330 nm or by measuring the fluorescence intensity at 470 nm. The PBR present in cow serum was eluted earlier from DEAE-Sephadex column to albumin major peak, while the reverse was the case with other ruminants. The PBR containing fractions from the DEAE-Sephadex column were pooled and further analysed on Sephadex G-100 column to get information regarding the molecular weight. The PBR from cow serum was eluted as a single peak in the mol wt region of approximately 20,000 (corresponds to RBP), whereas those from the other ruminants were resolved into two peaks corresponding to mol wt of approximately 75,000 (complexed RBP) and 20,000 (RBP), respectively. The electrophoresis of the material present in the mol wt region of 75,000 did indicate the presence of protein(s) migrating faster than albumin. From this data it is clear that only in cow plasma, RBP probably circulates in the free form, while in other ruminants it is mainly present as complexed RBP. This finding with cow plasma is in agreement with the observations of *Heller* (13). Further studies on RBP and complexed RBP were restricted to that present in goat plasma.

Complexed RBP from Goat Plasma

Complexed RBP was purified from goat plasma by repeated chromatography on DEAE-Sephadex A-50, Sephadex G-150 and finally anti-goat serum albumin, Sepharose-4B, to remove traces of albumin contamination. Complexed RBP, so obtained, was characterized as PA-RBP, based on its electrophoretic behaviour.

The physico-chemical properties of goat plasma RBP and complexed RBP are summarized in table I along with those reported for other systems. It is seen that in general they have similar properties. A higher value for $A_{280}:A_{330}$ ratio might arise due to a partial inactivation of the protein during isolation (7).

Dissociation of Retinol-Protein Complex

Dissociation of retinol from RBP and complexed RBP were carried out by shaking aqueous solutions of the appropriate concentration of proteins

Table I. Properties of RBP and complexed RBP from goat plasma compared with those from different animal species

Property	RBP									Complexed RBP	
	human (7)	monkey (7)	cow (13)	rat (7)	rabbit (24)	chicken (1)	dog (23)	pig (29)	goat (31)	chicken (1)	goat[1]
Mol wt (daltons) $M \times 10^{-3}$	20–22	20–21	20–21	20	20	19–20	19.9	21	20–21	76	75–77
Electrophoretic behaviour	MH	–	–	MH	MH	MH (16)	MH	–	MH	Dissociates	Dissociates
Electrophoretic mobility relative to albumin	α_1, α_2	α_1	α_2	β	α	α	α_1	α_2	α_1	α_1 and PA	α_1 and PA
Isoelectric point	4.4–4.8	4.4–4.8	–	–	–	–	–	–	–	–	–
UV absorption λ max, nm	280 330	280 330	279 329	280 330	280 330	280 330	280 330	279 329	280 330	280 330	280 330
$A_{280} : A_{330}$	1.0	–	1.06	–	1.05	1.07	1.72	–	2.02	2.0	3.0
$A^{1\%}_{1\,cm}$ 280 nm	17.5	–	17.5	19.2	19.0	19.2	–	–	18.9	20.2	13.48
Fluorescence											
excitation, λ max, nm	332	333	330	343	340	330	336	333	336	330	330
emission, λ max, nm	456	457	460	463	460	470	465	457	460	470	460
Nature of associated protein	TBPA	TBPA	Absent	TBPA	PA	PA	NC	NC	NC	–	–

MH = Exhibits microheterogeneity; TBPA = Thyroxine-binding prealbumin; PA = Prealbumin; NC = Not characterized.
[1] *Sreekrishna et al.* (unpublished).

(0.1–5 μM) present in 20 m*M* potassium phosphate buffer (pH 7.6), containing 0.2M NaCl with equal volume of n-heptane in dark at 26±2°C, under nitrogen in a stoppered test tube at a rate of 75±5 strokes/min. The aqueous phase was analysed at different time intervals for the concentration of residual holo-protein by measuring the fluorescence intensity at 460 nm, assuming that the fluorescence contribution of free retinol in aqueous phase, if any, is negligible. The dissociation behaviour of retinol from RBP and complexed RBP as a function of time as well as concentration revealed that (i) the equilibrium attains in both cases within 4 h, (ii) both the extent and rate of release of retinol from RBP alone is greater than that from complexed RBP, indicating that formation of complexed RBP stabilizes retinol-RBP interaction; a similar observation was made earlier with human RBP (10), and ciii) the extent of dissociation is strongly concentration dependent.

An attempt was made to calculate the dissociation constant K_D' from the limiting value of percent dissociation making use of an equation of the type: $K_D' = ([P]^2/[PR]\,[k+1])$ where [P] and [PR] are the equilibrium concentrations of holo and apo-protein; k is the partition coefficient of retinol between n-heptane and aqueous buffer. The values of K_D' were obtained as approximately $10^{-8}M$ and $10^{-9}M$ for retinol-RBP and retinol-complexed RBP, respectively. These values may differ from the true value of dissociation constant because of uncertainty of partition coefficient 'k' due to labile nature of retinol. Nevertheless, they indicate that complexed RBP has a nearly 10-fold greater affinity than RBP for retinol. The K_D' of $10^{-8}M$ so obtained for goat RBP is in agreement with the qualitative findings of *Heller* with human RBP (12). On the contrary, it differs significantly from that reported by *Muhilal and Glover* (21) and *Cogan et al.* (6) for human and chicken RBP (table II). Presumably this discrepancy may well be due to either species variation or differences in the methodology, or both. However, it should be pointed out that the uncertainty in the calculated value of dissociation constant prevails in both the methods due to unstable nature of retinol. The K_D' of retinol-albumin interaction (table II) suggests that goat RBP has nearly 30 times greater affinity for retinol than albumin. Obviously, this is what one would expect.

Specificity of Chicken Prealbumin with Respect to RBP and L-Thyroxine

Chicken plasma is known to contain three prealbumins (2). Although chicken RBP and PA-RBP have been purified and characterized (1, 14, 21, 24), the heterogeneity in the prealbumin of chicken serum has not been investigated in detail. The three prealbumins and RBP were purified using the method which consisted of DEAE-cellulose chromatography of serum followed by Sephadex G-100 gel filtration and preparative electrophoresis. The prealbumins were designated as

Table II. Interaction of retinol and its analogues with proteins: n, number of binding sites and K'_D, apparent dissociation constant

System	Method employed	Conditions	n	$K'_D \times 10^7$ M	Reference
Retinol-human plasma RBP	spectrofluorimetric titration	pH 7.5, 20°C	–	1.8	21
	spectrofluorimetric titration	0.005 *M* phosphate buffered saline, pH 7.4, 27°C	0.83	1.9	6
Retinol-chicken plasma RBP	spectrofluorimetric titration	0.005 *M* phosphate buffered saline, pH 7.4, 27°C	0.79	1.5	6
Retinol-goat plasma RBP	equilibrium partition	0.02 *M* phosphate buffer, pH 7.6 containing 0.2 M NaCl, 26 ± 2°C	–	0.1	[1]
Retinol-bovine serum albumin	spectrofluorimetric titration	0.02 *M* phosphate buffer, pH 7.6 containing 0.2 M NaCl, 26°C	0.71	3.3	[1]
Retinol-goat plasma complexed RBP	equilibrium partition	0.02 *M* phosphate buffer, pH 7.6 containing 0.2 M NaCl, 26 ± 2°C	–	0.01	[1]
Retinol-ovalbumin	spectrofluorimetric titration	0.02 *M* phosphate buffer, pH 7.6 containing 0.2 M NaCl, 26°C	0.59	23.2	[1]
Retinoic acid-human plasma RBP	spectrofluorimetric titration	0.005 *M* phosphate buffered saline, pH 7.4, 27°C	–	2.1	6
Retinoic acid-chicken plasma RBP	spectrofluorimetric titration	0.005 *M* phosphate buffered saline, pH 7.4, 27°C	–	2.2	6
Retinoic acid-human urinary RBP	equilibrium dialysis	Tris buffer, 4°C	–	11.0	11
Retinyl acetate-human plasma RBP	spectrofluorimetric titration	0.005 *M* phosphate buffered saline, pH 7.4, 27°C	–	2.2	6
Retinyl acetate-chicken plasma RBP	spectrofluorimetric titration	0.005 *M* phosphate buffered saline, pH 7.4, 27°C	–	1.7	6

[1] *Sreekrishna et al.* (unpublished).

PA_1, PA_2 and PA_3 in the decreasing order of their electrophoretic mobility. The prealbumins had mol wt in the range of 45,000–60,000, with high molar extinction coefficient at 280 nm, indicative of rich aromatic amino acid content. Purified chicken RBP exhibited microheterogeneity on polyacrylamide disc gel electrophoresis similar to those of other RBPs, but in contrast to the earlier findings of *Abe et al.* (1) with chicken RBP. While this work was being carried out, *Kopelman et al.* (16) also reported microheterogeneity in RBP isolated from retinol enriched chicken serum.

The affinities of PA_1, PA_2 and PA_3 to chicken RBP and *L*-thyroxine were determined by spectrofluorimetric titration based on the relative quenching of protein fluorescence upon addition of either RBP or *L*-thyroxine to constant amount of prealbumin (27). This data revealed that only PA_2 binds both RBP and *L*-thyroxine. PA_2 was further characterized as PA of the chicken PA-RBP complex by comparison of its electrophoretic mobility. PA-RBP complex also could bind thyroxine, indicating that PA has distinct sites for RBP and *L*-thyroxine and further, binding of RBP to PA does not inhibit the binding of *L*-thyroxine; a finding similar to that with human PA-RBP (10). The physiological significance of the transport of vitamin A and thyroxine by the interrelated carrier system needs to be investigated. Such studies might lead to a better understanding of the metabolic relationship that exists between vitamin A and thyroxine (3, 4, 5, 15).

Acknowledgement

The work from our laboratory reported here has been carried out with financial support from the Council of Scientific and Industrial Research, India. The authors wish to thank Hoffmann-La Roche, Bombay, India for the gift of synthetic vitamin A. The assistance of Mr. C. Venkateshan, Miss R.V. Jayamma and Miss V. Seetha is gratefully acknowledged.

References

1 *Abe, T.; Muto, Y., and Hosoya, N.:* J. Lipid Res. *16:* 200 (1975).
2 *Baker, C.M.A.; Manwell. C.; Lebisky, R.F., and Haper, J.A.:* Comp. Biochem. Physiol. *17:* 467 (1966).
3 *Bamji, M.S. and Sundaresan, P.R.:* J. Nutr. *74:* 39 (1961).
4 *Cama, H.R. and Goodwin, T.W.:* Biochem. J. *45:* 236 (1949).
5 *Cama, H.R.; Pillai, N.C.; Sundaresan, P.R., and Venkateshan, C.:* J. Nutr. *63:* 57 (1957).
6 *Cogan, U.; Kopelman, M.; Mokaday, S., and Shinitzky, M.:* Eur. J. Biochem. *65:* 71 (1976).
7 *Glover, J.:* Vitams Horm. *31:* 1 (1973).
8 *Glover, J.; Jay, C., and White, G.H.:* Vitams Horm. *32:* 215 (1974).

9 *Goodman, D.S.:* in *Galli, Jaicini and Pecile* Dietary lipids and postnatal development; p. 157 (Raven Press. New York).
10 *Gooaman, D.S.:* Vitams Horm. *32:* 167 (1974).
11 *Hase, J.; Kobashi, K.; Nakai, N., and Onosaka, S.:* J. Biochem. *79:* 373 (1976).
12 *Heller, J.:* J. biol. Chem. *250:* 3613 (1975).
13 *Heller, J.:* J. biol. Chem. *250:* 6549 (1975).
14 *Heller, J.:* Devl Biol. *51:* 1 (1976).
15 *Kishore, G.S.; Perumal, A.S., and Cama, H.R.:* Int. J. Vitam Nutr. Res. *41:* 172 (1971).
16 *Kopelman, M.; Cogan, U.; Mokaday, S., and Shinitzky, M.:* Biochim. biophys. Acta *439:* 442 (1976).
17 *Kopelman, M.; Cogan, U.; Mokaday, S., and Shinitzky, M.:* Biochim. biophys. Acta *439:* 449 (1976).
18 *Krishna Bhat, M.; Sreekrishna, K., and Cama, H.R.:* Indian J. Biochem. Biophys. (in press, 1977).
19 *Miller, S.B.:* Nature, Lond. *200:* 810 (1963).
20 *Mokaday, S. and Tal, M.:* Biochim. biophys. Acta *336:* 361 (1974).
21 *Muhilal, H. and Glover, J.:* Biochem. Soc. Trans. *3:* 744 (1975).
22 *Muto, Y. and Goodman, D.S.:* J. biol. Chem. *247:* 2533 (1972).
23 *Muto, Y.; Smith, F.R., and Goodman, D.S.:* J. Lipid Res. *14:* 525 (1973).
24 *Muto, Y.; Nakanishi, M., and Shidoji, Y.:* J. Biochem. *79:* 775 (1976).
25 *Nilsson, S.F.; Rask, L., and Peterson, P.A.:* J. biol. Chem. *250:* 8554 (1975).
26 *Oppenheimer, J.H.:* New Engl. J. Med. *278:* 1153 (1968).
27 *Peterson, P.A. and Rask, L.:* J. biol. Chem. *246:* 7544 (1971).
28 *Poulik, M.D.; Farrah, D.; Malek, G.H.; Shinnick, C.J., and Smithies, O.:* Biochim. biophys. Acta *412:* 326 (1975).
29 *Rask, L.:* Eur. J. Biochem. *44:* 1 (1974).
30 *Rask, L. and Peterson, P.A.:* J. biol. Chem. *251:* 6360 (1976).
31 *Sreekrishna, K; Podder, S.K., and Cama, H.R.:* Abst. Xth Int. Congr. Biochem. Hamburg; p. 203 (1976).
32 *Tylor, B.A.; Bailey, D.W., and Chery, M.:* Nature, Lond. *256:* 6451 (1975).

Dr. *K. Sreekrishna,* Department of Biochemistry, Indian Institute of Science, *Bangalore 560 012* (India)

Wld Rev. Nutr. Diet., vol. 31, pp. 59–64 (Karger, Basel 1978)

On the Systemic Mode of Action of Vitamin A

J. Ganguly, K. Sarada, M. Jayaram, P.S. Joshi, R.C. Das, S.K. Murthy, J.A. Thomas and M.K. Bhargava

Department of Biochemistry, Indian Institute of Science; Department of Pathology, St. John's Medical College, and Department of Pathology, Bangalore Medical College, Bangalore

Vitamin A is one of the earliest vitamins to be discovered; but, in spite of strenuous efforts made in many laboratories over a period of years, little is known regarding its systemic mode of action. Extensive information gathered by earlier investigators led to the generalisation that it is required in several major areas of physiology of higher animals, e.g., (i) vision, (ii) growth and (iii) reproduction. At the same time, numerous reports dealing with histopathological examination of tissues of vitamin A-deficient animals have consistently shown that the epithelial cells of intestinal mucosa, cornea, skin, trachea, etc., are the earliest to be affected by depletion of vitamin A. Probably the classical example here would be the vaginal cells. In a normal female rat they cycle every four to five days, but with the onset of vitamin A deficiency, these cells maintain a continuously cornified appearance. In fact, vaginal smear test is an accepted procedure for biological assay of vitamin A activity. One of the characteristic properties of the epithelial cells is that they undergo constant *in situ* differentiation.

On the other hand, it has been well established that the testes of the vitamin A-deprived rats do not grow and that such rats fail to fertilize normal females, while the ovaries of the deficient females do not develop properly. Spermatogenesis involves not only differentiation of the germinal epithelium, but several steps of mitosis also, while ovulation involves active mitosis of the theca and granulosa cells during the oestrous cycle. Similarly, development of rat foetus and chick embryo does not take place in retinol-deprived rats and chickens. Here also, both processes involve very rapid division and differentiation of cells.

These considerations had led *Ganguly* (3) to point out that all such diverse observations can be integrated on the basis of a unified hypothesis that vitamin A is required for division and differentiation of cells. During the past few years we have attempted to produce some evidence in support of such a concept by using regenerating rat liver and oestrogen-primed chick oviduct as typical model systems and some of our main observations are discussed here.

Regeneration of Rat Liver

Regenerating rat liver, following partial hepatectomy, has been recognised as a highly reproducible system for the study of growth and rapid cell division (1). We have shown that liver regeneration in terms of increase in net tissue weight as well as DNA, RNA and protein contents is markedly less in vitamin A-deprived rats, which could be restored to near normal levels by supplementation of the deprived rats with retinyl acetate immediately after partial hepatectomy (5). Histological examination showed that, after the hepatectomy, the mitotic index in the deficient livers was 1–2%, as compared to 1–4% in the corresponding normal controls. Moreover, the appearance of the endoplasmic reticulum differed markedly in the two groups in that, while it appeared essentially smooth in the depleted rats, in the normal animals it was mostly of the rough type (6).

Oestrogen-Primed Chick Oviduct

The other system we have used is the oestrogen-induced development of the oviduct of immature chicks. The magnum portion of the oviduct of immature chicks consists of a single layer of stratified columnar epithelial cells. Following oestrogen administration these primitive cells undergo initial rapid cell division, after which they differentiate into three types of cells; namely, the tubular gland cells, goblet cells, and ciliated epithelial cells (9, 10).

The chick oviduct offers a special advantage for studies of any role of vitamin A in cell division and differentiation. During its growth, the chick embryo draws upon the vitamin A laid down by the hen in the egg and, even after its development during the incubation period of 21 days, the freshly hatched chick can sustain itself for some more days by drawing upon the vitamin A still present in its liver as well as in the residual spare yolk (7). Therefore, the freshly hatched chick can be made deficient of vitamin A under well-controlled conditions by placing it on a suitable vitamin A-deficient diet.

We have shown that after six days of the hormone treatment the growth of the magnum portion of the oviduct in terms of increase in weight, length and in total DNA, RNA protein and phospholipid contents was strikingly less in the deficient birds, and that supplementation of the deficient birds with retinyl acetate during the hormone treatment reversed the effects of the deficiency almost fully (8). In contrast, when expressed per g of tissue, the differences between the depleted and normal groups were significant for proteins and phos-

Table I. Effect of vitamin A-nutritional status on the histomorphological patterns of the magnum of the oestrogen-primed chick oviduct

Treatment	Lobules per section		Acini		Oviduct wall	
	number	size	shape	number/ lobule	smooth muscle	connective tissue
Deficient	11.0 ± 0.2	+	elongated/oval	31.6 ± 4.2	++	++++
Retinyl acetate after depletion	9.4 ± 0.8	++++	circular	94.0 ± 4.5	++++	++++
Retinyl acetate from day 1, normal	11.7 ± 0.6	++++	circular	88.7 ± 3.6	++++	++++

Experimental conditions were as described in the text. The magnum portions were fixed in neutral formal saline and representative paraffin sections of 5 μ thickness were stained with (a) heamatoxylin and eosin, (b) van Gieson's stain and (c) Mason's trichrome with necessary controls. Quantitative assessment of the changes in some of the histomorphological parameters are expressed by using the notations +, ++, +++, ++++, keeping ++++ as an indicator for the morphological findings in the normal birds, which served as controls. The values are expressed as average ± SE.

pholipids, but those for RNA and DNA were not significant. It is thus obvious that the growth of the oviduct was due to an increase in its cell population.

Histomorphological examination of the magnum showed that, while the number of lobules per unit section was not significantly different in the various groups, their actual size differed markedly. It was even more striking that, while the average number of acini (tubular gland cells) per lobule was 88.7 ± 3.6 in the normal birds, the corresponding value for the deficient birds was only 31.6 ± 4.2. Here also, supplementation with retinyl acetate fully reversed the effect of the deficiency. It was equally striking that, while the deficiency markedly affected the formation of the smooth muscle, it had little effect on the formation of the connective tissue (table I).

It is, therefore, clear from these results that division and differentiation of the cells of the magnum depend upon adequate supply of retinol. But cell division is preceded by replication of cellular DNA. Therefore, the effect of deprivation of vitamin A on the incorporation *in vitro* of (^{3}H)-thymidine into DNA was investigated and it is shown in table II that the rate of incorporation of the labelled thymidine into the DNA of the deficient magnum was roughly 50%

Table II. Incorporation of (^{3}H)-thymidine into the DNA of the magnum of oestrogen-primed normal and vitamin A-deficient chick oviduct, and the effect of addition of retinol *in vitro*

Treatment	*In vitro* incorporation of (^{3}H)-thymidine (specific activity cpm/μg DNA) 48 h after 1st injection of estradiol	
	without retinol	with retinol (100 μg)
Retinyl acetate from day 1	6.81 ± 0.42	6.45 ± 0.31
Depleted	3.77 ± 0.27	5.39 ± 0.33

The experimental procedures were as described in the text. The values are means ± SD of six incubations from six birds.

of that in the normal control group. It was most significant that when retinol was added to the incubation medium at a concentration of 100 μg/ml, the thymidine incorporation into the deficient magnum was almost fully restored, while it had no such effects on the normal magnum.

Glycoproteins of the Oviduct

In recent years there has been considerable work demonstrating active participation of polyprenol phosphates in sugar-transfer reactions. Retinol is a tetraprenol and it is therefore a very attractive proposition that it might also participate in such reactions.

Chick oviduct is probably one of the most active tissues known for its ability to synthesize several glycoproteins, and we have, therefore, examined the contents of total sugar and free, as well as bound, sugar in the magnum of the normal and vitamin A-depleted birds treated with oestrogen. Our preliminary results have shown significant increase in the levels of free hexose and hexosamine in the depleted birds, with a corresponding decrease in the protein-bound sugars. We should, however, emphasize here that there were no significant differences in the amounts of total sugars in the tissues of the two groups of birds, and that the values were essentially comparable when expressed on the basis of per g tissue or per mg DNA.

At the same time, histochemical examination of the magnum revealed accumulation of striking amounts of alcian-blue positive materials (probably mucopolysaccharides) in the surface epithelial cells of the deficient magnum, with the normal birds showing very little of such materials. These materials were found to be localized on the luminal side of the cell cytoplasm.

From this work on the changes in free and bound sugar of the oviduct we have not been able to come to any definite conclusions regarding its role in sugar-transfer reactions. In addition, we should also point out several anomalous situations regarding participation of retinol in sugar-transfer reactions. Firstly, the role of polyprenols in such reactions is rather non-specific. In fact, according to *DeLuca et al.* (2) even under conditions where vitamin A participates in such reactions, dolichol also does so with considerable efficiency. Secondly, the amounts of dolichol found in animal liver are vastly in excess of the amounts of retinol present in the same tissue. Therefore, till some specificity with respect to retinol is demonstrated in these reactions, such an idea must remain unacceptable. Thirdly, such a mechanism cannot explain the physiological effects of retinoic acid, because it has not yet been demonstrated that retinoic acid can be reduced to retinol in the animal system, nor has it been shown that retinoic acid can directly participate in such reactions. Finally, while retinol is required in higher animals only, polyprenols also take part in sugar-transfer reactions in the lower organisms such as bacteria.

On the other hand, our electron microscopic examination of such an oviduct has revealed a markedly increased number of goblet cells in the deficient tissues treated with oestrogen. Earlier work of *Kohler et al.* (9) on the temporal relationship between the appearance of various types of cells in the oestrogen-primed chick oviduct showed that the tubular gland cells are the first to differentiate from the primitive epithelial cells, while the goblet and ciliated cells appear in significant numbers after the maturation of the gland cells takes place (normally around 7 to 8 days). But, in our work, goblet cells were found in larger numbers in the deficient birds, while in the normal tissues tubular gland cells predominated with occasional goblet cells. It is thus clear that depletion of vitamin A leads to a loss of control of the programmed differentiation of the epithelial cells of the oestrogen-treated oviduct magnum, and probably this is the first direct demonstration of involvement of retinol in the regulation of differentiation of epithelial cells. These considerations have led us to propose that retinol should be called a co-steroid hormone (4).

Acknowledgement

This work was supported by the PL–480 research grants FG-IN–460 and NIH–01–005–1 and, more recently, by a grant from the Department of Science and Technology, Government of India, New Delhi. Dr. *R.C. Das* wishes to thank the Council of Scientific and Industrial Research, New Delhi for a post-doctoral fellowship.

References

1 *Bresnick, E.:* Methods Cancer Res. *6:* 347 (1971).
2 *DeLuca, L.; Maestri, N.; Rosso, G., and Wolf, G.:* J. biol. Chem. *248:* 641 (1973).
3 *Ganguly, J.:* Medikon *6/7:* 23 (1974).
4 *Ganguly, J.; Sarada, K.; Joshi, P.S.; Das, R.C.; Murthy, S.K., and Bhargava, M.K.:* Indian J. Exp. Biol. (communicated).
5 *Jayaram, M.; Sarada, K., and Ganguly, J.:* Biochem. J. *146:* 501 (1975).
6 *Jayaram, M.; Sarada, K.; Ganguly, J., and Thomas, J.A.:* Ind. J. Exp. Biol. (communicated).
7 *Joshi, P.S.; Mathur, S.N.; Murthy, S.K., and Ganguly, J.:* Biochem. J. *136:* 757 (1973).
8 *Joshi, P.S.; Murthy, S.K., and Ganguly, J.:* Biochem. J. *154:* 249 (1976).
9 *Kohler, P.O.; Grimley, P.M., and O'Malley, B.W.:* J. Cell Biol. *40:* 8 (1969).
10 *O'Malley, B.W.; McGuire, W.L.; Kohler, P.O., and Korenman, S.G.:* Recent Prog. Horm. Res. *25:* 105 (1969).

Dr. *J. Ganguly*, Department of Biochemistry, Indian Institute of Science, *Bangalore 560012* (India)

Wld Rev. Nutr. Diet., vol. 31, pp. 65–70 (Karger, Basel 1978)

α-Retinol

G.A.J. Pitt

Department of Biochemistry, University of Liverpool, Liverpool[1]

α-Retinol is an isomer having an α-ionone ring instead of the β-ionone ring of retinol (fig. 1). It was first synthesized (22) when attempts were being made to identify the active derivative of retinaldehyde required for the regeneration of visual pigments, one hypothesis being that it might be α-retinaldehyde (10). The disproof of this hypothesis (18) and the failure to detect growth-promoting activity in α-retinaldehyde (1) temporarily diminished interest in α-retinol until *Houghton* (9) employed it for studying hypervitaminosis A.

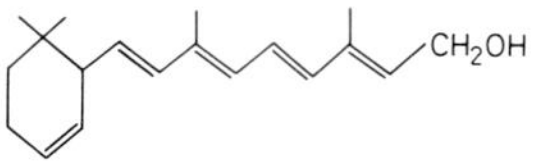

Dingle and Lucy (5) had investigated hypervitaminosis A as a possible approach to the mode of action of the vitamin. They had shown that the addition of large quantities of retinol produced marked effects on a number of systems *in vitro.* They were able to show that many of the characteristic effects of hypervitaminosis A both *in vitro* and *in vivo* could be ascribed to the excessive incorporation of retinol into the membranes of cells and organelles. They, therefore, advanced the hypothesis that the normal mode of action of the vitamin involved its incorporation into membranes which might be the physiological sites of action of the vitamin.

This hypothesis rested on the assumption that hypervitaminosis A was an exaggeration of the physiological action, an assumption strongly supported by the finding that over a range of compounds tested, the structural requirements for inducing hypervitaminosis A seemed to be the same as for curing vitamin A deficiency (4, 6, 13).

[1] We thank F. Hoffmann-La Roche and Co., Basel, Switzerland for the generous gift of (11, 12-$^3H_2$) retinyl acetate.

α-Retinol appeared to destroy this generalization. α-Retinol was very effective in inducing signs of hypervitaminosis A both *in vivo* and *in vitro.* When added in large quantities *in vitro,* it caused haemolysis of erythrocytes, swelling of mitochondria and the release of a protease from lysosomes. Feeding it in large amounts to rats resulted in the thinning of bones and fractures of long bones, the characteristic lesions of hypervitaminosis A.

All these effects it produced with approximately the same potency as retinol itself. In contrast, in rat growth tests it had only 2% of the activity of retinol (9, 20). I, (20, 21) therefore, concluded that some features of hypervitaminosis A were not related to the physiological mode of action of the vitamin. From their work on α-retinoic acid and other compounds, *Goodman et al.* (8) agreed with this.

By appearing to remove one of the major pieces of supporting evidence, this finding diminished, to some extent, the hypothesis, which nevertheless still had evidence in its favour (14, 23), that retinol operated in membranes.

One piece of evidence we had obtained on α-retinol did not, however, fit neatly into the pattern. Hypovitaminosis A is characterized by keratinizing squamous metaplasia, i.e., mucous epithelia change to keratinizing squamous epithelia (31); and in hypervitaminosis A one sees the opposite effect: keratinizing squamous epithelia undergo mucous metaplasia, i.e., they change to mucous epithelia (7, 28).

This can readily be demonstrated by sewing a wax pellet containing large amounts of retinol into a hamster cheek pouch. The normally squamous epithelium of the cheek pouch undergoes mucous metaplasia (12). At concentrations at which retinol is effective at initiating this change, α-retinol has no detectable activity (20). This is what was expected at the time: the physiological function of vitamin A involves a role in differentiation and as α-retinol does not maintain growth well, it was not thought it would induce mucous metaplasia.

When, however, levels of α-retinol higher than those first reported (20) were used, α-retinol was found (9) to have more activity in inducing mucous metaplasia than would have been expected from its very low potency in promoting growth.

Some years after these findings were made, *Sporn's* group investigated the effect of various compounds in curing vitamin A deficiency in hamster tracheas in organ culture (2, 26, 27). In the medium which was deficient in vitamin A, the tracheas began to show keratinizing metaplasia which could be cured by the addition to the culture medium of either retinol or α-retinol. α-Retinol was only slightly less effective than retinol. Although no relative potency figures were calculated, its activity was of the same order of magnitude as that of retinol (27).

Further, α-retinol had a high affinity for the cellular retinol-binding protein to which retinol has been found to be attached in a number of tissues (17).

Table I. Plasma vitamin A concentrations (expressed as ng retinol or α-retinol/100 ml) in vitamin A-deficient rats given a single dose of 40 μg (11-^{3}H)α-retinol or 1 μg (11–12-$^3H_2$) retinyl acetate

Dose	40 μg α-retinol			1 μg retinyl acetate		
time after dosing, h	total	alcohol	ester	total	alcohol	ester
4	468	286	181	150	130	20
8	205	84	116	364	354	10
24	165	35	126	166	163	3
72	48	12	35	103	103	0

Table II. Total vitamin A (expressed as ng retinol or α-retinol) in livers of retinol deficient rats given a single dose of 40 μg (11-^{3}H)α-retinol or 1 μg (11–12-$^3H_2$) retinyl acetate

Dose, time after dosing, h	40 μg α-retinol	1 μg retinyl acetate
4	4188	102
8	3488	48
24	1900	31
72	504	18

We have, therefore, an apparent paradox. α-Retinol has little growth-promoting activity when fed to animals on a diet deficient in vitamin A, a finding confirmed in other laboratories (3, 8, 25). In organ culture it is not very much less effective than retinol in discharging a physiological function of the vitamin; and in inducing hypervitaminosis A both *in vitro* and *in vivo* it also appears to be about as effective as retinol.

The clue to resolving this apparent paradox came when *Willetts* (29, 30) synthesized (11-^{3}H)α-retinol.

40 μg (11-^{3}H)α-retinol was given orally to each of 4 vitamin A-deficient rats. The rats were killed after 4, 8, 24 and 72 h. The amounts in the plasma were low (table I). The highest concentration was found after 4 h and reached only 468 ng/100 ml plasma; at later times the concentration fell until after 72 h it was only 48 ng/100 ml. In contrast, rats given, orally, the extremely small dose of only 1 μg (11, 12-$^3H_2$) retinyl acetate had higher plasma concentrations at all times from 8 h onwards (table I) even though the dose (equivalent to 0.8 μg retinol) was only 1/46 of that of α-retinol.

Table II shows that the low plasma concentrations of α-vitamin A were not due to there being less α-vitamin A in the liver.

Another noticeable difference (table I) was that in the rats given retinol almost all in the plasma was in the alcohol form; as expected, little was esterified. In the plasma of the rats given α-retinol the esterified form predominated over the free alcohol at all times from 8 h onwards (table I).

Larger doses of unlabelled α-retinol (5 mg/rat, spread over 3 days) were given to 3 rats which had been maintained on retinoic acid so that their bodies contained no retinol. Seven days after the last supplement the rats were exsanguinated. The total α-vitamin A content of the pooled plasma was 18 μg/100 ml, compared with 37 μg vitamin A/100 ml in the plasma of similar rats given equal doses of retinol. The plasma levels of α-vitamin A, therefore, remained below what might be expected, even though the doses were large enough to result in sizable liver stores, equivalent to a mean value of 763 μg α-retinol/rat (30). The presence of these substantial liver stores did not enable the plasma concentration of α-vitamin A to be maintained at a normal level for retinol. Although they did not determine the liver stores, *Goodman et al.* (8) also failed to raise the blood concentration with large doses of α-retinol.

The inability of the rat to maintain the concentration of α-vitamin A and its appearance in plasma in the esterified rather than the free alcohol form show that α-retinol is not being handled by the rat in the same way as is retinol.

Retinol is transported in the plasma on a carrier protein, retinol-binding protein (RBP) (16). *Muhilal and Glover* (15) tested α-retinol and found that, unlike retinol, it failed to combine *in vitro* with apo-RBP, i.e., RBP without retinol attached.

It is interesting that plasma RBP has a different and much narrower specificity than the cellular retinol-binding protein (17). Given that the specificity of RBP is such that it will not combine with α-retinol, all observations now fall into a consistent pattern.

Others had suggested that the low potency of α-retinol in promoting growth might have been due to failure of the plasma transport system (3, 8, 25). Our observations prove these suggestions and also explain why large oral doses of α-retinol are about as effective as retinol in inducing hypervitaminosis A, when small doses of α-retinol are very much poorer than retinol at maintaining growth.

Dietary α-retinol is carried to the liver in chylomicrons and stored there as esters. α-Retinol cannot, however, be put onto RBP, so the plasma concentration of α-retinol is low. Some enters the blood, mainly in the esterified form, probably attached to lipoproteins (11).

In hypervitaminosis A, the normal storage mechanism for esterfied vitamin A is overwhelmed and retinyl esters pass into the plasma in uncontrolled amounts attached to lipoproteins. They reach the tissues in relatively high concentrations and there cause hypervitaminosis A (11). High doses of α-retinol will have the same effects. The inability of α-retinol to combine with RBP will not diminish its ability to induce hypervitaminosis A; indeed it may even enhance it (11).

The obvious conclusion to be drawn from our findings and from other reports in the literature is that if a compound is to efficiently discharge the role of vitamin A in promoting growth, it must be bound to RBP. Presumably this is necessary for its effective delivery to tissues. For example, retinoic acid which does not normally bind to RBP (24) has much lower growth-promoting activity than retinyl acetate (which is readily converted to retinol). In contrast, in the α-compounds, α-retinyl acetate has even less growth-promoting activity than α-retinoic acid; both were very ineffective; neither binds to RBP.

My conclusion (20, 21) that many features of hypervitaminosis A were irrelevant to the physiological mode of action can be seen to have been rash. Now that we can correctly interpret the early work with α-retinol (20) there seems no reason to discard the hypothesis (5) that the membrane-seeking and potentially membranolytic action of retinol seen in hypervitaminosis A may represent an exaggeration of its physiological role.

There is little doubt that many compounds will behave similarly to α-retinol in that they will function as vitamin A if they can be delivered to the tissue where they have to operate, but if tested by orthodox rat-growth bioassay they will have little vitamin A activity. *Sporn et al.* have shown (26, 27) that a number of vitamin A analogues (retinoids) show vitamin A activity in tracheal organ culture. At least one of these besides α-retinol has no growth-promoting activity when fed to rats (8), and from past experience (19) one can confidently predict that many of the others will fail to promote growth.

Numerous rat-growth bioassays have been carried out over many years in attempts to identify the structural requirements for a molecule to show vitamin A activity (19). It is probable, in many cases, that what has been tested has been the structural specificity, not for the molecular mode of action of the vitamin in tissues, but rather of the retinol-binding protein necessary to transport it in plasma.

References

1 *Ames, S.R.; Swanson, W.J., and Harris, P.L.:* J. Am. chem. Soc. *77:* 4136 (1955).
2 *Clamon, G.H.; Sporn, M.B.; Smith, J.M., and Saffiotti, U.:* Nature *250:* 64 (1974).
3 *Clamon, G.H.; Sporn, M.B.; Smith, J.M., and Henderson, W.R.:* J. Nutr. *105:* 215 (1975).
4 *Dingle, J.T. and Lucy, J.A.:* Biochem. J. *84:* 611 (1962).
5 *Dingle, J.T. and Lucy, J.A.:* Biol. Rev. *40:* 422 (1965).
6 *Fell, H.B.; Dingle, J.T., and Webb, M.:* Biochem. J. *83:* 63 (1962).
7 *Fell, H.B. and Mellanby, E.:* J. Physiol. *119:* 470 (1953).

8 *Goodman, D.S.; Smith, J.E.; Hembry, R.M., and Dingle, J.T.:* J. Lipid Res. *15:* 406 (1974).
9 *Houghton, S.E.:* α-Retinol; Ph.D. Thesis, University of Liverpool (1969).
10 *Hubbard, R.; Gregerman, R.I., and Wald, G.:* J. gen. Physiol. *36:* 415 (1953).
11 *Krishna Mallia, A.; Smith, J.E., and Goodman, D.S.:* J. Lipid Res. *16:* 180 (1975).
12 *Lawrence, D.J.; Bern, H.A., and Steadman, M.G.:* Ann. Otol. Rhinol. Lar. *69:* 645 (1960).
13 *Lucy, J.A.; Luscombe, M., and Dingle, J.T.:* Biochem. J. *89:* 419 (1963).
14 *Mack, J.P.; Lui, N.S.T.; Roels, O.A., and Anderson, O.R.:* Biochim. biophys. Acta *288:* 203 (1972).
15 *Muhilal, H. and Glover, J.:* Biochem. Soc. Trans. *3:* 744 (1975).
16 *Muto, Y. and Goodman, D.S.:* J. biol. Chem. *247:* 2533 (1972).
17 *Ong, D.E. and Chytil, F.:* Nature *255:* 74 (1975).
18 *Oroshnik, W.; Brown, P.K.; Hubbard, R., and Wald, G.:* Proc. natn. Acad. Sci. USA, *42:* 578 (1956).
19 *Pitt, G.A.J.:* Proc. Nutr. Soc. *24:* 153 (1965).
20 *Pitt, G.A.J.:* Am. J. clin. Nutr. *22:* 1045 (1969).
21 *Pitt, G.A.J.:* J. Sci. Indust. Res. *29:* Suppl S 1 (1970).
22 *Robeson, C.D.; Cawley, J.D.; Weisler, L.; Stern, M.H.; Eddinger, C.C., and Chechak, A.J.:* J. Am. chem. Soc. *77:* 4111 (1955).
23 *Roels, O.A.; Anderson, O.R.; Lui, N.S.T.; Shah, D.O., and Trout M.E.:* Am. J. clin. Nutr. *22:* 1020 (1969).
24 *Smith, J.E.; Milch, P.O.; Muto, Y., and Goodman, D.S.:* Biochem. J. *132:* 821 (1973).
25 *Sneider, W.D.; Rosso, G.C.; Rogers, A.E.; Wolf, G.; Dowling, J.E., and Callahan, M.J.:* J. Nutr. *104:* 1662 (1974).
26 *Sporn, M.B.; Dunlop, N.M.; Newton, D.L., and Henderson, W.R.:* Nature *263:* 110 (1976).
27 *Sporn, M.B.; Clamon, G.H.; Dunlop, N.M.; Newton, D.L.; Smith, J.M., and Saffiotti, U.:* Nature *253:* 47 (1975).
28 *Sweeny, P.R. and Hardy, M.H.:* Anat. Rec. *185:* 93 (1976).
29 *Willetts, S.R.:* Retinol and α-Retinol, Ph.D. Thesis (University of Liverpool, 1973).
30 *Willetts, S.R.; Houghton, S.E.; Jones, G., and Pitt, G.A.J.:* Proc. Nutr. Soc. *35:* 142 A (1976).
31 *Wolbach, S.B.:* in *Sebrell and Harris* The vitamins; vol. 1, p. 106 (Academic Press, New York 1954).

Dr. *G.A.J. Pitt,* Department of Biochemistry, University of Liverpool, P.O.Box 147, *Liverpool L69 3BX* (England)

Wld Rev. Nutr. Diet., vol. 31, pp. 71–76 (Karger, Basel 1978)

Functional Aspects of the Plasma Retinol-Binding Protein[1]

Lars Rask and Urban Forsum

Institute of Medical and Physiological Chemistry, Biomedical Center and Department of Dermatology, University Hospital, University of Uppsala, Uppsala

Vitamin A is essential for the maintenance of normal physiological functions of epithelial tissues. Deficiency of the vitamin causes diminished growth, sterility, increased susceptibility to infection, blindness and, ultimately, death (15). The intestinal resorption of vitamin A was investigated by *Goodman et al.* (10). They found that the alcoholic form of vitamin A, retinol, is generated from both retinyl-esters and provitamin A compounds, carotenes, in the small intestine. The free retinol produced is subsequently re-esterified by long chain fatty acids within the mucosal cells and transported, bound to chylomicrons, via the lymphatics to the liver, where it is stored in the hepatocytes (18).

Retinol is then released into the plasma, bound to a specific carrier protein, the retinol-binding protein (RBP). RBP was first isolated from human plasma (11, 16) and human urine (17). Subsequently, it has been purified from the plasma of several species (1, 14, 18, 22, 27). RBP has a molecular weight of 21,000 and consists of a single polypeptide chain. In plasma, RBP of all species investigated is almost exclusively attached to thyroxine-binding prealbumin (1, 22, 27) which is composed of four identical subunits, each with a molecular weight of approximately 14,000 (2, 3, 13, 23).

RBP is synthesized in the hepatocytes. In vitamin A deficiency, when the liver has been exhausted of the vitamin, the plasma RBP concentration decreases drastically (14, 18). The main reason for that is, however, not a diminished *de novo* synthesis of RBP, but a decreased secretion of it into the plasma. The concentration of RBP is actually severalfold higher in the liver with vitamin A deficiency than under normal conditions. These observations warranted an investigation of the RBP-synthesis in the liver. RBP was quantified by means of a radio-immunoassay in different subcellular fractions. Rat liver was fractionated

[1] The work cited from the authors' laboratory has been supported by grants from the Swedish Medical Research Council.

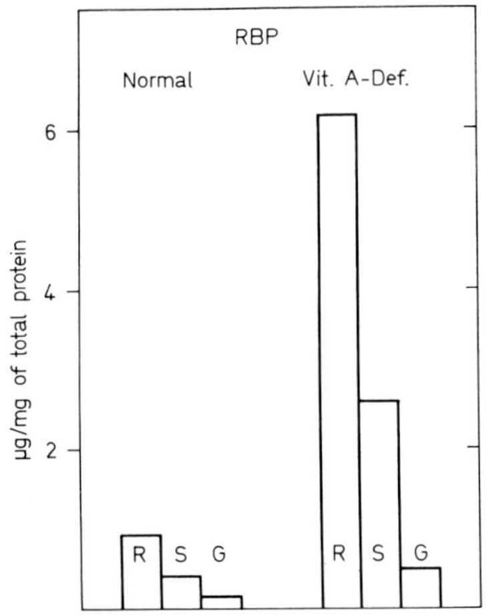

Fig. 1. The distribution of RBP in different subcellular fractions of rat liver under normal conditions and at vitamin A deficiency. RBP was quantified by means of a radioimmunoassay after solubilization with 1% Triton X-100 in 0.15 *M* NaCl, 0.02 *M* Tris-Cl, pH 8.0. R = rough endoplasmatic reticulum; G = Golgi fractions; S = smooth endoplasmatic reticulum.

by standard methods into rough and smooth endoplasmatic reticulum, Golgi fraction, plasma-membrane, and cell supernatant. The concentration of RBP relative to total protein content of the fractions was found to be highest in the rough endoplasmatic reticulum (fig. 1). RBP was undetectable in the plasma membrane fraction and in the supernatant. Albumin displayed a reversed distribution with the highest concentration in the Golgi fraction, lower in the smooth and still lower in the rough endoplasmatic reticulum. (Data not shown). In other respects RBP and albumin seem to behave in a similar manner. Both molecules are contained within the microsomes as soluble, secretory proteins. Furthermore, when the Golgi fraction was subfractionated, RBP and albumin were distributed in a similar way in contrast to, i.e., ceruloplasmin. In vitamin A deficiency, the concentration of RBP was found to be increased in all the three subcellular fractions studied (fig. 1). Studies under way may explain at what stage of the synthesis and secretion of RBP, vitamin A is introduced into the molecule and may resolve how the synthesis and secretion are regulated (25).

Retinol transported in plasma by the RBP-prealbumin complex is taken up by tissue cells, e.g., epithelial cells of the intestinal mucosa. In order to gain some insight into the vitamin A uptake system an *in vitro* system of dispersed monkey small intestinal cells was used to study the interaction of RBP and retinol with such cells (24). Monkey intestinal cells incubated with RBP containing (^{3}H)-retinol readily resorbed retinol. Vitamin A could even be taken up by the cells from RBP coupled to Sepharose-beads, which excluded the possibility that the RBP-molecule enters the cell when delivering its retinol molecule. Several lines of evidence, including inhibition experiments with fragments of antibodies against RBP, free retinol, and RBP with or without unlabelled retinol, strongly suggested that the plasma membrane of the intestinal cells contains some kind of receptor able to interact directly with RBP-molecules containing vitamin A. *Heller* reached a similar conclusion using a different experimental system (8). The demonstration of receptor structures for RBP on the cell surface has further implications. Firstly, it provides a possible explanation as to how different types of cells regulate their uptake of vitamin A. Cells not dependent on that vitamin may lack the receptor, while epithelial cells can be proposed to have it, at least during certain stages of their differentiation. Secondly, it provides a mechanism as to how the tissue cells avoid the toxicity of free vitamin A. Retinol is a highly surface-active substance, destroying cells if it is allowed to interact directly with them (7, 12, 24). When bound to RBP it is only delivered to the physiological sites on the cells, the receptors. Vitamin A toxicity can, therefore, be anticipated to occur when the RBP-prealbumin transport system has, for some reason, been overwhelmed.

When the RBP molecule has delivered its vitamin A to the tissue cells, it is modified in such a way that its affinity both for the receptor and for prealbumin decreases drastically (19, 24). The binding to prealbumin prevents the small molecule from being excreted through the kidney glomerulus. Consequently, the modified RBP-molecules which circulate free from prealbumin in plasma are rapidly filtrated through the kidney glomerulus and subsequently reabsorbed in the proximal tubulus. Recent studies have shown that the kidney has a key role in the regulation of the RBP metabolism (19).

The study of the vitamin A uptake to intestinal cells, and the fact that RBP is degraded in the kidney, show that the interaction between RBP and the tissue cells is only transient, which implies that it might be difficult to demonstrate physical binding of RBP to tissue cells under *in vivo* conditions. We, therefore, chose immuno-fluorescence microscopy as a method to survey different human and monkey tissues for the presence of RBP. The reason was that the preparation of tissues for this procedure actually freezes the cells almost instantaneously. If the vitamin A uptake process of certain cells is slow enough it might be possible to detect RBP-molecules remaining bound to those cells. Several epithelial tissues were investigated with indirect immuno-fluorescence microscopy. Figure 2A shows a transverse section of human skin stained with a non-immune rabbit serum followed by fluorescein conjugated goat anti-rabbit immunoglobulin. The only fluorescence observed is a weak autofluorescence from the collagen fibrills in the dermis. When an identical section was investigated by the same procedure for the presence of β_2-microglobulin, a constant chain of human histocompatibility antigens present on all nucleated cells (20),

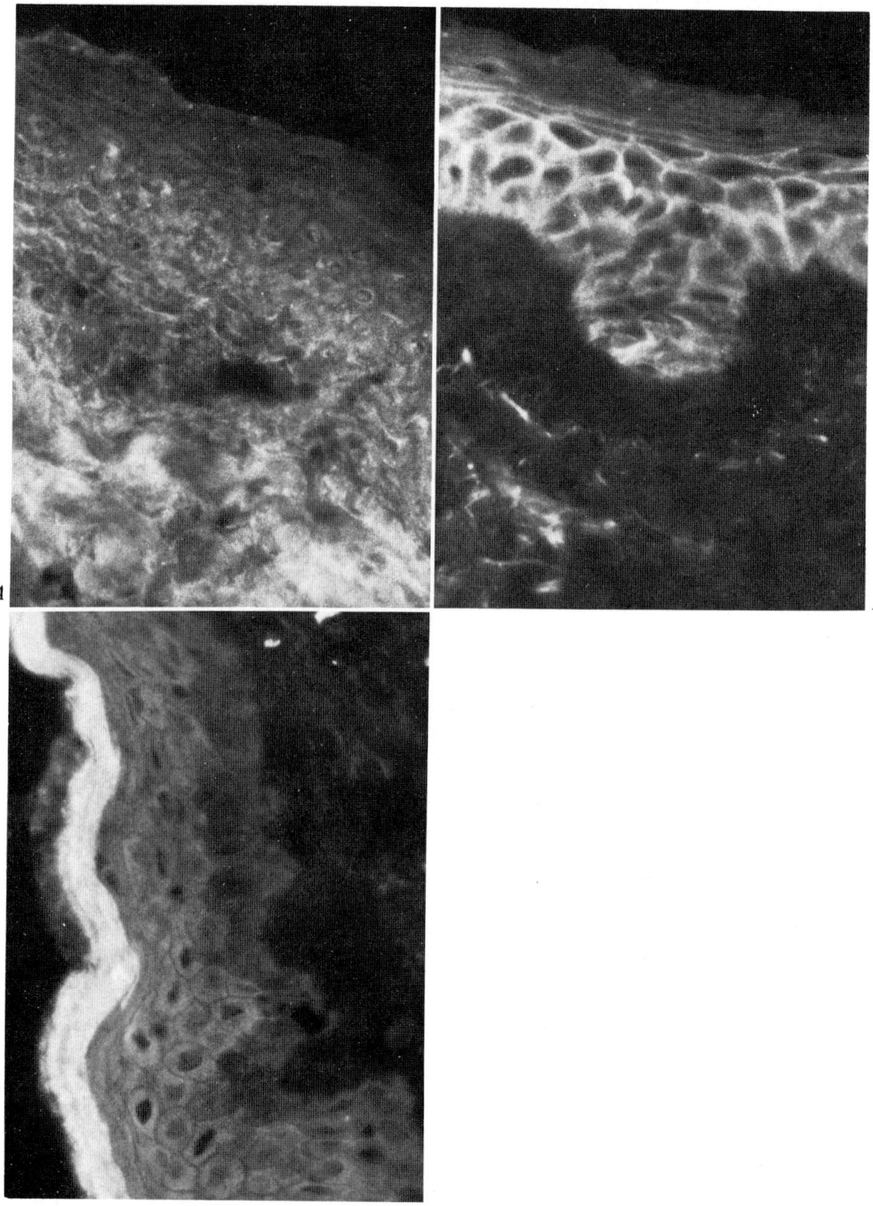

Fig. 2. Immuno-fluorescence micrographs of sections of human skin stained with: A = =non-immune rabbit serum; B = rabbit anti-β_2-microglobulin and, C = rabbit anti-RBP, followed by fluorescein conjugated goat anti-rabbit immunoglobulin.

all epidermal cells were brightly stained (fig. 2B). In contrast, a skin section treated with an anti-RBP serum showed an intense fluorescence confined to the external part of the epidermis, i.e., the internal part of *stratum corneum, stratum granulosum,* and the external cell layers of *stratum germinativum.* This finding may look astonishing. The cell layers shown to have RBP-molecules bound are about to keratinize or have already keratinized and it is well established that vitamin A prevents the keratinization of epithelial cells. An explanation of these apparently contradictory findings may be as follows: in epidermis, all mitoses occur in the most internal layer of *stratum germinativum.* Subsequently, the cells differentiate and concommittantly move outwards towards *stratum corneum.* These cells are dependent on vitamin A and have a fast turnover of RBP molecules at their receptors. However, at a certain stage of differentiation when the cells approach *stratum granulosum* and are about to keratinize, they lose their ability to take up vitamin A but still retain their receptors for RBP. As retinol remains in the RBP molecule, a sustained interaction between RBP and the cells is obtained which is visualized by the immunofluorescence technique. A similar pattern has not been found in tissues where almost all cells are vitamin A-dependent e.g., small intestinal epithelium and secretory glands (26).

What is then the actual physiological role of vitamin A in epithelial tissues? No unequivocal answer is at present available to that question. Particular interest has been placed on the demonstration of glycosylated retinyl-derivatives in different tissues (4, 9, 21). *DeLuca et al.*, showed earlier that the glycoprotein synthesis in small intestinal cells is affected by vitamin A deficiency (5, 6). Although it has been difficult to unambiguously demonstrate, it is tempting to speculate that the glycosylated retinyl derivatives are involved in the biosynthesis of carbohydrate-containing molecules, glycoproteins and/or glycolipids present on the cell surface. As entirely new techniques have become available for the study of cell membrane biochemistry during recent years, it may well be worthwhile to continue to extend these studies. It must, however, be emphasized that a possible role of vitamin A in glycosylation reactions does not exclude its participation in other biochemical events and that the vitamin may have different functions in different tissues.

References

1 *Abe, T.; Muto, Y., and Hosoya, N.:* Life Sci. *17:* 1579 (1976).

2 *Blake, C.C.F.; Swan, I.D.A.; Rerat, C.; Berthou, J.; Laurent, A., and Rerat, B.:* J. molec. Biol. *61:* 217 (1971).

3 *Branch, W.T., Jr.; Robbins, J., and Edelhoch, H.:* J. biol. Chem. *246:* 6011 (1971).

4 *DeLuca, L.; Rosso, G., and Wolf, G.:* Biochem. biophys. Res. Commun. *41:* 615 (1970).

5 *DeLuca, L.; Schumacher, M., and Wolf, G.:* J. biol. Chem. *245:* 4558 (1970).
6 *DeLuca, L.; Schumacher, M., and Nelson, D.P.:* J. biol. Chem. *246:* 5762 (1971).
7 *Dingle, J.T.; Fell, H.B., and Goodman, D.S.:* J. Cell Sci. *11:* 393 (1972).
8 *Heller, J.:* J. biol. Chem. *259:* 3613 (1975).
9 *Helting, T. and Peterson, P.A.:* Biochem. biophys. Res. Commun. *46:* 429 (1972).
10 *Huang, M.S. and Goodman, D.S.:* J. biol. Chem. *240:* 2839 (1965).
11 *Kanai, M.; Raz, A., and Goodman, D.S.:* J. clin. Invest. *47:* 2025 (1968).
12 *Mallia, A.K.; Smith, J.E., and Goodman, D.S.:* J. Lipid Res. *16:* 180 (1975).
13 *Morgan, F.J.; Canfield, R.E., and Goodman, D.S.:* Biochim. biophys. Acta *236:* 798 (1971).
14 *Muto, Y. and Goodman, D.S.:* J. biol. Chem. *247:* 2533 (1972).
15 *Olson, J.A.:* Fed. Proc. Fed. Am. Socs exp. Biol. *28:* 1670 (1969).
16 *Peterson, P.A.:* Abstr. of Uppsala Dissertations in Medicine *75:* (1969).
17 *Peterson, P.A. and Berggard, I.:* J. biol. Chem. *246:* 25 (1971).
18 *Peterson, P.A.; Rask, L.; Ostberg, L.; Andersson, L.; Kamwendo, F., and Pertoft, H.:* J. biol. Chem. *248:* 4009 (1973).
19 *Peterson, P.A.; Nilsson, S.F.; Ostberg, L.; Rask, L., and Vahlquist, A.:* Vitams Horm. *32:* 181 (1974).
20 *Peterson, P.A.; Rask, L., and Lindblom, J.B.:* Proc. natn. Acad. Sci. USA *71:* 35 (1974).
21 *Peterson, P.A.; Rask, L.; Ostberg, L.; Helting, T., and Fernstedt, Y.:* J. biol. Chem. *251:* 4986 (1976).
22 *Rask, L.:* Eur. J. Biochem. *44:* 1 (1974).
23 *Rask, L.; Peterson, P.A., and Nilsson, S.F.:* J. biol. Chem. *246:* 6087 (1971).
24 *Rask, L. and Peterson, P.A.:* J. biol. Chem. *251:* 6360 (1976).
25 *Rask, L.; Dallner, G., and Peterson, P.A.:* Manuscript in preparation.
26 *Rask, L.; Forsum, U.; Tjernlund, H.; Noren, P., and Peterson, P.A.:* Manuscript in preparation.
27 *Vahlquist, A. and Peterson, P.A.:* Biochem. *11:* 4526 (1972).

Dr. *L. Rask,* Institute of Medical and Physiological Chemistry, Biomedical Center and Department of Dermatology, University Hospital, University of Uppsala, *Uppsala* (Sweden)

Wld Rev. Nutr. Diet., vol. 31, pp. 77–82 (Karger, Basel 1978)

Mode of Action of Vitamin A

Studies on Lipid Metabolism

G.C. Ram and U.K. Misra

Department of Radioisotopes and Biochemistry, V.P. Chest Institute, University of Delhi, Delhi, and G.B. Pant University of Agriculture and Technology, Pantnagar

Generally, three models have been used to study the functions and mode of action of vitamin A, namely, (i) depletion-repletion models (ii) hypervitaminotic A models and (iii) isolated systems. All these models have their merits and limitations. We have studied the mode of action of vitamin A in cellular metabolism using acute and prolonged hypervitaminotic A models (1, 5, 6). These studies indicated that the effects of vitamin A are mediated through the adrenals, i.e., adrenocorticoids (4, 8, 10). There are several reports which show that vitamin A may be involved in the structural and functional integrity of biological membranes. The evidences to favour these are release of lysosomal and mitochondrial enzymes, rupture of erythrocytes, penetration of vitamin A into lecithin-cholesterol monolayers and presence of vitamin A in biological membranes (11). To study the membranolytic effect of excess vitamin A, we have chosen phenobarbital which is known to enhance the mass of endoplasmic reticulum and its constituents. Since phenobarbital enhances the proliferation of membranes and excess vitamin A labilises the membranes, vitamin A should minimise the membrane proliferation induced by phenobarbital, if both are given together. We have tested this hypothesis in liver of adult female rats by determining the following parameters: (a) distribution and synthesis of molecular species of phosphatidylcholine (PC) and (b) exchange of PC between microsomes and mitochondria.

Adult female rats weighing 100–120 g were divided into four groups of 4 rats each. To one group of rats 15 mg retinol in 0.2 ml of groundnut oil was fed daily for 4 days. To the second group of rats, phenobarbital dissolved in sterilised normal saline was given intraperitoneally (7.1 mg/100 g body weight) daily for 4 days. To the third group of rats, feeding of 15 mg retinol was immediately followed by intraperitoneal injection of phenobarbital (7.1 mg/100 g body weight) daily for 4 days. The fourth group was given the vehicle solution for 4 days. Food was given to rats in the evening. Following the phenobarbital injection on the night prior to killing, food was withheld from all the groups. Rats were injected intraperitoneally with a saline solution of $NaH_2(^{32}PO_4)$ (100 μCi/100 g body weight) and (methyl-^{14}C) *L*-methionine HCl (10 μCi/100 g body weight) 3 h and 90 min before sacrifice, respectively. Plasma, liver and its subcellular fractions were processed for the isolation of lipids. The molecular species of PC were isolated and estimated by means of silver nitrate impregnated thin layer chromatography (2).

In another set of experiments, female rats (110–130 g) were divided into two groups. To group one, 15 mg retinol dissolved in 0.2 ml groundnut oil was fed daily for 4 days. To the second group, only the vehicle solution was given for the same period. 17 h before sacrifice, $NaH_2(^{32}PO_4)$ (100 μCi/100 g body weight) was given intraperitoneally to rats of both groups. Exchange of PC between mitochondria and microsomal fractions was studied according to *Wirtz and Zilversmit* (12). Radioactivity measurements and other estimates have been reported earlier (10).

Either retinol feeding or phenobarbital administration increased liver weight, RNA content, triglycerides and free fatty acids. Both these agents, significantly increased liver microsomal protein, phospholipids, PC and phosphatidyl ethanolamine (9). When retinol and phenobarbital were administered together, their effects on liver and microsomal constituents were additive. Since increase in liver microsomal protein and phospholipids in phenobarbital-treated rats has been correlated with the proliferation of endoplasmic reticulum (13), it appears that retinol may also be causing proliferation of endoplasmic reticulum.

Molecular Species of PC in Liver

Retinol feeding increased the amounts of monoenoic and dienoic and decreased hexaenoic PC but did not affect the trienoic and tetraenoic species (table I). Phenobarbital administration significantly increased monoenoic, die-

Table I. Retinol and phenobarbital administration and molecular species of liver PC of female rats (mean ± SE)

PC species	Groups, μg PLP/liver			
	C	R	P	R + P
Monoenoic	246 ± 15	293 ± 9^s	393 ± 18^s	396 ± 13^s
Dienoic	522 ± 28	754 ± 31^s	703 ± 46^s	1123 ± 61^s
Trienoic	83 ± 5	105 ± 7	104 ± 8	140 ± 10^s
Tetraenoic	1168 ± 82	1185 ± 68	1796 ± 115^s	1837 ± 88^s
Hexaeonic	246 ± 16	182 ± 9^s	227 ± 16	236 ± 15

s = significant; C = control; R = retinol-fed; P = phenobarbital-treated; R ± P = retinol + phenobarbital treated; PLP = phospholipid.

noic and tetraenoic PC but did not affect the amounts of trienoic and hexaenoic PC as compared to controls. When both retinol and phenobarbital were given together, the dienoic and tetraenoic species were further elevated. These results indicate that retinol and phenobarbital effect the various pathways of PC synthesis differently.

Molecular Species of Mitochondrial and Microsomal PC

Retinol feeding significantly increased dienoic PC, decreased tetraenoic PC and did not affect other species of PC of liver microsomes. Also, in mitochondria, retinol feeding increased dienoic PC, decreased monoenoic and hexaenoic PC and did not affect other species of PC. A decrease in brain polyunsaturated fatty acids in hypervitaminotic A rats (7) and in mitochondria of vitamin A-deficient rats has been observed and this has been associated with permeability (3).

The incorporation of $NaH_2(^{32}PO_4)$ into dienoic PC was significantly increased whereas it was decreased into trienoic, tetraenoic and hexaenoic PC of retinol fed rats (1). The specific activity (cpm/μg PLP) of monoenoic PC was decreased in retinol-fed or phenobarbital-treated rats. When both retinol and phenobarbital were given together, the total activity as well as the specific activity of monoenoic PC was reduced, suggesting that its synthesis and turnover was depressed (table II).

Phenobarbital decreased both the total activity and specific activity of dienoic PC. When retinol and phenobarbital were given together, the total and specific activities of dienoic PC were reduced, but the relative percentage radioactivity distribution of (^{32}P) into dienoic PC was increased (table II). These results show that retinol stimulated the synthesis of dienoic PC whereas phenobarbital depressed it. Retinol reduced the incorporation of (^{32}P) into tetraenoic PC whereas phenobarbital had no effect. Rats given retinol and phenobarbital together also showed reduced label in tetraeonic PC. Administration of retinol and phenobarbital either alone or in combination also reduced the incorporation of (^{32}P) into hexaenoic PC.

Retinol significantly increased the incorporation of (^{32}P) into dienoic PC and decreased into tetraenoic PC of liver microsomes. However, unlike whole liver, retinol did not affect the incorporation into hexaenoic PC of microsomes. (Data not shown here.) However, in mitochondria, incorporation of (^{32}P) into hexaenoic PC was also reduced. Thus the decreased amounts and the decreased (^{32}P) incorporation into mitochondrial hexaenoic PC suggest that retinol reduced both the exchange of hexaenoic PC from microsomes to mitochondria as well as the turnover rates of hexaenoic PC. The total activity of dienoic PC in mitochondria of retinol fed rats was, however, higher suggesting an increased

Table II. Retinol and phenobarbital administration and synthesis of molecular species of liver PC from $NaH_2(^{32}PO_4)$ in female rat (mean ± SE)

PC species	Groups, cpm/liver × 10^2			
	C	R	P	R + P
Monoenoic	7,511 ± 291	6,750 ± 119	7,368 ± 781	3,983 ± 26^S
Dienoic	18,497 ± 796	21,653 ± $1,041^S$	13,690 ± $1,414^S$	11,502 ± $1,076^S$
Trienoic	1,263 ± 60	1,035 ± 67^S	1,179 ± 129	986 ± 93^S
Tetraenoic	10,748 ± 847	7,333 ± 773^S	8,207 ± 498	4,022 ± 408^S
Hexaenoic	3,538 ± 324	1,623 ± 175^S	2,254 ± 233^S	1,275 ± 157^S

s = significant; C = control; R = retinol fed; P = phenobarbital; R + P = retinol + phenobarbital.

Table III. Retinol and phenobarbital administration and synthesis of molecular species of liver PC from (methyl-^{14}C) methionine in female rats (mean ± SE)

PC species	Groups, cpm/liver × 10^2			
	C	R	P	R + P
Monoenoic	629 ± 21	362 ± 23^S	498 ± 42^S	507 ± 19^S
Dienoic	2,284 ± 155	2,543 ± 203	2,021 ± 98	4,077 ± 363^S
Trienoic	350 ± 35	411 ± 22	368 ± 42	532 ± 49^S
Tetraenoic	7,803 + 636	8,566 + 654	12,550 ± 750^S	13,753 ± 588^S
Hexaenoic	4,291 + 336	3,836 + 119	6,380 + 439^S	3,765 + 253

s = significant; C = control; R = retinol-fed; P = phenobarbital; R + P = retinol + phenobarbital.

exchange proportional to their increased synthesis in microsomes. It is also likely that decreased amount of hexaenoic PC could be due to enhanced degradation by mitochondrial phospholipase in retinol-fed rats.

The incorporation of (methyl-^{14}C) *L*-methionine hydrochloride into tetraenoic and hexaenoic PC of retinol-fed rats was not significantly different from the controls (table III). Administration of phenobarbital significantly increased the label in hexaenoic PC but no alteration was noted when retinol and phenobarbital were given together (table III). Phenobarbital significantly increased the incorporation of (methyl-^{14}C) methionine into tetraenoic PC. Same pattern was obtained when retinol and phenobarbital were given together (table III). Thus, phenobarbital either alone or with retinol enhances the synthesis of PC by N-methylation pathway.

Table IV. Retinol feeding and phospholipid exchange between liver microsomes and mitochondria

	Percent exchange[1]					
	control			retinol fed		
	MICRO	MITO	SUP	MICRO	MITO	SUP
Exchange between (^{32}P)-labelled microsomes and non-labelled mitochondria						
PL	68 ± 1.0	26 ± 0.7	2.2 ± 0.6	65 ± 1.0	28 ± 0.8	3.4 ± 0.3
PC	66 ± 1.0	26 ± 1.0	2.7 ± 0.5	61 ± 1.0^{S}	31 ± 0.9	3.6 ± 0.3
Exchange between (^{32}P)-labelled mitochondria with non-labelled microsomes						
PL	42.8 ± 0.8	51 ± 0.3	–	40 ± 0.4	54 ± 0.7	–
PC	49 ± 1.1	44 ± 1.8	–	50 ± 1.7	45 ± 1.9	–

Phospholipid exchange between (^{32}P)-labelled microsomes of control rats and unlabelled mitochondria of retinol fed rats

	Percent exchange[1]			
	under standard conditions		under present conditions	
	MICRO	MITO	MICRO	MITO
PL	68 ± 1.0	25.7 ± 0.7	57 ± 0.2^{S}	36.2 ± 0.3^{S}
PC	66 ± 1.2	26.7 ± 1.1	57 ± 0.2^{S}	37.2 ± 0.2^{S}

s = significant; PL – total phospholipid; PC – phosphatidyl choline.

[1] Percent exchange was calculated as: $\frac{\text{Total activity after incubation} \times 100}{\text{Total activity before incubation}}$

Retinol feeding altered the amounts of labelling of mitochondrial PC. Since mitochondria depend on microsomes for the supply of PC by an exchange process, the exchange of PC and its molecular species was studied between microsomes and mitochondria and vice versa (table IV). Retinol feeding significantly increased the transfer of (^{32}P)-labelled PC from microsomes to mitochondria (table IV), which is suggestive of impaired permeability of mitochondria. Retinol feeding did not affect the transfer of mitochondrial PC to microsomes as compared to the control. In order to find out the effect of retinol on the mitochondrial membrane integrity, the labelled microsomes of control rats were incubated with unlabelled mitochondria of retinol-fed rats and exchange of PC was studied. The transfer of PC from control microsomes to mitochondria of retinol-fed rats was significantly increased. These results indicate that retinol feeding profoundly affected the integrity of mitochondrial membranes.

Acknowledgement

Dr. Ram is grateful to CSIR, New Delhi, for the award of Senior Research Fellowship. Vitamin A used was kindly provided by Hoffmann-La Roche, Bombay.

References

1 *Ahuja, H.C.:* Thesis, University of Delhi (1973).
2 *Arvidson, G.A.E.:* Eur. J. Biochem. *4:* 478 (1968).
3 *Liquori, G.; Carbini, L., and Padelino, A.:* Acta vitam. enzym. *28:* 195 (1975).
4 *Mathur, A.K.; Ramanathan, R., and Misra, U.K.:* Int. J. Vitam. Nutr. Res. *44:* 19 (1974).
5 *Misra, U.K.:* Biochem. J. *95:* 30 p (1965).
6 *Misra, U.K.:* Nature, Lond. *209:* 910 (1966).
7 *Misra, U.K.:* Can. J. Biochem. *44:* 1539 (1966).
8 *Misra, U.K. and Srivastava, N.:* Int. J. Vitam. Nutr. Res. *44:* 230 (1974).
9 *Ram, G.C. and Misra, U.K.:* Int. J. Vitam. Nutr. Res. *44:* 301 (1974).
10 *Ram, G.C. and Misra, U.K.:* Int. J. Vitam. Nutr. Res. *45:* 3 (1975).
11 *Roels, O.A.; Anderson, O.R.; Lui, N.S.T.; Shah, D.O., and Trout, M.E.:* Am. J. clin. Nutr. *22:* 2000 (1969).
12 *Wirtz, K.W.A. and Zilversmit, D.B.:* J. biol. Chem. *243:* 3596 (1968).
13 *Young, D.L.; Powell, G., and McMillan, W.O.:* J. Lipid Res. *12:* (1971).

Dr. *G.C. Ram,* Department of Radioisotopes and Biochemistry, V.P. Chest Institute, University of Delhi, *Delhi* (India)

Wld Rev. Nutr. Diet., vol. 31, pp. 83–88 (Karger, Basel 1978)

Metabolic and Turnover Studies on Retinol and Retinoic Acid

P.R. Sundaresan

Lipids Laboratory, Research Institute, St. Joseph Hospital, Lancaster, Pa.

Previous reports on the distribution and metabolism of retinol when injected either in the form of chylomicrons containing newly absorbed retinol (4) or as a Tween emulsion (19) have led to a renewed interest in the metabolism of small doses of retinol. We have carried out extensive studies on the distribution and metabolism of retinol using double-labelled (6,7-$^{14}C_2$, 11,12-$^{3}H_2$) retinol in physiological doses in vitamin A-deficient rats.

Distribution of Radioactive Retinol and its metabolites in Tissues of Rats Injected with 6,7-$^{14}C_2$, 11, 12-$^{3}H_2$ Retinol

The highest concentration of radioactivity was observed in the adrenals. This was followed by kidney, spleen, liver, intestine and blood. The total radioactivity in ng of retinol equivalents/tissue was highest in urine followed by liver, kidney, blood and intestine. The $^{14}C/^{3}H$ ratios in intestine, lungs, heart and feces were similar to the ratio of the injected material. However, the ratios in the adrenals, kidney, spleen, blood and urine were very different from that of injected retinol.

Alumina column chromatography of kidney and intestinal extracts revealed that the principal form of vitamin A in the kidney is retinol, while that in the intestines is retinyl palmitate. The main radioactive fraction in the liver has a $^{14}C/^{3}H$ ratio of only 0.4. This compound did not react with ethanolic HCl to yield anhydroretinol. One of the possibilities for the low $^{14}C/^{3}H$ ratio is isotopic discrimination. If more of the ^{14}C-labelled or non-tritiated molecules were utilized, more tritiated molecules would accumulate in the liver causing a lower $^{14}C/^{3}H$ ratio than 1. Since this compound did not react with ethanolic HCl, it is possible that retinol with a low $^{14}C/^{3}H$ ratio was converted to a metabolite with a low $^{14}C/^{3}H$ ratio (15).

Distribution of Retinol and Retinyl Esters in Intestinal Mucosa and Jejunal Mucinous Adenocarcinoma

Histological and biochemical studies (1, 18) have indicated that vitamin A is necessary for the maintenance of normal mucus secreting epithelial phenotype. It was of interest to determine whether transformed tissues of similar phenotype have the same nutritional requirement for vitamin A. The concentration of retinyl esters and retinol were assayed fluorometrically (17) in normal and transformed intestinal mucosa.

Normal intestinal mucosa contained about ten times as much retinol as the mucinous adenocarcinoma. The small amount of vitamin A in the tumor (83.4 ng/g wet weight) probably represents vitamin A in the tumor tissue at its fifth passage. The low levels of vitamin A in the tumor cells may be the result of a decreased requirement for the vitamin after five passages, as some changes do take place in the differentiating character of the tumor cells due to transplantation, or may also be the result of their conversion to unknown metabolites or to retinyl phosphate and its derivatives (3) which would not be detected by the method employed in this study.

Zinc, a Factor Affecting the Metabolism of Vitamin A

Recent studies have indicated that zinc may interfere with the synthesis in the liver of retinol-binding protein (10). More recently, *Huber and Gershoff* (6) found that zinc deficiency decreased the alcohol dehydrogenase and retinal reductase of the retina but not of the liver of adult rats. Further, the plasma vitamin A has been found to be depressed not only in zinc-deficient animals but also in those severely restricted in food and growth (11). Since retinal reductase (alcohol:NAD oxidoreductase, EC 1.1.1.1) and and retinal oxidase (EC 1.2.1.3) are intimately involved in vitamin A metabolism (12), it was of interest to study the effect of zinc deficiency on these enzymes. No significant difference is noticed in the activity of retinal reductase among the zinc-sufficient; the pair-fed and zinc-deficient groups. However, the liver retinal oxidase activity in the zinc-deficient group is significantly higher than either the pair-fed ($p < 0.05$) or the zinc-sufficient ($p < 0.05$) groups. Thus, the activity of retinal oxidase in the zinc-deficient group increases 1.84-fold over that of the zinc-sufficient group and 1.43-fold over that of the pair-fed group. The lack of effect on liver retinal reductase activity in zinc-deficient compared to pair-fed animals suggests that retinal reductase-dependent storage of vitamin A in liver may not be affected. Thus, no difference in the total vitamin A levels of the liver was observed in the zinc-deficient compared to pair-fed animals. In contrast, zinc deficiency seems to have a profound effect on the activity of liver retinal oxidase. The increase in retinal oxidase activity in the zinc-deficient group seems to indicate increased utilization of retinal through conversion to retinoic acid. This may be an adaptive mechanism to maintain a normal flow of retinal to retinoic acid in the presence of reduced growth and/or food intake in zinc-deficient animals. In contrast to the liver, retinal reductase and oxidase activities in the testes are decreased in zinc-deficient compared to pair-fed and zinc-sufficient animals. Thus, zinc may play an important role in the metabolism of vitamin A both in the liver and the testes.

Metabolic Studies on Retinoic Acid

Previous studies from our laboratory indicated the existence of six or more metabolites of retinoic acid in the urine, based on the assumption that the radioactivity in the urine from ($15\text{-}^{14}C$)retinoic acid represented a molecule with an intact side chain and a substituted cyclohexene ring (13). These results were confirmed in another study in which a mixture containing either ($15\text{-}^{14}C$), ($14\text{-}^{14}C$) or ($6,7\text{-}^{14}C_2$)-labelled and ($11,12\text{-}^{3}H_2$)-labelled retinoic acids in a total amount of 10 μg was employed (14). Distribution of radioactivity in ether-soluble, acidic and water-soluble fractions of urine indicated that the ether-soluble fractions had similar but higher $^{14}C/^{3}H$ ratios. Thin-layer chromatography of the ether-soluble fractions indicated a metabolite which was common to the three ^{14}C-labelled retinoic acids. However, this metabolite had $^{14}C/^{3}H$ ratio of 2, indicating loss of tritium at 11,12 double bond of retinoic acid. It was speculated that a metabolic attack at 11,12 double bond had taken place possibly through hydroxylation as postulated by *Morton* (7).

Recent studies by *Rietz et al.* (8) seem to support the above hypothesis. These investigators have isolated two main metabolites from the urine of rats and humans treated with high doses of unlabelled retinoic acids. Metabolite II appears to have been derived from metabolite I by loss of one methyl group. (fig. 1).

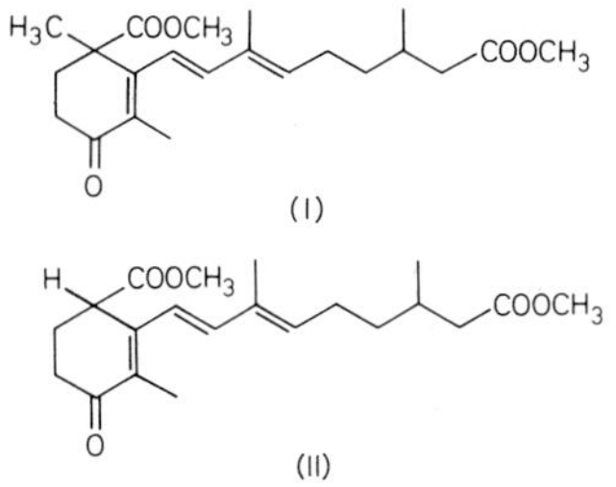

Fig. 1. Structures of urinary metabolites (I and II) of retinoic acid and retinol from rat and human urine.

Rate of Metabolism of Retinol in Retinoic Acid-Supplemented Rats

Previous work by *Sewell et al.* (9) and *Hayes et al.* (5) had indicated continuous mixing and dynamic exchange of vitamin A in the liver, blood and the target organs for vitamin A. It was found that although the concentration of retinol in the liver remained constant, the amount of radioactivity in liver retinol declined exponentially both in rats and steers when administered a tracer dose of retinol. In our laboratory, we carried out studies on the half-life and metabolism of vitamin A in vitamin A-deficient rats maintained on weekly retinoic acid supplementation after a single dose of 340 μg of (6,7-$^{14}C_2$)-retinol (sp. activity 17.4 μCi/mg) intraperitoneally (17).

The half-life and metabolism time for vitamin A in liver were estimated as 7 and 10 days, respectively. These results are in agreement with those obtained by *Dowling and Wald* (2) after plotting their data semilogarithmically.

The urinary excretion of radioactivity plotted on a semilogarithmic scale for 10 weeks can be accounted for by three different pools (fig. 2). The first pool with a rapid fall in daily excretion has a very short half-life (0.75 day). After the first week, the daily excretion of radioactivity reached a low but gradually declining level and this process continued for 5 weeks. The nature of urinary excretion of this pool is a zero order process. After this period of slow excretion, the radioactivity in urine began to fall off more rapidly beginning with the sixth week until the tenth week of the experiment, apparently in a logarithmic fashion. It is assumed that this pool begins from day 43 and does not contribute much to pool 2. Pool 3 has a half-life of 13 days. Weekly oral feeding of retinoic acid seems to significantly decrease the excretion of radioactivity from retinol in the urine. The effect was noticeable at 5 days after the oral dose of retinoic acid. However, the urinary excretion returned to the original level of excretion on the sixth day after supplementation. This data suggested that the urinary metabolites of retinol and retinoic acid are probably identical and that retinoic acid is in the pathway of retinol metabolism. The fecal excretion of radioactivity also revealed 3 pools, as in the case of urinary excretion.

Vitamin A in the liver declines exponentially with time. The specific activities of retinyl esters indicate slow equilibration of retinyl esters in liver from first through fourth week after dose of radioactive retinol. The blood levels of retinol at 8 days after injection indicated that normal levels were reached during the first week after a dose of retinol. The specific activity of retinol did not change throughout the experiment.

Our results demonstrate that there is retinol in the tissues even in the vitamin A-deficient rats 4 weeks after weaning; that there are three distinct metabolic reactions of retinol: an early rapid one (perhaps representing metabolism of excess retinol), metabolism of retinol derived from what has been stored, and metabolism after the stores have been depleted from the liver.

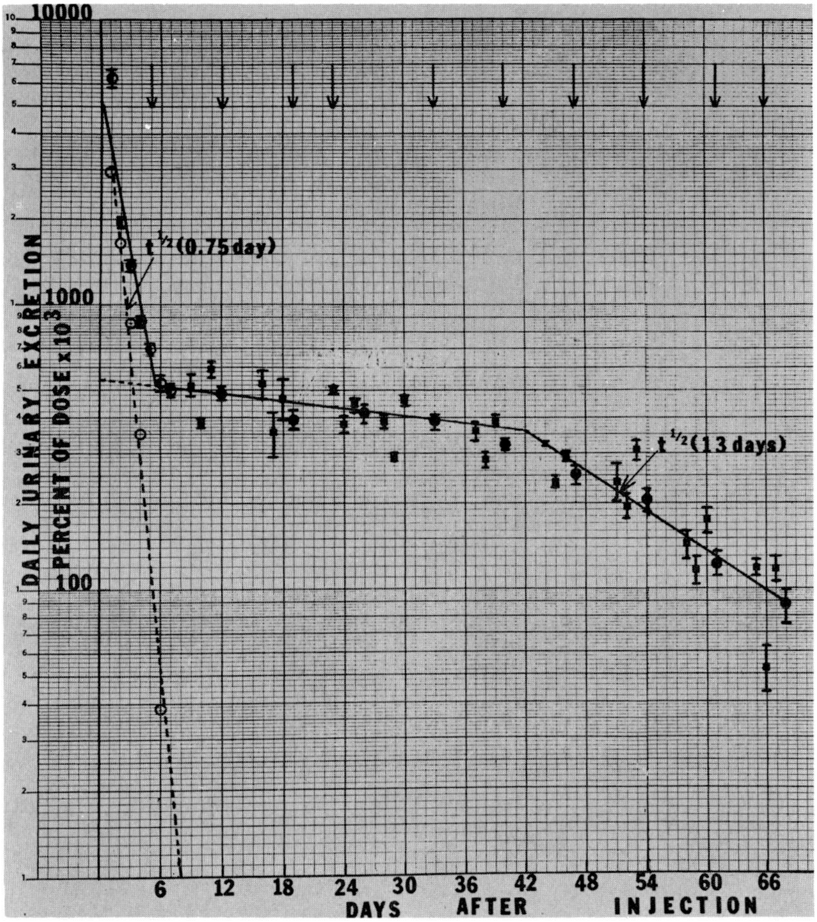

Fig. 2. Adapted from *Sundaresan* (17). The total daily average radioactivity for days 1–7 (◐——◐) and the total daily average radioactivity for weeks 2 through 10 (•——•) represented on days 12, 19, 26, 33, 40, 47, 54, 61 and 68 were plotted on a semilogarithmic graphy: ○——○ represents the corrected urinary ^{14}C activity due to the rapidly declining pool; ↓ at the top of the figure represents the day on which the rats received 100 μg of retinoic acid in peanut oil. The total daily urinary ^{14}C activity at days 4, 5 and 6 after retinoic acid feeding are indicated by each week.

Acknowledgement

The author thanks Drs. *Luigi M. DeLuca,* National Cancer Institute and *J.C. Smith, Jr.*, Veterans Administration Hospital, Washington, for their active collaboration, and *Fred. O. Cope* and *G.M. Sundaresan* for their expert technical assistance in some of the research described herein. This work is supported in part by US Public Health Service Grant AM 13557 from the National Institute of Arthritis, Metabolism and Digestive Diseases, Bethesda, Maryland.

References

1 *DeLuca L.M.; Schumacher, M.; Wolf, G., and Newberne, P.M.:* J. biol. Chem. *245:* 4551 (1970).
2 *Dowling, J.E. and Wald, G.:* Proc. natn. Acad. Sci. USA *44:* 648 (1958).
3 *Frot-Coutaz, J.P.; Silverman-Jones, C.S., and DeLuca, L.M.:* J. Lipid. Res. *17:* 220 (1976).
4 *Goodman, D.S.; Huang, H.S., and Shiratori, T.:* J. Lipid Res. *6:* 390 (1965).
5 *Hayes, B.W.; Mitchell, G.E.; Little, C.O., and Sewell, H.B.:* J. Anim. Sci. *26:* 855 (1967).
6 *Huber, A.M. and Gershoff, S.N.:* J. Nutr. *105:* 1486 (1975).
7 *Morton, R.A.:* Vitams Horm. *18:* 566 (1960).
8 *Rietz, P.; Wiss, O., and Weber, F.:* Vitams Horm. *32:* 237 (1974).
9 *Sewell, H.B.: Mitchell, G.E.; Little, C.O., and Hayes, B.W.:* Int. Z. VitamForsch. *37:* 301 (1967).
10 *Smith, J.E.; Brown, E.D., and Smith, J.C., Jr.:* J. Lab. clin. Med. *84:* 692 (1974).
11 *Smith, J.C., Jr.; Brown, E.D.; McDaniel, E.W., and Chen, W.:* J. Nutr. *106:* 569 (1976).
12 *Sundaresan, P.R.:* J. Sci. & Ind. Res. *313:* 581 (1972).
13 *Sundaresan, P.R. and Bhagavan, H.N.:* Biochem, J. *122:* 1 (1972).
14 *Sundaresan, P.R. and Sundaresan, G.M.* Int. J. Vitam. Nutr. Res. *43:* 61 (1973).
15 *Sundaresan, P.R. and Sundaresan, G.M.:* Biochem. J. *152:* 99 (1975).
16 *Sundaresan, P.R. and DeLuca, L.M.:* J. natn. Cancer Inst. *58:* 1643 (1977).
17 *Sundaresan, P.R.:* J. Nutr. *107:* 70 (1977).
18 *Wolbach, S.B. and Howe, P.R.:* J. exp. Med. *42:*753 (1925).
19 *Wolf, G.; Kahn, S., and Johnson, B.C.:* J. Am. chem. Soc. *79:* 1208 (1957).

Dr. *P.R. Sundaresan,* Division of Toxicology, Bureau of Foods, Food and Drug Administration, Building FOB–8, *Washington, DC 20204* (USA)

Wld Rev. Nutr. Diet., vol. 31, pp. 89–94 (Karger, Basel 1978)

Biosynthesis of Dehydroretinol[1]

A.B. Barua
Department of Chemistry, Gauhati University, Gauhati

Except at the terminal carbon atom 15, any structural change in vitamin A considerably reduces growth-promoting power. The only change in the C_1-C_{14} portion of retinol which does not reduce growth-promoting activity to a very low level is further dehydrogenation and the naturally occurring compounds of this type, are those of vitamin A_2 or 3-dehydroretinol, or simply dehydroretinol, series with an extra double bond in the β-ionone ring (27). Dehydroretinol commonly has about half the activity of the corresponding A_1 compounds (29, 30). Dehydroretinol, first observed in fish liver oil (18), is mainly found in freshwater fish, but occurs to a small extent in marine fish and certain amphibia. The distribution and chemistry of dehydroretinol have been described (14, 21) but the biosynthesis of dehydroretinol is not yet clearly known.

There are several possibilities for obtaining the extra double bond in the β-ionone ring of dehydroretinol from a carotenoid precursor: (i) by desaturation (dehydrogenation) of carotenes containing at least one unsubstituted β-ionone ring such as β-carotene, α-carotene, γ-carotene or retinol; (ii) from xanthophylls such as lutein and 5, 6-epoxylutein, which can be dehydroxylated into a carotenoid containing a 3, 4-dehydro-β-ionone ring; (iii) from other carotenoids which already possess a 3, 4-dehydro-β-ionone ring such as 3, 4-dehydro-β-carotene, anhydrolutein, etc.

Dehydroretinol from Carotene and Retinol by means of Desaturation Mechanism

As early as 1939, *Morton and Creed* (23) observed that both retinol and dehydroretinol content increased when vitamin A-deficient fish were given a diet enriched with carotene. This experiment was aimed at studying the structure of

[1] Dedicated to the memory of late Prof. *R.K. Barua.*

vitamin A_2 and according to *Morton* (24) 'this experiment does not necessarily imply that carotene is the main natural provitamin responsible for the liver reserves of fishes'. According to *Grangaud and Moatti* (15), only a small amount of dehydroretinol is formed from dietary β-carotene in *Gombusia holbrooki.*

The conversion of β-carotene into dehydroretinol may take place by two routes. First β-carotene can be converted into 3, 4-dehydro-β-carotene (or 3, 4, 3′, 4′-bis-dehydro-β-carotene) which is then cleaved into dehydroretinol. Alternatively, retinol can first be formed, and then undergo dehydrogenation into 3, 4-dehydroretinol. As there are no reports on the presence of 3,4-dehydrocarotene in fish it may be assumed that β-carotene is first cleaved into retinol which in turn is dehydrogenated into dehydroretinol. *Morcos and Salah* (22) studied the conversion of retinol to dehydroretinol in two species of Nile river fish, but could not show dehydrogenation of vitamin A_1 to A_2. *Naito and Witt* (25), on the other hand, have been able to detect tritium-labelled dehydroretinol in the eyes of green gills following injection of tritium-labelled retinol. *Braekkan et al.* (11) and *Lambertson and Braekkan* (20) studied the uptake and storage of vitamin A in rainbow trout and observed the transformation of retinol into dehydroretinol, but concluded that the fish possess a dehydrogenation system of limited capacity. The vitamin $A_1 \rightleftharpoons A_2$ interconversion has also been reported by *Yoshikami et al.* (31).

Present Study with β-Carotene and Retinol

Surveys of vitamin A content in North-East Indian freshwater fish (3, 5), revealed that all species contain both retinol and dehydroretinol, and in some retinol is practically absent. Some of these species, especially *Saccobranchus (Heteropneustus) fossilis,* were found to be very sturdy and thrive under adverse conditions for several months. Attemps were made, by two different methods, to study the origin of vitamin A_2 in this species of fish as it contained more dehydroretinol than retinol (sometimes retinol is absent).

In the first method, vitamin A stored in the livers of vitamin A-deficient fish, kept on a diet of rice supplemented with minced goat meat and β-carotene administered orally or intraperitoneally, was analysed. The experiments indicated absorption and storage of β-carotene in the liver, but neither retinol nor dehydroretinol could be detected in the liver (6). In similar experiments on fish not made vitamin A-deficient but dosed with retinol, very little dehydroretinol, which was probably present originally, was detected. When the experiment was carried out on vitamin A-deficient fish, no dehydroretinol could be detected after 15 days of feeding the fish with retinyl acetate.

In the second method, the intestinal conversion of β-carotene to vitamin A was followed. Freshly caught *S. fosillis* were allowed to starve for 15–20 days when their alimentary canals were found to be free of carotenoids, vitamin A and other food particles. In such fish, β-carotene suspended in Tween-80 was directly administered into the alimentary canal, killed 30 min to 20 days after dosing, and only the alimentary canals were analysed for vitamin A. Out of nearly 100 such experiments carried out so far, retinoic acid could be detected and isolated in twelve experiments, whereas retinol was detected in only two experiments; in the rest of the experiments neither retinoic acid nor retinol could be detected (9). Further, in experiments where retinoic acid was detected, it appeared within 4–6 h after dosing with β-carotene; no retinoic acid has so far been detected in experiments where the fish were killed before or after this period (4–6 h).

Dehydroretinol from Xanthophylls and Other Carotenoids Possessing 3, 4-Dehydro-β-Ionone Ring

Karmakar and Petracek with *Zechmeister* (19, 26) showed that 3′-hydroxy-3,4-dehydro-β-carotene (anhydrolutein) is 10% as active as β-carotene. A smooth conversion of anhydrolutein to dehydroretinol was shown in chicks (12, 13) and rats (28). It was speculated that freshwater fish might be able to convert lutein or similar xanthophyll into a suitable precursor for dehydroretinol but the occurrence of anhydrolutein in the natural food of the fish has not yet been reported, nor the conversion of xanthophylls into vitamin A studied in fish.

Astaxanthin (3,3′-dihydroxy-4,4′-diketo-β-carotene) is the only natural xanthophyll that has been shown to be converted into both retinol and dehydroretinol; it has been claimed that carotene is an intermediate in this transformation (16, 17).

We have studied the conversion of xanthophylls into dehydroretinol in *S. fosillis.* Experiments similar to those performed with β-carotene by the liver storage test method were carried out using zeaxanthin; neither absorption nor conversion of zeaxanthin to vitamin A was observed (6).

The presence of considerable quantities of lutein in the livers of freshly caught *S. fosillis* and several other freshwater fish tempted us to examine the fate of lutein in the vitamin A-depleted fish. Accordingly, lutein mixed with minced meat was given orally to vitamin A-deficient fish and the livers analysed for vitamin A. Evidence of formation of dehydroretinol was obtained in most of the experiments (6). From the liver oil of lutein-dosed fish dehydroretinyl ester, anhydrolutein ester and a compound exhibiting λ-max 328–330 nm (designated 'compound 330') were isolated by chromatography. A compound showing λ-max 330 nm was reported earlier in the liver oil of *Wallago attu* and *Ophicephalus striatus* (1) but the nature of the compound was not studied. The presence of such a compound has been frequently observed by us in several other freshwater fish liver oils. It has now been characterized as 3-hydroxyretinol occurring as a diester (10). The naturally occurring 3-hydroxyretinol has been found to be identical with a synthetic sample prepared from methyl retinoate and from zeaxanthin (4). 3-Hydroxyretinol absorbs at 328 nm and the antimony thrichloride blue colour shows λ-max 675 nm. Positive evidence in favour of a 3-hydroxyretinol structure was obtained when the naturally occurring diester produced 3-hydroxyretinal after saponification, followed by oxidation with manganese dioxide. 3-Hydroxyretinal, thus obtained from 'compound 330', was identical in all respects with 3-hydroxyretinal prepared from zeaxanthin (4).

The 3-hydroxyretinol structure was further supported by converting it into anhydrovitamin A_2; two anhydrovitamins A_2 were formed, one was the usual 3-ethoxyanhydrovitamin A, which was easily separated from the other strongly absorbed one and now characterized as 3-hydroxyanhydrovitamin A (8) and identical with the naturally occurring anhydrovitamin A_2 (1, 2).

Savithry et al. (28) were unable to detect any hydroxyretinol in rats fed with anhydrolutein and concluded that the cleavage occurs at the ring substituted end. However, we have been able to isolate both dehydroretinol and 3-hydroxyretinol from lutein- and anhydrolutein-dosed fish. It, therefore, appears that the mechanism of cleavage of carotenoids into vitamin A is different in fish.

Anhydrolutein, an Intermediate in the Transformation of Lutein into Dehydroretinol

Liver oils of freshly caught *S. fossilis* or lutein-dosed vitamin A-depleted fish contained anhydrolutein and it appears to be an intermediate in the transformation of lutein into dehydroretinol. In order to verify this, anhydrolutein was administered to vitamin A-deficient fish (7) and it was found to be converted into dehydroretinol and some 3-hydroxyretinol (diester).

Intestinal Conversion of Lutein into Dehydroretinol

Experiments similar to those described on the intestinal conversion of β-carotene into retinoic acid were performed on *S. fosiilis* using lutein (9). Unlike β-carotene, lutein was found to be converted into dehydroretinol in most of the experiments within 5–6 h after dosing. The intestinal extract contained dehydroretinyl ester, dehydroretinol and 3-hydroxyretinol (diester). In none of the experiments has dehydroretinoic acid been detected.

General Conclusions

The formation of retinoic acid from β-carotene in apparently healthy fish is an interesting observation. Is our failure to detect both retinol and retinoic acid in many of the experiments due to formation of solely retinoic acid which disappeared quickly (as glucuronide) before it could be isolated? Is this hidden form of vitamin A (21) abundantly present and very active in freshwater fish which contain little or no retinol?

Lutein has been found to be an effective precursor for dehydroretinol in *S. fossilis* and anhydrolutein is an intermediate in this transformation. This observation shows that the freshwater fish has an enzyme system capable of removing the allylic hydroxyl group at 3′-position of lutein. Thus, xanthophylls can serve as effective precursors of dehydroretinol in freshwater fish (14). It will be of importance to study if, like retinol, there are other precursors for dehydroretinol.

For the first time the natural occurrence of 3-hydroxyretinol has been reported as an intermediate in the biosynthesis of dehydroretinol from lutein and anhydrolutein. The occurrence of 3-hydroxy-anhydrovitamin A in fish liver oil has also been established. The presence of these hydroxy analogs of vitamin A in the liver oils of several freshwater fish can easily be explained if lutein is considered as the provitamin A_2. Based on our observations, the following biosynthetic pathway for dehydroretinol from lutein is suggested:

Lutein ⟶ Anhydrolutein ↗ Dehydroretinol
Lutein ⟶ Anhydrolutein ↘ 3-Hydroxyretinol

Acknowledgement

The work presented in this paper has been carried out by several of my colleagues, without whose able and diligent participation this work would not have been possible. Special mention should be made of Dr. *R.C. Das*, Dr. *H. Tombi Singh*, Mrs.*Kamna Verma*, Mr. *U.C. Goswami* and Mr. *S.R. Das*. Grateful acknowledgement is due to Professor *J. Ganguly* of the Indian Institute of Science, Bangalore, for some useful discussion, especially during the work on 3-hydroxyretinol and the intestinal conversion of carotenoids to vitamin A.

References

1 *Balasundaram, S.; Bamji, M.S.; Cama, H.R.; Sundaresan, P.R., and Varma, T.N.R.:* J. biol. Chem. *233:* 827 (1958).
2 *Barua, R.K. and Nayar, P.G.:* Curr. Sci. *32:* 257 (1963).

3 *Barua, R.K. and Nayar P.G.:* Indian J. Chem. *2:* 254 (1964).
4 *Barua, R.K. and Barua, A.B.:* Biochem. J. *101:* 250 (1966).
5 *Barua, A.B. and Singh, H.T.:* Indian J. Biochem. Biophys. *9:* 128 (1972).
6 *Barua, A.B.; Singh, H.T., and Das, R.C.:* Br. J. Nutr. *30:* 1 (1973).
7 *Barua, A.B. and Das, R.C.:* Br. J. Nutr. *33:* 319 (1975).
8 *Barua, A.B. and Das, S.R.:* (unpublished work).
9 *Barua, A.B. and Goswami, U.C.:* Biochem. J. *166:* 133 (1977).
10 *Barua, A.B.; Das, R.C., and Verma, K.:* Biochem. J. *168:* 557 (1977).
11 *Braekkan, O.R.; Ingibrigtsen, O., and Mykelstad, H.:* Int. Z. VitamForsch. *39:* 123, (1969).
12 *Budowoski, P.; Ascarelli, I.; Gross, J., and Nir, I.:* Science, N.Y. *142:* 969 (1963).
13 *Budowoski, P. and Gross, J.:* Nature *206:* 1254 (1965).
14 *Ganguly, J. and Murthy, S.K.:* in *Sebrell and Harris* The vitamins; 2nd ed., p. 148 (Academic Press, New York).
15 *Grangaud, R. and Moatti, J.P.:* Compt. Renol. *152:* 1235 (1958).
16 *Grangaud, G.; Vignais, P.; Massonet, R., and Moatti, J.P.:* Compt. Rend. *243:* 1170 (1956).
17 *Grangaud, R. and Moatti, J.P.:* Séanc. soc. biol. *152:* 1235 (1958).
18 *Heilbron, I.M.; Gillam, A.E., and Morton, R.A.:* Biochem. J. *25:* 1352 (1931).
19 *Karmakar, G. and Zeichmeister, L.:* J. Am. chem. Soc. *77:* 55 (1955).
20 *Lambertson, G. and Braekkan, O.R.:* Acta chem. scand. *23:* 1063 (1969).
21 *Moore, T.:* Vitamin A (Elsevier, Amsterdam 1957).
22 *Morcos, S.R. and Salah, M.K.:* Nature *167:* 117 (1951).
23 *Morton, R.A. and Creed, R.H.:* Biochem. J. *33:* 318 (1939).
24 *Morton, R.A.:* Absorption spectra of vitamins and hormones (Adam Hilger, London 1942).
25 *Naito, K. and Wilt, F.H.:* J. biol. Chem. *237:* 3060 (1962).
26 *Petracek, F.j. and Zeichmeister, L.:* J. Am. chem. Soc. *78:* 1427 (1956).
27 *Pitt, G.A.J.:* in *Isler* Carotenoids, p. 717 (Birkhäuser, Basel).
28 *Savithry, K.N.; Krishna Mallia, A., and Cama, H.R.:* Indian J. Biochem. Biophys. *9:* 325 (1972).
29 *Shantz, E.M. and Brinkmann, J.H.:* J. biol. Chem. *183:* 467 (1950).
30 *Sundaresan, P.R. and Cama, H.R.:* Br. J. Nutr. *15:* 225 (1961).
31 *Yoshikami, S.; Pearlman, J.T., and Crescitelli, F.:* Vision Res. *9:* 633 (1969).

Dr. *A.B. Barua,* Department of Chemistry, Gauhati University, *Gauhati 781 014* (India)

Wld Rev. Nutr. Diet., vol. 31, pp. 95–99 (Karger, Basel 1978)

Prevention of Vitamin A Deficiency

S.G. Srikantia

National Institute of Nutrition, Indian Council of Medical Research, Hyderabad

Vitamin A deficiency is one of the major public health nutritional problems in many developing countries and is an important cause of preventable blindness. Apart from India, its occurrence has been reported in Bangla Desh, Burma, Pakistan, Philippines, Sri Lanka and Thailand. It is also frequently seen in several countries in the Middle East, Central and South America. Although the number of children who go blind as a result of vitamin A deficiency in India is not accurately known, it is estimated that about 12,000–15,000 pre-school age children of poor income groups lose their eyesight every year as a result of vitamin A deficiency.

Dietary inadequacy of vitamin A is the single most important factor in the development of the deficiency state. Among additional contributory factors are the poor hepatic reserves with which the infant is born consequent to inadequate dietary intake of the mother during pregnancy, low intakes of vitamin A in breast milk and frequent episodes of infection to which children of the poor socioeconomic group are exposed.

The diets which infants of poor economic groups receive when they are weaned are almost exclusively vegetable-based and, therefore, contain little preformed vitamin A. Their entire vitamin A intake is in the form of pro-vitamin A – β-carotene. In several carefully conducted surveys among pre-school children in India, mean daily intake of the vitamin has been found to be 130 μg, or less, per day. This represents only about 40% of the recommended intake for this age group (6). Since the diets provide β-carotene and not vitamin A, the actual availability of β-carotene in these diets may be even lower, as there is little or no fat in the diet – a factor known to influence absorption and utilization of carotene. A number of observations in experimental animals and in man have indicated the existence of a close inter-relationship between protein nutritional status and vitamin A metabolism. Since the protein nutritional status of many older infants and pre-school children, belonging to the poor income groups, is sub-optimal, it is believed that this is an important contributory factor in the development of vitamin A deficiency. However, as indicated earlier, the single most important factor in the development of the disease appears to be inadequate intake of dietary vitamin A.

The most rational approach, therefore, to the control and prevention of this condition would to be improve the diets so as to ensure adequate intake of the vitamin. Preformed vitamin A is present only in foods of animal origin which are expensive and beyond the reach of most of the population segments. Green leafy vegetables are rich and inexpensive sources of vitamin A, but their use, particulary among rural people, is limited for socio-cultural reasons. It has been suggested that should such population groups be persuaded to include green leafy vegetables in their habitual diet, its impact may be somewhat limited because of the coexisting protein calorie malnutrition.

A study was therefore undertaken to determine the effects of including a commonly used green leafy vegetable, amaranth, in the diets of children. A group of rural children was given 30 g of amaranth daily which provided about 1000 μg of β-carotene along with their habitual diet. These children suffered from mild and moderate forms of protein-calorie malnutrition as judged by a deficit in weight for age. At the end of three weeks of feeding, levels of serum vitamin A were significantly higher than levels seen in another group of similar children who did not receive amaranth. Also, in two children, Bitot's spots disappeared following the ingestion of amaranth (4). This observation is of considerable practical public health significance, since it is clear that notwithstanding the known inter-relationship that exists between protein nutritional status on the one hand and metabolism of vitamin A on the other, undernourished children of the type who were investigated, and who constitute a very high proportion of the child population in rural areas, are able to utilise dietary β-carotene satisfactorily.

Improvement of dietary intake of vitamin A, even through the use of inexpensive foodstuffs, is unlikely to occur as an isolated phenomenon, since it calls for social evolution and must, therefore, be considered as a long-term measure. Till such time as this goal can be achieved, the conventional method of administration of vitamin A to segments of the population at high risk, which is currently being practised, not only needs to be continued but intensified as a short-term method. This physiologically sound approach, however, has limited application, since maternal and child health centres, hospitals and other health units, through which regular periodic distribution of vitamin A supplements can be attempted, cover but a very small fraction of the population. Also, even among those who attend such centres, frequent visits cannot be ensured with regularity. This is one of the reasons that the problem of vitamin A deficiency continues to be one of public health in developing countries. Other more effective measures would, therefore, appear to be necessary.

Fortification of a suitable food with vitamin A is one of the methods by which additional amounts of vitamin A can be delivered to large population groups in a country and such an approach has, in fact, been developed and implemented recently in Guatemala (1). Sugar was chosen as the vehicle to carry vitamin A and studies carried out at INCAP have shown that the added vitamin A is stable, does not alter consumer acceptance, and that bioavailability of the vitamin is satisfactory. While this approach has been successful in Guatemala, it may not be so in other situations. One of the crucial factors in using food fortification as a public health measure is the proper choice of the food item which can be fortified. In India, a suitable vehicle is common salt and attempts to fortify this commodity with vitamin A have not been successful because of the rapid rate at which the added vitamin A was lost (5).

It has long been known that the human liver has a very large capacity for storing vitamin A, and can release it for utilisation as the need arises. One of the approaches that could make an impact on widespread vitamin A deficiency would be to develop a method by which liver reserves of vitamin A can be built up. Such a method, however, must be capable of being implemented within the existing resources and health infrastructure of the developing country. The use of a single large dose of vitamin A given preferably once a year has been suggested as a public health measure for the control of vitamin A deficiency. This approach has a sound theoretical basis and the National Institute of Nutrition, Hyderabad, undertook field trials to determine whether such an approach would be feasible. Practical aspects that have to be considered in this context are (i) the size of the dose, (ii) the type of preparation to be used, (iii) the route of administration and (iv) the frequency with which it has to be administered. The dose must be large enough to be useful but should not produce acute hypervitaminosis A. The preparation should result in as large a hepatic storage as possible, and the dose should be administered as infrequently as possible, preferably not more than once a year.

Studies carried out at the National Institute of Nutrition have provided answers to all these questions. With a single dose of 90,000 μg of vitamin A, given orally as a water-miscible preparation, 25% of a large goup of pre-school children developed transient signs of acute vitamin A toxicity. The same amount given as an oil soluble preparation reduced the incidence of toxic signs to about 4% (9). Clinical studies showed that oily preparations of vitamin A administered intramuscularly failed to produce significant elevation of serum vitamin A levels, while water-miscible preparations did (7). Experimental studies in rats revealed that much of the intramuscularly administered oily preparation could be recovered from the site of injection, providing partial explanation for the observation in children. Although with the water-miscible preparation, serum levels of the vitamin increased, the liver stores were not satisfactory. The best hepatic storage was achieved with oral administration of an oil-soluble preparation of vitamin A (7). The extent of absorption and retention of a massive single dose of vitamin A (90,000 μg) was investigated in children using tritiated retinol. About 70% of the vitamin was absorbed and a little less than 50% of the total dose retained (13). Following the administration of a large dose of vitamin A, levels of serum vitamin A in a group of children were found to be significantly higher than basal levels both at 6 and 12 months after dosing (7).

In view of the known toxic effects of large doses of vitamin A, studies were also carried out to determine the extent to which a massive dose influenced the urinary excretion of two lysosomal enzymes – aryl sulphatase and acid phosphatase. While 50% of the children showed no changes, others showed an increase in the urinary excretion of these two enzymes, which, was transient, however, indicating that there was no significant lysosomal injury (12). There appeared to be no correlation between the development of clinical toxic signs and the increase in the urinary excretion of these enzymes.

One of the epidemiological features of vitamin A deficiency is that the corneal lesions, which lead to blindness, are rarely seen after the age of 5 years, although the incidence of other ocular signs like conjunctival xerosis and Bitot's spots progressively increase with age. Pre-school children thus constitute the segment at highest risk. A pilot study was, therefore, carried out involving about 2500 pre-school children in several villages in and around Hyderabad. These children, aged 1–5 years, received 90,000 μg of vitamin A once every year, after a baseline survey of the prevalence of vitamin A deficiency signs was conducted. The study was carried out over a period of 5 years and an evaluation of the study showed that the incidence of ocular signs of vitamin A deficiency was reduced by about 75%. During the entire five-year period, not a single new case of keratomalacia was seen in these areas (10). Estimation of serum vitamin A in some of these children showed that even at the end of 6 months, levels of vitamin A were significantly higher than in children who had not received a massive dose (8).

Based on the results of this pilot study, this approach has now been taken up as a national programme for the control of blindness due to vitamin A deficiency. In this programme, instead of 90,000 μg given once a year, 60,000 μg are given once every 6 months to children from 1–5 years of age. This modification was introduced not only to further reduce the incidence of acute toxicity, but also to ensure that levels of serum vitamin A would be more uniformly elevated. The programm is in operation in several states of India, where vitamin A deficiency is widespread, and approximately 4 million children are being covered. Evaluation done in two states, Karnataka and Kerala, has shown that it is administratively possible to implement this programme with the existing health infrastructure. It also showed that as in the case of the pilot study carried out by the National Institute of Nutrition, there was a reduction in the prevalence of vitamin A deficiency signs to the extent of 75%.

The extent of reduction in the prevalence of ocular signs of vitamin A deficiency, particularly Bitot's spots, before and after the implementation of the programme has been used for the evaluation of the programme. It is not always possible to obtain satisfactory baseline data on the prevalence of deficiency signs, particularly in large scale operations and this is one of the major difficulties in the proper evaluation of many nutrition programmes, including the vitamin A prophylaxis programme. A simple and reliable method has now been developed by which the effectiveness of the vitamin A prophylaxis programme can be evaluated, even in the absence of baseline data. The method makes use of the wellknown relationship between age on the one hand and the incidence of ocular signs of vitamin A deficiency on the other (11).

Two other Asian countries, Bangla Desh (2) and Indonesia (3), have also implemented a similar vitamin A prophylaxis programme, and the experience of both countries is similar to that in India, a considerable impact having been made on the extent of vitamin A deficiency.

References

1 *Arroyave, G.:* Personal communication (1972).
2 *Kamel, W.W.:* Vit. A xerophthalmia and blindness; vol. 1 (Published by the Office of Nutrition, Technical Assistance Bureau, A.I.D., U.S. Dept. of State, 1973).
3 *Karjadi, D.:* Personal communication (1972).
4 *Lala, V.R. and Vinodini, R.:* Am. J. clin. Nutr. *23:* 110 (1970).
5 *National Institute of Nutrition:* Indian Council of Medical Research, Hyderabad, Annual Report (1972).
6 *Pralhad Rao, N.; Darshan Singh, and Swaminathan, M.C.:* Indian J. med. Res. *57:* 2132 (1969).
7 *Srikantia, S.G. and Vinodini, R.:* Am. J. clin. Nutr. *23:* 114 (1970).
8 *Susheela, T.P.:* Indian J. med. Res. *57:* 2151 (1969).
9 *Swaminathan, M.C.; Susheela, T.P., and Thimmayamma, B.V.S.:* Am. J. clin. Nutr. *23:* 119 (1970).
10 *Swaminathan, M.C.:* Proc. Ist Asian Congr. Nutr. (1971).
11 *Vijayaraghavan, K.; Naidu, A.N.; Rao, N.P., and Srikantia, S.G.:* Am. J. clin. Nutr. *28:* 1189 (1975).
12 *Vinodini, R. and Mohanram, M.:* Int. J. Vitam. Nutr. Res. *41:* 321 (1971).
13 *Vinodini, R., and Sivakumar, B.:* Indian Pediat. *9:* 307 (1972).

Dr. *S.G. Srikantia,* National Institute of Nutrition, Indian Council of Medical Research, *Hyderabad 500 007* (India)

Wld Rev. Nutr. Diet., vol. 31, pp. 100–106 (Karger, Basel 1978)

Vitamin A Nutrition in Relation to Gangliosides and Myelination in the Developing Brain

P. V. Bhat and P.B. Rama Rao

Biochemistry and Applied Nutrition Discipline, Central Food Technological Research Institute, Mysore

Malnutrition is a major contributory factor to the high mortality and morbidity in early childhood in the developing countries. Several studies are available on the effects of protein-calorie deficiency or undernutrition on the central nervous system (CNS), but the effect of specific vitamin inadequacy, or excess, on brain development of the newborn has not been well studied. The effects of vitamin A deficiency on the CNS include disproportionate growth of the surrounding bone, increased cerebrospinal fluid pressure, lesions of the spinal cord, degeneration of myelin (9) and paralysis in young rats (10). Whether these effects of vitamin A deficiency on CNS are direct or indirect is a point of interest. A stimulating hypothesis is that the CNS could have a specific requirement for vitamin A or its metabolite. Here, the specific effect of vitamin A deficiency on brain development was investigated with particular reference to brain lipids and myelination.

Albino rats of Wistar strain were used and the composition of the vitamin A-deficient diet has been described (2). Control groups of rats were given an oral supplement of 100 IU vitamin A/rat (diet B_1) whereas the experimental group (diet B_2) were given 10 IU vitamin A/rat/day. 'Undernutrition' was produced in an additional control group by increasing the litter size to 15 pups/mother rat as against 5 pups/mother in the other two groups. Protein was determined according to *Clausen* (4) and vitamin A was assayed according to *Ames et al.* (1). Lipid extraction and other methodology has been described (2, 3).

Brain Gangliosides

On day 17 after birth the rats were sacrificed and the gangliosides isolated, separated and estimated (12, 14). The body and brain weights in undernourished and 'low' vitamin A groups were significantly lower than in controls (table I).

Table I. Brain gangliosides: effect of vitamin A inadequacy and undernutrition (mean ± SEM)

	Dietary group		
	control, B_1	experimental, B_2	undernourished[1]
Body weight, g	22.6 ± 0.24	17.8 ± 0.02	15.25 ± 0.2
Brain weight, g	1.09 ± 0.005	0.9 ± 0.01	0.82 ± 0.02
Liver vitamin A stores IU/g liver	56.8 ± 1.04	Not detectable	57.0 ± 1.58
Brain gangliosides, /μg NANA/g tissue			
Total gangliosides	376 ± 16.2	301 ± 6.1[1]	399.8 ± 16
GM_1	44.4	43.6	6.2
GD_{1a}	201.9	163.6	226.6
GD_{1b}	62.7	38.3	54.1
GT_1	76.6	54.5	88.5

[1] B_1 vs B_2 ganglioside content $p < 0.01$.

The observations to be emphasized are the significant decrease in total ganglioside and of GD_{1a} and GD_{1b} in the group receiving lower amounts of vitamin A. It is of interest to note that the liver convent of vitamin A in the undernourished and control groups were the same and it was below the detectable limit (< 30 IU/g) in the experimental group.

The decrease in GD_{1a} and GD_{1b} observed only in the group given 'low' vitamin diet, but not in the undernourised group, suggests that it is not a non-specific effect of 'undernutrition' of the new born. *Vanier et al.* (14) have pointed out that the onset of myelination in the phase 10–20 days takes place when the pattern of GD_{1a} as the major component is established. The decrease observed in GD_{1a} concentration at day 17 after birth in rats from the 'low' vitamin A group indicate a possible effect on the multiplication of glial cells.

(1-^{14}C) glucosamine (3.5 μCi/rat) was injected intraperitoneally to 10-day old rats of control and vitamin A low groups. 24 h after injection the specific radioactivity of brain total gangliosides in the experimental group was 68 cpm/μg N-acetyl neuraminic acid (NANA). This was significantly lower than the specific activity of 107 cpm/μg NANA in the control group. In rats sacrificed 72 h after the injection, however, the specific activity of ganglioside NANA was the same in both the groups.

Sialidase activity in brain homogenates with endogenous ganglioside as substrate was assayed according to *Heijlman and Roukema* (7). This enzyme activity was lower in vitamin A-low group compared to controls until the 9th day after birth, became comparable by day 14 and was twice as high as controls by 21st day. (Data not given here). *Tulsiani and Carubelli* (13) have reported that the activities of brain neuraminidases remained fairly constant in post-weaning rats irrespective of whether they were maintained on vitamin A-deficient or adequate diets. It must be emphasised, however, that in the present study change in particulate neuraminidase activity due to vitamin A deficiency was studied in the preweaning rat.

The present observations of lowered initial rates of incorporation of ($1\text{-}^{14}C$) glucosamine into brain gangliosides and decreased sialidase activity up to 9 days postnatally in vitamin A low group, suggest that vitamin A is required for normal development of brain gangliosides.

Studies on Myelin and Associated Basic Proteins

Rats of control and experimental groups were injected intraperitoneally with ($1\text{-}^{14}C$)-DL-leucine on day 15 after birth and sacrificed subsequently. After separation of the acid extractable proteins (AEP) by disc gel electrophoresis (8), bands P_1, P_2 and P_3 were stained, solubilized in hydrogen peroxide and ^{14}C-activity determined. A progressive decrease in the ^{14}C-incorporated into these proteins was observed in both the groups (table II). The rate of decrease of specific activity of P_1, P_2 and P_3 (for 8 days) after injection of leucine was greater in the control than in the experimental group.

Gaitonde and Martenson (6) showed that in the rat, the synthesis of basic encephalitogenic protein is closely associated with myelination and that the basic myelin proteins P_1 and P_2 could be detected by day 10 after birth. In contrast, we observed that P_3, possibly a histone, was the only protein detected at this point postnatally, and in rats from mothers fed 'low' vitamin A diets the pattern of accretion of these basic proteins was altered (unpublished results). Injected ($1\text{-}^{14}C$)-leucine was incorporated into these proteins, but the *in vivo* rate of loss (^{14}C) from these proteins in 8 days after injection of labelled leucine was greater in the control group. This indicates that early vitamin A deficiency altered the catabolic rate of brain basic proteins. *Dallman and Spirito* (5) have suggested that in protein-malnourished rats, conservation of brain protein may occur through utilization of amino acids from degradation of protein elsewhere in the body.

Crude myelin was isolated essentially as described by *Clausen* (4) and the protein and lipid constituents were determined. Data in table III shows that the yield of myelin was less in undernourished and 'low' vitamin A groups than in controls. No significant changes were observed in protein and lipid components of the isolated myelin.

Table II. Incorporation of (1-^{14}C)-leucine into acid extractable proteins of rat brain: effect of maternal diet 'low' in vitamin A

Dietary group	Age of rat at the time of sacrifice, days	Specific radioactivity, cpm/100 μg protein			
		AEP	P_1	P_2	P_3
B_1, control	16 (3)[1]	3394	1846	800	1631
	19 (2)	2489	1040	805	1202
	21 (2)	2042	800	605	1008
	23 (3)	1435	612	308	822
B_2, 'low' vit. A	16 (3)	4262	1700	1140	1411
	19 (2)	3253	1602	1100	1300
	21 (2)	2594	1312	918	1134
	23 (2)	2080	1090	815	1025

15 day-old female rats were injected with 10μCi of (1-^{14}C)-leucine (IP) and sacrificed at the age indicated. Liver vitamin A store in B_1 = 118 IU/g mean value; B_2 = not detectable <30 IU/g.

[1] Figures in parentheses indicate number of animals sacrificed.

Table III. Data on yield of myelin and its composition in 19 day-old rats

Dietary group	Myelin		
	yield mg/brain, wet wt.	yield mg/g brain	protein mg/100mg dry myelin
1 'Undernourished' (15)[1]	2.10[2]	1.82	29.2
	2.15	1.90	28.8
2 Diet B_1 (5)	2.90	2.82	29.4
	3.10	2.91	31.0
3 Diet B_2 (5)	2.25	2.00	29.4
	2.18	2.02	29.2

[1] Number of rats/group.
[2] Myelin and constitutents: values given are duplicate determination. Brain tissues from male and female rats were pooled separately, myelin isolated and the constitutents determined.

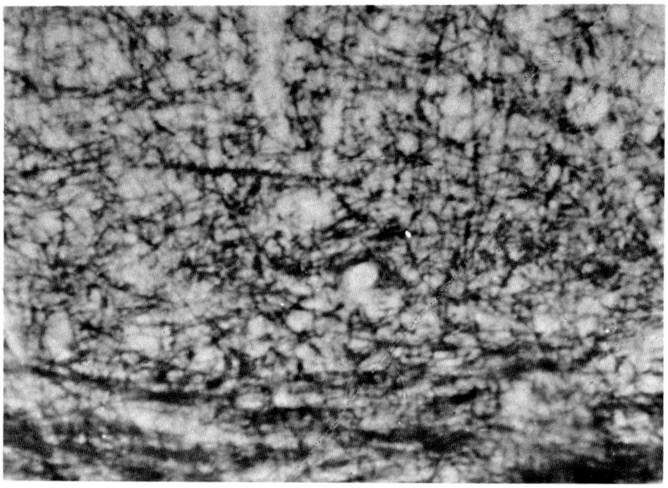

Fig. 1. Myelin stain (ferric alum, hematoxylin) × 100 cerebral cortex of 19 day-old rat from B_1, control.

Whole brains were fixed in 10% formalin and frozen sections (15 μm thick) stained for myelin (11). Coronal sections from the frontal lobe of the control rats of vitamin A supplemented group (B_1) show uniform staining and distribution of myelinated nerve fibres (fig. 1). In contrast, in the undernourished and the vitamin A-deficient group (B_2), demyelination was evident (fig. 2, 3). Similar histological examination of the cerebral cortex for myelin in the 50-day old rats, maintained on a vitamin A low diet, showed evidence of poor myelination, and supplementation with vitamin A to the deficient rat after weaning (day 21) did not show histological evidence of proper myelination. Though the present studies do not delineate a specific functional role for vitamin A or its metabolites, they strongly suggest that vitamin A is an important nutrient affecting, directly or indirectly, the normal myelination processes in the developing brain.

Studies on metabolism of retinol, (6, 7-$^{14}C_2$) and retinol-15-^{14}C have shown the presence of retinol and an unidentified metabolite in lipid extracts of rat brain (unpublished results). Further work on the specific functional significance of retinol/metabolites in relation to ganglioside synthesis and myelin proteins would be of interest.

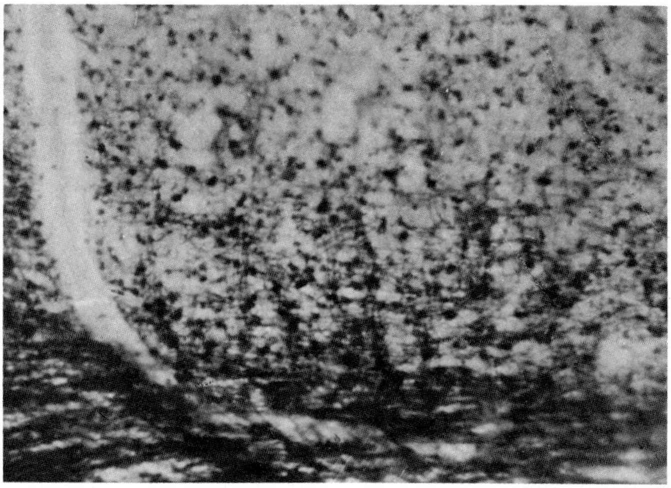

Fig. 2. Myelin stain × 100: cerebral cortex of 19 day-old rat from group B_2, 'low' vitamin A diet.

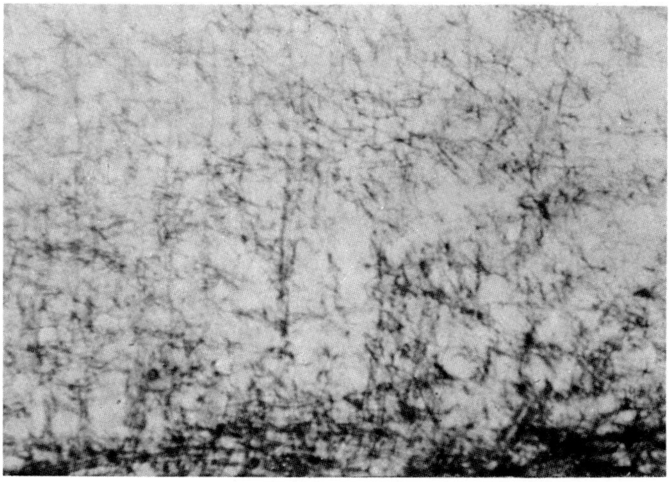

Fig. 3. Myelin stain × 100: cerebral cortex of 19 day-old rat from the 'undernourished' group.

Acknowledgement

We wish to place on record the active collaboration of Paul Jayaraj in carrying out the histological and tissue autoradiography aspects of these investigations. A part of this work on histology of myelin is included in this paper.

References

1 *Ames, S.R.: Risley, H.A., and Harris, P.L.:* Anal. Chem. *26:* 1378 (1954).
2 *Bhat, P.V. and Rama Rao, P.B.:* Environ. Physiol. Biochem. *2:* 147 (1972).
3 *Bhat, P.V. and Rama Rao, P.B.:* Arogya, J. Health Sci. *11:* 96 (1976).
4 *Clausen, J.:* Eur. J. Biochem. *7:* 575 (1969).
5 *Dallman, P.R. and Spirito, R.A.:* J. clin. Invest. *51:* 2175 (1972).
6 *Gaitonde, M.K. and Martenson, R.E.:* J. Neurochem. *17:* 551 (1970).
7 *Heijlman, J. and Roukema, P.A.:* J. Neurochem. *19:* 2567 (1972).
8 *Martenson, R.E.: Diebler, G.E., and Kies, M.W.:* J. Neurochem. *18:* 2417 (1971).
9 *Mellanby, E.:* J. Physiol., Lond. *XXIV:* 61 (1926).
10 *Rogers, Jr. W.E. and Bieri, J.G.:* Proc. Soc. exp. Biol. Med. *132:* 622 (1969).
11 *Spielmeyer:* in *Lillie* Histopathologic technique and practical histochemistry; 3rd ed., p. 490 (McGraw Hill, New York 1965).
12 *Suzuki, K.:* Life Sci. *3:* 1227 (1964).
13 *Tulsiani, D.R.P. and Carubelli, R.:* Nut. Rep. Int. *8:* 349 (1973).
14 *Vanier, M.T.; Holm, M.; Ohman, R., and Svennerholm, L.:* J. Neurochem. *18:* 581 (1971).

Dr. *P.V. Bhat,* Dermatology Branch, National Institute of Health, *Bethesda, MD 20014* (USA)

Wld Rev. Nutr. Diet., vol. 31, pp. 107–112 (Karger, Basel 1978)

Alterations in Structure and Function Relationship in Cellular and Subcellular Membranes in Vitamin A-Deficient Rat

H.R. Adhikari, R.S. Mullick, U.K. Vakil and A. Sreenivasan

Biochemistry and Food Technology Division, Bhabha Atomic Research Centre, Bombay

Vitamin A appears to be required for the maintenance of membrane integrity. Thus, both hypo- and hyper-vitaminosis A cause release of intracellular hydrolases from lysosomes (17), swelling of mitochondria (8, 14), hemolysis of erythrocytes (9) and changes in the enzyme activities associated with oxidative phosphorylation (19). It has been demonstrated that vitamin A forms an integral part of liver plasma membrane, endoplasmic reticulum and erythrocyte ghosts (15). We have now studied the effect of vitamin A deficiency on the lipid composition of some of the biomembranes isolated from rat liver and its significance in the maintenance of structure and function.

Effect of Protein Status on Subcellular Distribution of Vitamin A

We compared the subcellular distribution pattern of orally fed ^{3}H-retinol in livers of protein-depleted and control rats. Animals maintained on vitamin A-free diet for 4 to 5 weeks, were divided into two groups and fed either a 3%, or pair-fed with a 20%, protein diet. After 3 weeks, each animal was administered orally 5 μCi (^{3}H)-retinol along with 100 μg unlabelled retinol and sacrificed at different time intervals. The results on the distribution of the label in liver fractions are shown in table I. The radioactivity was measured at 48 h after ^{3}H-retinol administration, when it reached maximum in both the groups. About 20% less activity was recovered from protein-depleted rat liver compared to control. The radioactivity was mainly associated with cell-sap and nuclear fractions. The important point here is that about 10% of nuclear activity was recovered from the plasma-membrane, accounting for about 1% of the total activity. Normal plasma membrane contained twice as much activity as in protein deficiency. We also found that 60% of the label was accounted for by retinol and the rest was confined to retinyl ester and retinoic acid. These observations point

Table I. Effect of protein status on subcellular distribution of ^{3}H-retinol in liver

Liver fraction	Radioactivity recovered, cpm x 10^{-2}/whole liver	
	20% casein	3% casein
Homogenate	3020.0	2410.0
Nuclei	371.5	161.4
Mitochondria	141.9	101.2
Cell-sap	2307.0	1988.0
Plasma membrane	30.0	16.0

Liver homogenate (20%) was fractionated by modified differential centrifugation method (1). Nuclear pellet was layered over a discontinuous sucrose density gradient and centrifuged at 100,000 g for 2 h and plasma membrane separated. The purity of the preparation was checked by measuring 5'-nucleotidase activity, using 5'-AMP as substrate (6). Total vitamin A was extracted with chloroform:methanol (2:1) mixture and radioactivity counted in Beckman LS-100 liquid scintillation counter.

to a role of retinol in membrane structure. As a first step towards elucidating this, the effect of vitamin A deficiency on the nature and amount of lipids in intact mitochondria, as well as in lysosomal and plasma membranes, were then studied.

Effect of Vitamin A Deficiency on Lipid Composition of some Biological Membranes

Weanling male rats (body wt 30–35 g), having low reserves of liver vitamin A, were obtained from dams fed on marginal levels of the vitamin. They were maintained on 20% casein diet devoid of vitamin A. Control rats were administered orally 50 IU of retinyl palmitate/day and pair-fed with deficient ones. At the end of 8 weeks, liver mitochondria were prepared. The liver lysosomal membrane was isolated by washing intact lysosomes with 0.15 *M* NaCl, followed by Na-deoxycholate treatment (16). It was ascertained that this highly purified preparation was practically free of all the membrane-bound enzymes. The purity was also established by ultrastructural criteria.

Results on lipid composition are summarised in table II. Total lipids and phospholipids in all the membranes were significantly low, whereas cholesterol and triglyceride levels increased in vitamin A deficiency compared to pair-fed controls. Cholesterol accumulation in membranes may be explained by the known decrease in cholesterol side chain cleavage enzyme activity in vitamin A deficiency (13). It can be noticed that cholesterol:phospholipid molar ratio was

Table II. Effect of vitamin A deficiency on lipid composition of membranes (μg/mg protein)

Lipid component	Plasma membrane		Lysosomal membrane		Mitochondria	
	control	vitamin A-deficient	control	vitamin A-deficient	control	vitamin A-deficient
Total lipids	305.0	227.6	658.2	416.0	228.0	129.8
Triglycerides	15.2	19.6	10.6	17.2	7.6	12.5
Total phospholipids	170.0	105.0	405.0	270.0	155.0	87.5
Cholesterol	38.6	52.1	42.6	57.2	6.9	11.5
Cholesterol: lipid P molar ratio	0.45	1.00	0.22	0.41	0.10	0.25
Individual phospholipids:						
Cardiolipin	2.0	1.7	8.7	7.2	18.0	11.7
Phosphatidyl serine	4.7	3.7	17.0	18.5	ND[1]	ND[1]
Sphingomyelin	44.2	29.5	43.5	22.0	4.0	1.2
Phosphatidyl choline	72.2	42.5	190.5	123.0	73.7	32.7
Phosphatidyl ethanolamine	43.7	26.0	188.7	85.0	55.0	39.0
Lysolecithin	1.5	2.2	4.7	7.5	2.2	3.0

Lipid extracts were analysed for total lipids. Cholesterol was estimated by colorimetric method described by *Sperry and Webb* (20) and phospholipids, as outlined by *Bartlett* (3). Triglycerides and individual phospholipids were separated by TLC on silica gel-G plates, using chloroform:methanol:water (80:20:2 v/v) as solvent system. Spots were identified by exposure to I_2 vapour.

[1] not detected.

markedly increased in vitamin A deficiency. This ratio has been implicated as a governing factor in maintaining the integrity of biological membranes and influencing their osmotic permeability (10).

Lysolecithin concentration was consistently higher in vitamin A deficiency in all the membranes studied. Its addition to liposomes is shown to bring about distinct ultrastructural derangements (18). Thus, increase in this potent lytic agent may accentuate the fragility of biomembranes in vitamin A deficiency.

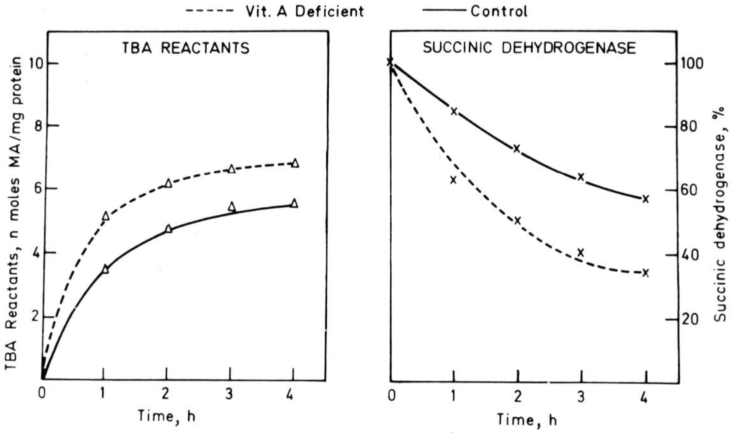

Fig. 1. Measurement of TBA reactants and succinic dehydrogenase activity in isolated mitochondria. Isolated liver mitochondria were suspended in Tris buffer pH 7.5 and incubated at 37°C under O_2. Aliquots were withdrawn at intervals and TBA reactants measured at 535 nm. Results were expressed on the basis of molar extinction coefficient of malonaldehyde formed (2). Succinic dehydrogenase activity was determined by spectrophotometric method (4).

The membranes of the vitamin A-deficient group also contained much lower content of polyunsaturated fatty acids (PUFA) and showed a lower peroxidizable index which indicates more susceptibility of PUFA of cell membranes to autoxidation in this group.

Measurement of Peroxidative Products in Isolated Mitochondria

Production of malonaldehyde, diene conjugates and lipofuscin compounds was measured and used as criteria for peroxidative changes. Isolated intact mitochondria were used, since any disturbance in oxidative metabolism is most pronounced in this organelle (22).

It can be observed (fig. 1) that concentration of malonaldehyde, a peroxidative decomposition product of PUFA from subcellular membrane (21), was increased at much faster rate with time in vitamin A-deficient rat liver mitochondria compared to control one. This coincided with concomitant decrease in membrane-bound succinic dehydrogenase activity. The level of conjugated diene peroxides, formed as a consequence of peroxidation of lipids, was increased in vitamin A-deficient rat plasma, but they were not detected in lipid extracts of liver mitochondria. We also examined Schiff-base type fluorescent products, formed by combination of malonaldehyde with primary amino groups of structural proteins (5). These chromophores, with characteristic excitation and emis-

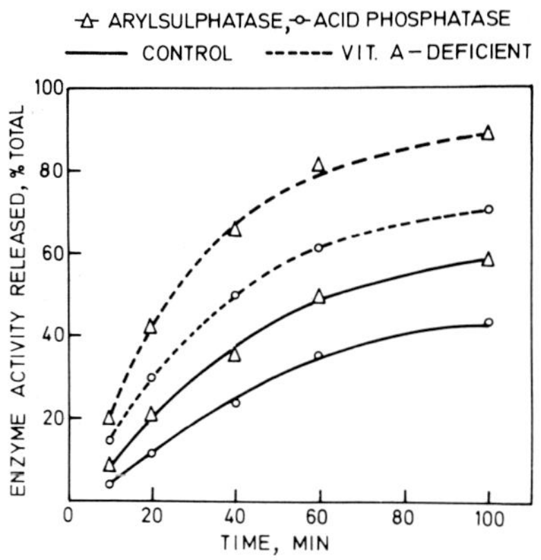

Fig. 2. Effect of vitamin A deficiency on the structural latency of lysosomal enzymes. Isolated lysosomes were incubated as described in the text. Activities of acid phosphatase and aryl sulfatase were measured at pH 5.0, using Na-β-glycerophosphate and p-nitrocatechol sulfate as substrates, respectively (11). Enzyme activities in lysosomal pellet and supernatant together were taken as total.

sion maxima at 360 and 430 nm, respectively, are common in biological systems and possibly reflect membrane damage (7). Initially, the quantitites of chromophores were almost the same, but after incubation for 4 h, about 50% more product was accumulated in vitamin A-deficient group. The accumulation of peroxidative products suggests rapid peroxidative changes in vitamin A deficiency, which in turn cause functional and morphological aberrations in the mitochondria.

Effect of Vitamin A Deficiency on the Structural Latency of Lysosomal Enzymes

Altered membrane properties in vitamin A deficiency were also studied with rat liver lysosomes, isolated by a modified method of *Roels et al.* (11). They were suspended in 0.25 *M* sucrose (pH 7.0) and incubated for about 3 h at 37°C. Aliquots were withdrawn at indicated time, centrifuged and bound and free enzyme activities measured in the pellet and supernatant, respectively. At 100 min, in the vitamin A-deficient sample, aryl sulfatase was recovered completely from soluble phase, compared to only 60% in pair-fed controls (fig. 2). However, about 40 and 70% of acid phosphatase was released from control and deficient groups, respectively. These observations suggest that the rate of release of enzymes from lysosomes is higher in vitamin A deficiency because of increased cell permeability.

In Vitro *Binding of Aryl Sulfatase B with Lysosomal Membrane*

Binding of aryl sulfatase B *in vitro* to isolated liver lysosomal membranes took place optimally at pH 5.0. The enzyme-membrane complex dissociated gradually with increasing buffer molarity from 0.01 to 0.1 *M*. Such experiments showed that aryl sulfatase B binding to lysosomal membrane of vitamin A-deficient rats was only about 60% of controls. We also noted a 40% decrease in lysosomal sialic acid content in vitamin A-deficient group. Pre-treatment of lysosomal membrane with neuraminidase decreased the binding irrespective of the source of the membrane. These results support the view that the positively charged aryl sulfatase binds to lysosomal membrane through the negatively charged groups (12) and suggest a damage of lysosomal membrane in vitamin A deficiency.

References

1 *Adhikari, H.R.; Vakil, U.K., and Sreenivasan, A.:* Indian J. Biochem. Biophys. *8:* 157 (1971).
2 *Ambe, K.S. and Tappel, A.L.:* J. Food. Sci. *26:* 448 (1961).
3 *Bartlett, G.R.:* J. biol. Chem. *234:* 466 (1959).
4 *Caplan, A.I. and Greenawalt, J.W.:* J. Cell Biol. *36:* 15 (1968).
5 *Chio, K.S. and Tappel, A.L.:* Biochemistry *8:* 2821 (1969).
6 *Coleman, R.; Michell, R.H.; Finean, J.B., and Hawthorne, J.N.:* Biochim. Biophys. Acta *135:* 573 (1967).
7 *Dillard, C.J. and Tappel, A.L.:* Lipids *6:* 715 (1971).
8 *Dingle, J.T.; Lucy, J.A., and Fell, H.B.:* Biochem. J. *79:* 497 (1961).
9 *Dingle, J.T. and Lucy, J.A.:* Biochem. J. *84:* 611 (1962).
10 *Finkelstein, A. and Cass, A.:* Nature, *216:* 717 (1969).
11 *Guha, A. and Roels, O.A.:* Biochim. biophys. Acta *111:* 364 (1965).
12 *Henning, R.; Plattner, H., and Stoffel, W.:* Biochim. biophys. Acta *330:* 61 (1973).
13 *Jayaram, M.; Murthy, S.K., and Ganguly, J.:* Biochem. J. *136:* 221 (1973).
14 *Lucy, J.A.; Luscombe, M., and Dingle, J.T.:* Biochem. J. *89:* 419 (1963).
15 *Mack, J.P.; Lui, S.T.N.; Roels, O.A., and Anderson, R.O.:* Biochim. biophys. Acta *288:* 203 (1972).
16 *Pappu, A.S.; Adhikari, H.R.; Vakil, U.K.; Fatterpaker, P.; Sreenivasan, A., and Bachhawat, B.K.:* Indian J. Biochem. Biophys. (communicated).
17 *Roels, O.A.; Trout, M., and Guha, A.:* Biochem. J. *93:* 23C (1964).
18 *Sessa, G. and Weissmann, G.:* J. Lipid Res. *9:* 310 (1968).
19 *Seward, C.R.; Vaughan, G., and Hove, E.L.:* J. biol. Chem. *241:* 1229 (1966).
20 *Sperry, M.W. and Webb, M.:* J. biol. Chem. *187:* 97 (1950).
21 *Tappel, A.L.:* Fed. Proc. Fed. Am. Socs exp. Biol. *32:* 1870 (1973).
22 *Weinbach, E.C.; Sheffield, H., and Garbus, J.:* Proc. natn. Acad. Sci. USA *50:* 561 (1963).

Dr. *H.R. Adhikari*, Biochemistry and Food Technology Division, Bhabha Atomic Research Centre, *Bombay 400 085* (India)

Wld Rev. Nutr. Diet., vol. 31, pp. 113–118 (Karger, Basel 1978)

Early Effects of Hypervitaminosis A on Hepatic Gluconeogenesis[1]

Vishwa Nath Singh, Malathy Singh and K.N. Dileepan

Department of Biochemistry, Vallabhbhai Patel Chest Institute, University of Delhi, Delhi

Oral administration of large doses (30,000 IU/day) of retinol to young rats for 2 days (early hypervitaminosis A) was shown to cause, among other changes, a marked stimulation of gluconeogenesis (17).

Hepatic gluconeogenesis is generally regulated through, either the supply of non-carbohydrate precursors, or gluconeogenic activity of the liver. Among the precursors, amino acids from muscle are of major quantitative significance. The gluconeogenic activity of the liver is determined by several factors, the important ones being (i) activities of the rate-limiting gluconeogenic enzymes, (ii) $NADH/NAD^+$ ratio, (iii) rate of fatty acid oxidation, and (iv) transport of pyruvate into the mitochondria. In the present study, effect of early hypervitaminosis A on these aspects of the regulatory mechanisms of hepatic gluconeogenesis was, therefore, undertaken in order to gain some insight into the mechanism by which retinol stimulates hepatic gluconeogenesis. Some of the findings have been published earlier (17).

Young male albino rats weighing 70–90 g were divided into two groups: (i) 'control' and (ii) 'retinol-fed'. Each retinol-rat was fed, with the help of a canula, 30,000 IU of retinyl palmitate in 0.4 ml ethyl oleate once daily for 2 days. The control animals received appropriate volume of ethyl oleate (the vehicle solution) in lieu of retinyl palmitate. Animals were starved for about 18 h before they were killed for the studies. Other experimental protocols and procedure for processing tissues are described elsewhere (17).

Assays of pyruvate carboxylase (EC 6.4.1.1), PEP-carboxykinase (EC 4.1.1.32), fructose 1,6-bisphosphatase (Fru-P_2ase; EC 3.1.3.11), glucose 6-phosphatase (Glc 6-Pase; EC 3.1.3.9), alanine amino-transferase (EC 2.6.1.2) and aspartate aminotransferase (EC 2.6.1.1) have been described in detail in one of our

[1] This investigation was supported by a grant from the Indian Council of Medical Research New Dehli, India.

Table I. Effect of hypervitaminosis A on the levels of amino acids in blood, liver and skeletal muscle

	Amino acids level[1]		% alteration
	control	retinol-fed	
Blood	15.06 ± 0.50[2]	8.82 ± 0.66 $p < 0.01$	– 41
Liver	0.18 ± 0.01	0.14 ± 0.01 $p < 0.01$	– 16
Skeletal muscle	1.48 ± 0.60	0.98 ± 0.24 $p < 0.05$	– 21

[1] Values are given as mg amino nitrogen/100 ml blood.
[2] Mean ± S.E. of 8 rats.

earlier publications (17). Assays of serine dehydratase (EC 4.2.1.13) (18), tyrosine aminotransferase (EC 2.6.1.5) (13), ornithine aminotransferase (EC 2.6.1.13) (12), tryptophan pyrrolase (EC 1.13.1.12) (4) were performed in appropriate cell-free preparations.

Pyruvate kinase (EC 2.7.1.40) was assayed by measuring pyruvate formed from phosphoenolpyruvate (11). Glucokinase (EC 2.7.1.2) and hexokinase (EC 2.7.1.1) were assayed simultaneously by the method of *Sharma et al.* (15). Phosphofructokinase (EC 2.7.1.11) was assayed by measuring formation of NADH through a coupled enzyme reaction (9).

Trichloroacetic acid-soluble fraction of blood, liver and skeletal muscle were used for estimation of amino nitrogen (6).

Citric acid level in the liver was estimated by the method described by *Stern* (3). Levels of NAD^+ and NADH in the liver were determined by a fluorometric method (10).

The methods for estimation of DNA and protein in the liver have been described earlier (17).

Excessive intake of retinol caused marked lowering of the level of free amino acids in the blood (table I). Levels of amino acids in the liver and skeletal muscle were also decreased, but decreases were less marked.

The early effects of hypervitaminosis A on activities of the key enzymes of gluconeogenic and glycolytic pathways and some important amino acid metabolizing enzymes of the liver are summarized in tables II and III. Excess retinol enhanced the activities of PEP-carboxykinase, Fru-P_2ase and Glc 6-Pase but decreased those of pyruvate kinase and phosphofructokinase (table II). Among the amino acid metabolizing enzymes, activities of alanine aminotransferase and

Table II. Effect of hypervitaminosis A on the activities of key enzymes of gluconeogenic and glycolytic pathways in the liver

Enzyme	Units[1] /mg DNA	
	control	retinol-fed
Gluconeogenic enzymes		
Pyruvate carboxylase	2.98 ± 1.11	3.20 ± 0.11[2]
PEP-carboxykinase	5.21 ± 0.46	8.65 ± 0.61 $p < 0.001$
$Fru\text{-}P_2ase$	3.01 ± 0.28	4.46 ± 0.34 $p < 0.001$
Glc 6-Pase	10.03 ± 0.61	13.90 ± 0.63 $p < 0.01$
Glycolytic enzymes		
Glucokinase	0.71 ± 0.13	0.70 ± 0.07
Hexokinase	0.22 ± 0.04	0.24 ± 0.03
Phosphofructokinase	0.89 ± 0.09	0.66 ± 0.05 $p < 0.05$
Pyruvate kinase[3] (–FDP)	7.15 ± 0.68	5.28 ± 0.54
Pyruvate kinase[4] (+FDP)	12.42 ± 0.83	8.72 ± 0.65 $p < 0.01$

[1] One unit of pyruvate carboxylase and PEP-carboxykinase catalyzes incorporation of 1 μmole $H^{14}CO_3$ into acid-stable compounds and oxalacetate respectively. One unit of $Fru\text{-}P_2ase$ or Gluc 6-Pase liberates 1 μmole Pi/min. One unit of a glycolytic enzyme catalyzes the formation of 1 μmole of product/min.
[2] Values are mean ± S.E. of 6 rats.
[3] Activity measured in the absence of any added FDP.
[4] Activity measured in the presence of added FDP (50 μ*M*).

ornithine aminotransferase were markedly increased and that of tryptophan pyrrolase decreased in retinol-fed rats (table III). Activities of pyruvate carboxylase, glucokinase, hexokinase, tyrosine aminotransferase, aspartate aminotransferase and serine dehydratase remained unaltered.

Hypervitaminosis A decreased the level of NAD^+ and increased the levels of NADH and citrate (table IV).

According to the current concept of regulation of gluconeogenesis, stimulation of this process in the liver could be brought about either by a direct enhancement of the gluconeogenic activity in the liver or through augmented supply of precursors from extrahepatic tissues like muscle and adipose (2).

Table III. Effect of hypervitaminosis A on activities of some important amino acid metabolizing enzymes of the liver

	Units[1] /mg DNA	
	control	retinol-fed
Ala aminotransferase(6)[3]	6.99 ± 0.51[2]	13.7 ± 0.82 $p < 0.001$
Orn aminotransferase(6)	1.54 ± 0.02	0.77 ± 0.07 $p < 0.01$
Tyr aminotransferase(8)	8.54 ± 0.47	1.37 ± 0.32 $p > 0.05$
Asp aminotransferase (6)	25.21 ± 2.10	22.61 ± 1.94 $p > 0.05$
Ser dehydratase(14)	1.08 ± 0.41	0.99 ± 0.40 $p > 0.05$
Trp pyrrolase(8)	1.76 ± 0.28	1.00 ± 0.12 $p < 0.01$

[1] One unit of ala aminotransferase and asp aminotransferase catalyzes the formation of 1 μmole of pyruvate and oxalacetate, respectively, per min. One unit of ser dehydratase and tyr aminotransferase catalyzes formation of 1 μmole of pyruvate and p-hydroxyphenyl pyruvate, respectively, per min. One unit of orn aminotransferase produces 1 μmole of pyrroline-5-carboxylate/min. One unit of tryptophan pyrrolase produces 1 μmole of kynurenine/h.

[2] Mean ± S.E.

[3] Figures in parentheses indicate number of rats used.

Table IV. Effect of hypervitaminosis A on levels of NAD^+, NADH and citrate in the liver

Estimation	μmoles/mg DNA	
	control	retinol-fed
Citrate	120 ± 10[1]	170 ± 10 $p < 0.01$
NAD^+	113 ± 13	93 ± 5 $p < 0.01$
NADH	35 ± 3	46 ± 6 $p < 0.01$
$NADH/NAD^+$	0.32 ± 0.03	0.51 ± 0.08 $p < 0.01$

[1] Mean ± S.E. of 6 rats.

Among the substrates for hepatic gluconeogenesis, amino acids are of major quantitative importance and there are indications that their supply could regulate the rate of gluconeogenesis in the liver (2). In the present investigation, excessive intake of retinol decreased the levels of free amino acids in the plasma, liver and muscle. If one considers the level of amino acids in the blood to reflect the rate of mobilization of these acids from muscle, retinol-mediated stimulation of hepatic gluconeogenesis could not be attributed to an increased supply of amino acids from extra-hepatic tissues. In fact, the decrease in the amino acid level may be a consequence of increased gluconeogenesis.

Besides other factors, increase in the activities of enzymes catalyzing the first step in the catabolism of amino acids and the key enzymes of the gluconeogenic pathway between pyruvate and glucose has been implicated in the stimulation of hepatic gluconeogenesis by dietary and hormonal factors (14). Thus, marked increase in the activities of alanine aminotransferase, ornithine aminotransferase, PEP-carboxykinase, Fru-P_2ase and Glc 6-Pase noted in the present study, may be responsible for the stimulation of gluconeogenesis in hypervitaminosis A. The increase in PEP-carboxykinase activity is of particular interest because enhanced activity of this enzyme has been associated with stimulation of gluconeogenesis under a variety of conditions (5). Likewise, pronounced increase in the activity of alanine aminotransferase is of special significance because it catalyzes the first (possibly a rate-limiting) step in the gluconeogenesis from alanine, which is considered to be the major carbon source for this pathway (2, 8).

Coupling of pyruvate kinase to PEP-carboxykinase and pyruvate carboxylase and of phosphofructokinase to Fru-P_2ase creates futile cycles between pyruvase and PEP and Fru-P_2 and F6P, respectively. Thus, in order to achieve an effective increase in the flux rate of metabolites in the direction of gluconeogenesis, enhancement in the activites of gluconeogenic enzyme must be accompanied with a reciprocal change in the activities of pyruvate kinase and phosphofructokinase. Decrease in the activities of hepatic pyruvate kinase and phosphofructokinase, noted in the present study, is expected to reinforce the effects of increased activities of key gluconeogenic enzymes and lead to more effective stimulation of the gluconeogenic flux rate in hypervitaminosis A.

Increased level of citrate in the liver is expected to facilitate gluconeogenesis in hypervitaminosis A by inhibiting phosphofructokinase (7) and activating Fru-P_2ase (1).

A marked increase in the NADH:NAD^+ ratio in hypervitaminosis A, noted in the present study, is expected to shift the equilibrium of the malate dehydrogenase catalyzed reaction in the mitochondria towards malate and facilitate the transfer of carbon skeleton as well as reducting equivalents from inside the mitochondria to cytosol, where PEP-carboxykinase and other enzymes, catalyzing subsequent steps of gluconeogenesis (oxalacetate to glucose) are located.

In the cytosol, NADH will facilitate glyceraldehyde-3-P dehydrogenase – catalyzed reaction in the direction of gluconeogenesis (1,3-diphosphoglycerate to glyceraldehyde-3-P). In addition, NADH is expected to spare pyruvate for gluconeogenesis by inhibiting pyruvate dehydrogenase (16).

References

1 *Datta, A.G.; Abrams, B.; Sasaki, T.; van den Berg, J.W.O.; Pontremoli, S., and Horecker, B.L.:* Arch. Biochem. Biophys. *165:* 641 (1974).
2 *Exton, J.H.; Mallette, L.E.; Jefferson, L.S.; Wong, E.H.A.; Friedmann, N.; Miller, T.B., Jr., and Park, C.R.:* Adv. Hormone Res. *26:* 411 (1970).
3 *Stern, J.R.:* Meth. Enzym. *3:* 425 (1957).
4 *Knox, W.E.; Yip, A., and Reshef, L.:* Meth. Enzym. *17,* part A: 415 (1970).
5 *Lardy, H.A.:* Harvey Lect. *60:* 261 (1966).
6 *Lee, Y.P. and Takahashi, T.:* Analyt. Biochem. *14:* 71 (1966).
7 *Mansour, T.E.:* Curr. Topics Cell. Reg. *5:* 1 (1972).
8 *Marliss, E.; Aoki, T.T.; Felig, P.; Pozefsky, T., and Cahill, G.F., Jr.:* Adv. Enzyme Res. *8:* 3 (1970).
9 *Meyer, W.L. and Kunin, A.S.:* Arch. Biochem. Biophys. *129:* 431 (1969).
10 *Pande, S.V.; Bhan, A.K., and Venkitasubramanian, T.A.:* Analyt. Biochem. *8:* 446 (1964).
11 *Passeron, S.; deAsua, L.J., and Carminatti, H.:* Biochem. biophys. Res. Commun. *27:* 33 (1967).
12 *Peraino, C., and Pitot, H.C.:* Biochim. biophys. Acta *73:* 222 (1963).
13 *Rosenberg, J.S. and Litwack, G.:* J. biol. Chem. *245:* 5677 (1970).
14 *Scrutton, M.C. and Utter, M.R.:* Ann. Rev. Biochem. *37:* 249 (1968).
15 *Sharma, C.; Manjeshwar, R., and Weinhouse, S.:* J. biol. Chem. *238:* 3840 (1963).
16 *Singh, M.; Singh, V.N., and Venkitasubramanian, T.A.:* Biochim. biophys. Acta *218:* 183 (1970).
17 *Singh, M.; Singh, V.N., and Venkitasubramanian, T.A.:* Arch. Biochem. Biophys. *173:* 82 (1976).
18 *Suda, M. and Nakagawa, H.:* Meth. Enzym. *17,* part B: 346 (1971).

Dr. *V.N. Singh,* Department of Biochemistry, Vallabhbhai Patel Chest Institute, University of Delhi, *Delhi 110007* (India).

Wld Rev. Nutr. Diet., vol. 31, pp. 119–124 (Karger, Basel 1978)

Labilizing Effects of Radiolytic Products of β-Carotene and Vitamin A on Liver Lysosomes *in vitro*

V. Ninjoor, Brij Bhushan and G.B. Nadkarni

Biochemistry and Food Technology Division, Bhabha Atomic Research Centre, Bombay

The involvement of vitamin A and its congeners in determining the structural stability of a variety of membrane-limited organelles including lysosomes has been well documented (17, 19). Our earlier studies showed that irradiation of tissues such as liver caused a rapid release of bound lysosomal hydrolases accompanied by an increase in the accumulation of hydrolytic end-products (11). These observations suggested that radiation could promote formation of radiation degradation products (RDPs) of vitamin A, which may have a capacity to disrupt lysosomes. We now report the isolation of RDPs of vitamin A and β-carotene and their influence on liver lysosomes.

Methods

Male albino rats of Wistar strain (body weight, 250–300 g) were reared on a stock diet (15). Liver homogenate (10), mitochondrial lysosome rich fraction F_3 (18) and heterogeneous forms of lysosomes (12), pellet before lysosome (PBL) and lysosome (L) were prepared. The particulate fractions were then suspended in 0.7 *M* sucrose.

β-Carotene was purified over an 8% deactivated alumina column using petroleum ether as solvent (8). Solutions of β-carotene, vitamin A alcohol and acetate, each at a concentration of 1×10^{-3} *M* in isooctane, were exposed to γ-radiation at a dose of 1.0 Mrad in a ^{60}Co-γ-cell-220 (AECL), Canada, dose rate: 0.56 *M*rad/h at room temperature with air as gas phase. Separation of irradiation products of vitamin A acetate was carried out as described earlier (11). The highly polar RDP of β-carotene was separated essentially according to this procedure, except an 11% deactivated alumina column was used instead of 6%. The loss in vitamin A and β-carotene by γ-radiation and the amount of RDPs formed were determined spectrophotometrically. The amount of RDPs formed was computed using $E^{1\%}_{1\,cm}$ values of β-carotene (2200) and vitamin A (1650) and expressed as equivalent of the parent molecules. The R_f values of RDPs were measured by thin layer chromatography on silica gel using solvent systems comprising acetone and petroleum ether.

RDPs of β-carotene or vitamin A were added to liver homogenate or the particulate fraction (20 μg dissolved either in 2 μl ethanol or dioxane/ml tissue suspension) and the release of marker enzymes was measured. Acid ribonuclease (EC 2.7.7.16), acid phosphatase (EC 3.1.3.2) and aryl sulphatase (EC 3.1.6.1) were assayed according to the methods described (1). Protein content of tissue suspensions was measured employing *Miller*'s method (9).

Results and Discussion

The characteristic spectra of irradiated vitamin A acetate and the isolated RDPs are shown in figure 1. There was a complete loss in the absorption peak at 325 nm and an increased absorption in the lower UV region. The destruction in vitamin A acetate was found to be 89%. Four polar RDP fractions of vitamin A were obtained. The highly polar RDP (FR IV) eluting with 50% diethyl ether in petroleum ether had a maximum yield of 10% and exhibited an absorption maximum at 240 nm, with an inflection at 280 nm. Irradiated β-carotene also resulted in 4 fractions. In contrast to the characteristic peak of β-carotene at 478, 450 and 425 nm, the highly polar RDP isolated from the irradiated sample showed an absorption maximum at 220 nm and an inflection at 270 nm. The yield was 15% as revealed by spectrophotometric measurements. The R_f value of the product was 0.1 as against 0.9 for β-carotene.

The RDP formed either from vitamin A acetate or alcohol did not respond positively for carbonyls (14), furfural (6), vitamin A aldehyde (5), 5,6- and 5,8-epoxides (7) and thiobarbituric acid reacting compounds (3). Some of the properties of the RDPs of vitamin A acetate are summarised in table I.

The data on the comparative labilizing activity of vitamin A acetate, alcohol and their corresponding RDPs on rat liver particulate enzymes are given in figure 2. RDP accomplished lysosome labilization more readily than vitamin A alcohol. Also, while vitamin A acetate did not appreciably cause lysosomal fragility, the RDP isolated from the irradiated parent molecule accomplished lysosome labilization as efficiently as that of RDP from retinol. Similarly, β-carotene which has never been implicated in causing disturbance in the lysosomal integrity, after irradiation induced alterations in the stability of liver lysosomes. When the isolated RDP of β-carotene was tested on rat liver lysosome-rich fraction for its membrane disrupting property, it caused the release of marker enzymes from the mitochondria-lysosome rich fractions as seen in figure 3. The responses of heterogeneous forms of lysosomes PBL and L towards the RDPs of vitamin A and β-carotene are shown in figure 4. Again, the products showed their labilizing action on both the populations of lysosomes. These results show that while vitamin A acetate or β-carotene were ineffective in damaging the lysosomal integrity, the RDPs derived from these compounds were potent labilizers of hepatic lysosomes.

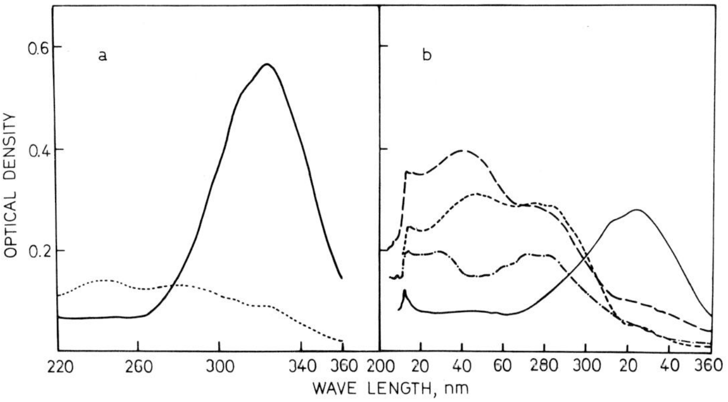

Fig. 1. Spectral patterns of γ-irradiated (1.0 *M*rad) solutions of vitamin A acetate: (a) characteristic spectra of unirradiated (continuous line) and irradiated (dotted line) vitamin A acetate; (b) absorption spectra of fractions isolated from irradiated solution of vitamin A acetate —·— FRI; —— FRII (untransformed vitamin A); ---- FRIII; and – – – FRIV (highly polar fraction).

Table I. Some characteristic properties of RDP isolated from irradiated vitamin A

Test	Characteristics	
	Vitamin A acetate	RDP
Elution property	1% diethyl ether in petroleum ether	50% diethyl ether in petroleum ether
R_f value	0.84	0.03
Carr-Price reaction	Transient blue	Reddish violet light green
TBA	No reaction	No reaction
Furfural test	No reaction	No reaction
Epoxide	No absorption maxima at 280 nm	No absorption at 280 nm
UV-spectra	CH_3OH λ-max 325 nm	CH_3OH λ-max 244, 280 nm
UV-spectra (alcoholic HCl)	CH_3OH λ max 325 nm	CH_3OH λ-max 422, 365, 346 and 330 nm
IR-spectra	Frequency 1748 cm^{-1} Frequency 1235 cm^{-1} Frequency –	1754 cm^{-1} 1236 cm^{-1} 3546 cm^{-1}
Acetic anhydride + pyridine	No esterification	Esterifies
Yield	–	10%

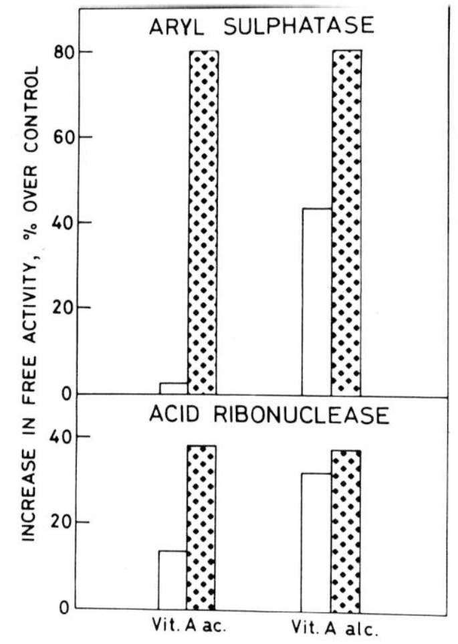

Fig. 2. Comparative labilizing activity of vitamin A and its RDPs on rat liver lysosomes. The ordinate shows increase in free activities of enzymes. Shaded areas show the corresponding effect due to RDPs.

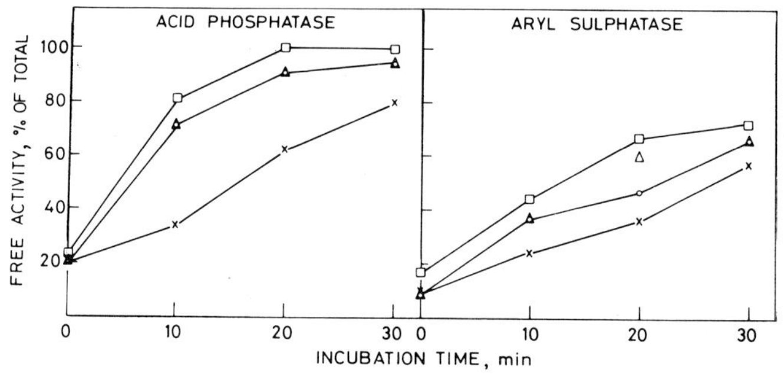

Fig. 3. Influence of RDP of β-carotene on the release of lysosomal enzymes. The mitochondria-lysosome rich fraction was incubated at 37°C with either β-carotene or its polar RDP. β-Carotene added was 100 μg/ml and the polar RDP added was 15 μg/ml.
X——X No addition ▲——▲ β-Carotene ■——■ RDP.

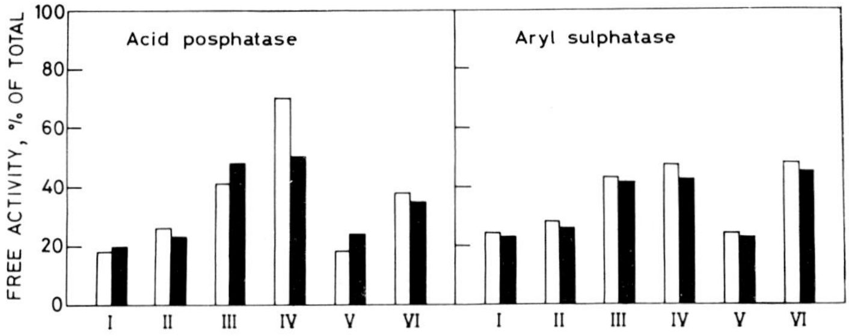

Fig. 4. Influence of vitamin A, β-carotene and their respective RDPs on the structural integrity of heterogeneous populations of lysosomes. I = no addition; II = vitamin A acetate; III = vitamin A; IV = RDP of vitamin A; V = β-carotene; and VI = RDP of β-carotene; □ = lysosome (L) ■ = pellet before lysosome (PBL).

The degree of lysosomal damage induced by vitamin A and its congeners seemed to depend on the type of derivatives employed (4, 16). The RDPs were able to exert their labilizing influence on lysosomes in liver homogenate, mitochondria-lysosome rich fraction, and also on heterogeneous forms of the organelles as evidenced by a faster release of the marker enzymes. Although the two forms of lysosomes have been shown to respond differently to physiological stress conditions (13), the response of PBL and L populations to the RDPs remained similar. However, in contrast to vitamin A alcohol or the RDP of vitamin A, the compound isolated from irradiated β-carotene labilized lysosomes only after incubation suggesting that the RDP of β-carotene was less effective in labilizing lysosomes.

Photo-oxidation of vitamin A has been known to produce a dimer, kitol (2). However, the exact chemical compositions of the RDPs derived from vitamin A and β-carotene respectively are yet to be elucidated. Preliminary chemical tests and the examination of UV and IR spectra of the RDP of vitamin A indicated hydroxylation of the molecule accompanied by a marked loss in the conjugated double bonds while the RDP of β-carotene showed extensive deconjugation (unpublished data). In the absence of precise information on the structural aspects of RDPs, their action on lysosomes could be explained only on the basis of a hypothesis proposed by *de Duve et al.* (4) for other fat-soluble compounds. These products could disrupt the integrity of lysosomes by directly interacting with the lipoprotein membranes or may induce extensive lipid peroxidation which could lead to membrane damage.

References

1 *Barrett, A.J.:* in *Dingle* Lysosomes, a laboratory handbook, p. 46 (Elsevier Publishing, New York 1972).
2 *Canet, M.M. and Mani, D.L.:* J.C. Bull Chem. Soc. France *11:* 4639 (1968).
3 *Dahle, L.K., Hill, E.G., and Holman, R.T.:* Archs Biochem. Biophys. *98:* 253 (1962).
4 *De Duve, C.; Wattiaux, R., and Wibo, M.:* Biochem. Pharm. *9:* 97 (1962).
5 *Futterman, S. and Saslow, L.D.:* J. biol. Chem. *236:* 1652 (1961).
6 *Gattermann, L.:* Laboratory methods of organic chemistry; p. 376 (MacMillan, London 1932).
7 *Jungalwala, F.B. and Cama, H.R.:* Biochem. J. *95:* 17 (1965).
8 *Kumta, U.S.; Sawant, P.L., and Ramakrishnan, T.V.:* Radiat. Botany *10:* 161 (1970).
9 *Miller, G.L.:* Analyt. Chem. *31:* 964 (1959).
10 *Ninjoor, V.; Saroja, S.; Padwal-Desai, S.R.; Sawant, P.L., Kumta, U.S., and Sreenivasan, A.:* Br. J. Nutr. *23:* 755 (1969).
11 *Ninjoor, V.; Brij Bhushan, Warrier, S.B.K.; Harikumar, P., and Kumta, U.S.:* Acta Vitam. Enzym. *26:* 181 (1972).
12 *Ninjoor, V. and Kumta, U.S.:* Indian J. Biochem. Biophys. *11:* 221 (1974).
13 *Ninjoor, V.; Harikumar, P.; Brij Bhushan; Warrier, S.B.K., and Kumta, U.S.:* Indian J. Biochem. Biophys. *12:* 9 (1975).
14 *Owen, T.C., Jr.:* An introductory laboratory text book; p. 144 (Marcel Dekker, New York 1969).
15 *Padwal-Desai, S.R.; Ninjoor, V.; Ramakrishnan, T.V.; Sawant, P.L.; Kumta, U.S., and Sreenivasan, A.:* Br. J. Nutr. *23:* 745 (1969).
16 *Perumal, A.S.; Lakshmanan, M.R., and Cama, H.R.:* Biochim. biophys. Acta *170:* 399 (1968).
17 *Roels, O.A.:* in *Dingle and Fell* Lysosomes in biology and pathology, vol. 1; p. 257 (North Holland Publishing, Amsterdam 1969).
18 *Sawant, P.L.; Shibko, S.; Kumta, U.S., and Tappel, A.L.:* Biochem. biophys. Acta *85:* 82 (1964).
19 *Seeman, P.;* in *Bolis et al.* Permeability and function of biological membranes; p. 40 (North Holland Publishing Co., Amsterdam 1970).

Dr. *V. Ninjoor,* Biochemistry and Food Technology Division, Bhabha Atomic Research Centre, *Bombay 400 085* (India)

Wld Rev. Nutr. Diet., vol. 31, pp. 125–129 (Karger, Basel 1978)

Studies on Vitamin A Absorption in Children

B. Sivakumar and Vinodini Reddy
National Institute of Nutrition, Indian Council of Medical Research, Hyderabad

Vitamin A deficiency is a major public health problem among children belonging to the poor sections of the population in our country. One of the important causes of the widespread prevalence is the inadequate dietary intake of the vitamin (6). Under these conditions, three considerations prompted us to investigate the quantitative aspects of vitamin A absorption in children in various physio-pathological states; (i) no reliable quantitative data were available on the absorption of vitamin A in human beings; (ii) computation of daily requirements would need correct information on the magnitude of intestinal absorption of vitamin A, and (iii) factors like infections and intestinal infestations, which are known to influence the absorption of other nutrients, may have a contributory role to play in the etiopathogenesis of vitamin A deficiency.

The most effective method of combating vitamin A deficiency would be to ensure that adequate amounts of vitamin A are present in the diet. As a short term prophylactic measure, however, administration of a single oral massive dose of 60 mg retinol once in six months has been suggested by our institute (12, 13). This is being implemented in our country in as many as nine states covering 4 million children. In addition, other countries have also adopted such a programme. The details of absorption and retention of such a large dose of vitamin A palmitate and the efficacy of the dose are reported elsewhere in the symposium. There is some experimental evidence to show that vitamin E promotes the absorption, storage and utilization of vitamin A (3, 9). There have been suggestions that inclusion of vitamin E in the massive dose of vitamin A may facilitate the accumulation of larger liver stores in children (11). In Indonesia and other South-East Asian countries prophylaxis programmes are being executed with 40 mg of added vitamin E. If such a procedure can successfully decrease the frequency of vitamin A administration, say, from twice a year as is being done now, to once a year, the advantages in the field are obvious. A study was undertaken, therefore, to test the effect of various amounts of vitamin E on the absorption and retention of vitamin A massive dose.

Vitamin A deficiency is commonly associated with protein-energy malnutrition in children. The incidence of vitamin A deficiency signs in children with kwashiorkor has been found to be as high as 36% (14). It has been shown that protein deficient rats suffer from impaired absorption of vitamin A in the gut (5). Earlier, *Arroyave et al.* (1) concluded that the malnourished children had poor absorption. Later, *Vinodini Reddy and Srikantia* (15) demonstrated a satisfactory rise in serum levels of kwashiorkors after a test dose of vitamin A, indicating normal absorption. Hence, we have also examined the extent of vitamin A absorption in kwashiorkor using labelled vitamin A.

Repeated attacks of infections like gastroenteritis, bronchopneumonia and intestinal infestation with round worms *(Ascaris lumbricoides)* are frequently seen among poor children. Infections were known to have adverse effects on nitrogen balance. In subjects whose dietary intake of protein is marginal, infections can precipitate clinical signs of protein deficiency. However, there is little information regarding the effect of infections in aggravating the deficiency of vitamin A. An attempt was, therefore, made to assess the absorption of vitamin A in children during infection.

Absorption of Vitamin A in Normal Children

Physiological Dose

When the label was given to normal children along with 1000 μg of vitamin A, less than 5% of the label was found in the feces indicating that the intestinal absorption is almost complete. There was no significant difference between the absorption and retention of retinyl palmitate and retinyl acetate.

Enterohepatic circulation of vitamin A metabolites has been demonstrated in the rat (10). But the very small amount of label excreted in feces of these subjects suggests that the amount of vitamin A excreted in bile may be negligible.

Massive Dose

When the label was given along with 60,000 μg of vitamin A, both retinyl palmitate and acetate were absorbed and retained in body to the same extent. This net retention is equivalent to that of 28,200 μg of retinol.

Effect of Vitamin E on Vitamin A Absorption

Supplementation of the massive dose of vitamin A acetate with 40 and 100 mg vitamin E acetate did not influence the absorption and retention of vitamin A. However, the children receiving 500 mg vitamin E showed a significant increase in the absorption. These subjects also excreted higher amounts of the label in urine and as a result the amount retained was not different from that seen in those which did not receive any vitamin E.

In experimental animals, very high amounts of vitamin E have been shown to have a beneficial effect on the absorption and storage of vitamin A (3, 8). Other investigators who worked with smaller doses of vitamin E failed to demonstrate any such beneficial effect of vitamin E in rats (2, 7). The present studies confirm these findings in humans.

Absorption of Vitamin A in Protein-Energy Malnutrition

In children with kwashiorkor, 90% of retinyl palmitate label administered was absorbed from the gut. This was not significantly different from the 96% absorption observed in normal children. The urinary excretion of the label was lower than in normal children. These results indicate that vitamin A absorption is not significantly altered in kwashiorkor.

Absorption of Vitamin A in Children with Infections

The mean level of absorption in children with bronchopneumonia was 74% as compared to 99% in the control group. These differences were found to be statistically significant. The duration of illness did not appear to be related to the extent of reduction in absorption. The urinary excretion of the label was not altered. However, the percentage of the dose retained was significantly lower in children with respiratory infection. None of these children had abnormal bowel movements and the fat content of the feces was less than 5 g/24 h.

Normal children receiving antibiotics did not show any abnormal excretion of the label in urine and feces, thus eliminating the possibility of the drugs having influenced the absorption of vitamin A. The mechanism by which infections depress the absorption of vitamin A needs further study.

In children with acute gastroenteritis also, there was an appreciable decrease in the intestinal absorption of vitamin A. The defective absorption in this condition could be due either to the infection or to the excessively rapid passage of the intestinal contents or due to both the factors.

Repeated attacks of respiratory infections and diarrhea may thus enhance the vitamin requirements by interfering with intestinal absorption of the vitamin.

Absorption of Vitamin A in Children with Ascariasis

In children with round worm infestation, the mean absorption was only 80% of the dose – a value that is significantly lower than that observed in normal children. There was, however, no difference between the two groups with respect to the urinary excretion of the label. The net retention of the vitamin was, therefore, less in children with ascariasis.

Fecal fat estimations indicated that the malabsorption is not due to steatorrhea and unaltered label excretion patterns in piperazine administered normals excludes a role for the drug in bringing about the observed defects in absorption of vitamin A in ascariasis.

The number of worms passed by the children following anthelminthic treatment ranged from 4–275. There was no correlation between expelled worm load and the magnitude of depression in vitamin A absorption. It is possible that the presence of worms may lead to an alteration in the structural integrity of the mucosa and intestinal motility (14).

Only trace amounts of label were detected in the homogenates of the worms. The mean content of vitamin A estimated spectrophotometrically was 0.33 μg/worm – a value much higher than that suggested by the trace amounts of label. This was probably due to the accumulation of the vitamin in the body of the worm over a long period of time and the amount of vitamin A lost as a result of the worm taking up the vitamin A may be considered too small to have contributed directly to the impaired absorption.

The more striking observation made here is that during infections and intestinal infestation by round worms there was gross impairment in the absorption of vitamin A. Repeated bouts of such diseases, as commonly seen in poor children who are already subsisting on marginal intakes of the vitamin, may precipitate clinical signs of vitamin A deficiency. So, while undertaking community prophylactic measures against vitamin A deficiency, one has to improve the general health and include deworming and agents for curing infections in an integrated approach.

References

1 *Arroyave, G.; Viteri, F.; Behar, M., and Scrimshaw, N.S.:* Am. J. clin. Nutr. *7:* 185 (1959).
2 *Bacharach, A.L.:* J. Pharm. Pharmac. *13:* 138 (1940).
3 *Cawthorne, M.A.; Bunyan, J.; Diplock, A.T.; Murrel, E.A., and Green, J.:* Br. J. Nutr. *22:* 133 (1968).
4 *Chandra, H.; Venkatachalam, P.S.; Belavadi, B.; Vinodini Reddy and Gopalan, C.:* Indian J. Ch. Health *9:* 589 (1960).
5 *Deshmukh, D.S.; Malathi, P., and Ganguly, J.:* Biochem. J. *90:* 98 (1964).
6 *Gopalan, C.; Venkatachalam, P.S., and Belavadi, B.:* Am. J. clin. Nutr. *8:* 833 (1960).
7 *Hebert, J.W. and Morgan, A.F.:* J. Nutr. *50:* 175 (1953).
8 *Hickman, K.C.D.; Kaley, M.W., and Harris, P.L.:* J. biol. Chem. *152:* 321 (1944).
9 *Moore, T.:* Biochem. J. *34:* 1321 (1940).
10 *Olson, J.A.:* Vitams Horm. *26:* 1 (1968).

11 *Olson, J.A.:* Israel J. med. Scis *8:* 1199 (1972).
12 *Srikantia, S.G. and Vinodini Reddy:* Am. J. clin. Nutr. *23:* 114 (1970).
13 *Swaminathan, M.C.; Susheela, T.P., and Thimmayamma, B.V.S.:* Am. J. clin. Nutr. *23:* 119 (1970).
14 *Tripathy, K.; Duque, E.; Bolanos, O.; Latero, H., and Mayoral L.G.:* Am. J. clin. Nutr. *25:* 1276 (1972).
15 *Vinodini Reddy and Srikantia, S.G.:* Am. J. clin. Nutr. *18:* 105 (1966).

Dr. *B. Sivakumar,* National Institute of Nutrition, Indian Council of Medical Research, *Hyderabad 500007* (India)

Wld Rev. Nutr. Diet., vol. 31, pp. 130–134 (Karger, Basel 1978)

Evaluation of Vitamin A Status in Children

James Allen Olson

Department of Biochemistry and Biophysics, Iowa State University, Ames, Iowa

Vitamin A deficiency is a widespread nutritional problem in the world (14). Each year 50,000–100,000 children lose their sight primarily because of vitamin A deficiency. Methods for diagnosing deficiency fall into clinical, biochemical, physiological and dietary. Clinical diagnosis, which is most commonly used, focuses on the eye: conjunctival xerosis with or without Bitot's spots (XIB and XIA), corneal xerosis (X2), corneal ulceration with xerosis (X3A), keratomalacia (X3B) and corneal scars (X5). Other signs, such as xerophthalmia fundus (XF), may also be noted. As with all procedures, however, clinical methods have limitations: the milder signs often tend to be nonspecific, whereas the more severe signs (X2, X3A and X3B) are rare and fleeting. Biochemical analysis has mainly been limited to plasma vitamin A determinations, although studies of liver stores of vitamin A and of plasma retinol-binding protein (RBP) are increasing. Plasma values are affected by a variety of factors (9, 11, 12). Retinol-binding protein concentrations, which are relatively low at birth and then increase through adolescence to adult levels are significantly affected by protein status as well as by the availability of vitamin A. Physiological indicators, such as night blindness and an abnormal electroretinogram, are highly effective procedures for adults under laboratory conditions (5), but are inappropriate and awkward for use with small children in a village setting. Dietary data, unless carefully gathered over a significant period, usually reflect only current intake patterns. In addition, the actual intake of vitamin A equivalents is often difficult to calculate from the diet because of inadequate knowledge about the carotenoid content and composition of foods and their absorption efficiency. Consequently, whereas the diagnosis of a clear case of acute vitamin A deficiency is relatively uncomplicated, adequate measures do not exist for determining marginal vitamin A status, or indeed the vitamin A status generally. Attempts to do so by the use of isotope dilution techniques (4) and by the analysis of urinary excretion products (13) have been successful only in highly controlled animal experiments.

Although the liver has long been known as the major storage organ for vitamin A in mammals (3), analysis of vitamin A in the liver has not generally been used as an indicator of vitamin A status. Although the transport of vitamin A in the plasma and its rate of uptake by peripheral tissues is of prime nutritional importance, the concentration of vitamin A in the liver is nonetheless the single best measure of vitamin A status.

But what indeed is vitamin A status? In order to avoid arbitrary designations, vitamin A status may be defined in terms of the period of time during which a person on a vitamin A-free diet is free of any overt signs of the deficiency state. This span of time might be termed the protection period. Obviously the greater the initial stores of vitamin A and the slower the depletion rate, the longer this protection period will be. To employ this concept operationally, however, two relationships must be defined: first, the manner in which vitamin A concentrations in the liver vary with the protection period; and second, how long an acceptable protection period should be.

In order to define the first relationship, some assumptions need to be made: (i) that the recommended daily allowance for small children of 400 μg of retinol or its equivalent (4.8 mg of mixed carotenoids) is a relatively accurate measure of need, but is not a firmly defined value; it is, rather, a fairly liberal estimate of the actual need of a normally growing child in a satisfactory environment (5); (ii) that the storage efficiency of dietary vitamin A is 20%; this value actually varies from 20–80% in various studies (5, 7); (iii) that the liver depletion rate is first-order down to a vitamin A level equivalent to the utilization rate and then is linear thereafter (3, 5, 8); (iv) that the half-time of depletion ($t_{1/2}$) is 50 days in preschool children (1), and (v) that the ratio of liver mass to body weight in small children is 0.03.

The method of calculation is simple. The minimal daily requirement of vitamin A from liver stores, which might also be termed the utilization rate, for a preschool child is 20% × 400 μg/day, or 80 μg/day. If the body weight of a child is 15 kg, the liver weight will be 450 g and at a vitamin A concentration of 100 μg/g, the total liver stores of vitamin A will be 45,000 μg. Three half-lives of 50 days would deplete the stores to 5125 μg, which would then be used up in 64 days at a linear rate of 80 μg/day. The protection period for an initial vitamin A concentration of 100 μg/g would, therefore, be 3 × 50 + 64 days, or 214 days.

The relative stability of the calculated protection period in the face of significant changes in the values of several important factors is shown by the following examples. If the actual requirement is 200 μg/day rather than 400 μg/day, the utilization rate would be 40 μg/day. The protection period for an initial liver concentration of 100 μg/g would then be 264 days rather than 214 days. A 2-fold change in utilization rate thus gives only a 24% change in protection period. Similarly, if the storage efficiency is 50% rather than 20%, the utilization rate would be 200 μg/day. The calculated protection period for an initial liver vitamin A concentration of 100 μg/g is then 156 days rather than 214 days. Thus 2½-fold change in storage efficiency gives only 27% change in the protection period. At lower initial concentrations of vitamin A in the liver, however, the calculated protection period is affected more by changes in the presumed requirement and storage efficiency.

At very low liver concentrations of vitamin A, i.e., 5 μg/g, the value of the calculated protection period (28 days) in a nutritional sense is problematical. Although the total amount of vitamin A in the liver of our 15 kg child (2250 μg) would still far exceed that in the plasma, even at a respectable level of 30 μg/100 ml (225 μg), a number of other factors come into play at very low concentrations. First of all, all of the remaining vitamin A may not be in a form suitable for mobilization as an RBP-complex. Alternatively, other unsaturated compounds in the liver, which do react in conventional vitamin A assays, might significantly contribute to the observed readings, thus giving a falsely high vitamin A value. Both of these considerations would decrease the length of the protection period. Differences in the concentrations of vitamin A in various parts of the liver, which may be as great as two-fold, would also markedly influence the length of the protection period. And finally, the amount of mobilizable vitamin A and, to a lesser degree, carotenoids in other tissues will affect the length of the protection period when liver stores are nearly depleted. Since discrete eye lesions have been observed in children whose liver stores were 7 μg/g or less (2), values in this range must be viewed with alarm.

The selection of a suitable protection period is a social and not a scientific decision. In my view 100 days is a suitable period, long enough to provide children with a reserve which might sustain them over a seasonal change of diet or a span of ill health, but not so long that a significant proportion of otherwise healthy children would be considered as marginally nourished in vitamin A. A liver store of 20 μg/g vitamin A should provide protection for a bit over 100 days and any value above 20 μg/g can be considered as acceptable. In a somewhat arbitrary manner, values between 10–20 μg/g can be considered as marginal, values between 5–10 μg/g as poor and values less than 5 μg/g as very poor.

Before this approach to vitamin A status is applied to a field situation, its predictive value might be tested against a public health case. As a result of extensive and crucial experimentation in the use of massive doses of vitamin A to prevent the signs of vitamin A deficiency near Hyderabad, a single oral dose of 200,000 IU of retinyl palmitate in oil was administered at 180 day intervals (10). If 20% of this dose were stored, 12,000 μg would initially be found in the liver in addition to any endogenous reserves. The protection period would, therefore, be around 125 days. If, on the other hand, 50% of the dose were stored and the daily dietary requirement was only 200 μg (a reasonable assumption in view of a somewhat reduced growth rate in many of these children), the protection period would be 175 days. Therefore the calculated and selected protection periods agree very well within reasonable limits.

The procedure for obtaining suitable samples of liver should be briefly mentioned. The biopsy of liver patients, although a relatively simple and safe procedure when performed with cause by highly skilled technicians under controlled conditions in a hospital, is both unfeasible and ethically uncertain when considered as a survey technique under field conditions. Necessarily, therefore, autopsy specimens must be employed. Happily vitamin A is remarkably stable in liver, even after partial autolysis or after being frozen for long periods. Since most children die from accidents or acute disease, such as pneumonia, dehydration and gastroenteritis, the prevalence of chronic liver problems, which are known to affect liver stores of vitamin A adversely, is rare. Finally, most children who die from infectious disease or dehydration are a representative portion of a larger group who somehow manage to survive similar stresses. The group which is studied tends to be closely representative of a much larger group of surviving children who are subject to similar stresses and inadequate food intake patterns. On the other hand, the sample is clearly not random and consequently each study must be scrutinized for bias which might infer the presence of a more serious problem than exists in a given society.

The use of autopsy samples for the evaluation of vitamin A status in very young children was conducted in 1974–1975 in Salvador, Brazil. Salvador is a city of about two million people and the capital of the State of Bahia. Red palm oil, one of the richest commercial sources of α- and β-carotene, is frequently used in the Bahian cuisine. Here poverty abounds, children are weaned between 3–6 months, families are large and conventional post-weaning foods consist mainly of cassava gruel and molasses.

With the cooperation of Dr. Maria Theresa Pacheco of the Institute de Medicinal Legal, Prof. Zilton Andrade of the Hospital Edgard Santos and Prof. Francisco Tripoli and Dr. Luis Erlon Rodrigues of the Department of Biochemistry of the University of Bahia, liver samples were obtained from the right central lobe at autopsy, frozen at $-20°C$, and analyzed for vitamin A and carotene by a combined spectrophotometric and Carr-Price method. Of the 135 liver samples analyzed, 101 came from children up to eight years of age. From the fetal period up to 2 months of age, median vitamin A values expressed as retinol were around 30 μg. From 2–6 months, median values fell to 12 μg/g, and between 6–12 months reached an amazingly low median value of 7 μg/g. Therefore, the median increased to around 20 μg/g at 1–4 years and then approached or exceeded adult levels (50–100 μg/g) beyond 4 years. It is instructive to consider these same data from a different viewpoint, namely the percentage of each group with liver stores of vitamin A less than 5 μg/g. Very few children fell into this category up to 1 month of age, but the percentage then increased dramatically, reaching a maximal level of about 40% between 3–12 months of age and then declined again. As far as causes of death are concerned, the present sample agrees very closely with the distribution found among nearly 8000 children between the ages of 1–4 years who died in Salvador in 1973. With regard to our previously suggested criteria for defining the presence of a public health problem, preschool children in the Salvador region are very much at risk. Happily, the Brazilian government is now taking steps to alleviate vitamin A malnutrition in northeastern Brazil by a variety of programmes.

Acknowledgement

Supported by grants-in-aid from the Rockefeller Foundation (GA-HS-7521) and from the US Department of Agriculture (616-15-173), and by travel support from the National Science Foundation.

References

1 *Hayes, B.W.; Mitchell, G.E., Jr.; Little, C.O., and Sewell, H.B.:* J. Anim. Sci. *26:* 855 (1967).
2 *McLaren, D.S.:* Trans. R. Soc. trop. Med. Hyg. *60:* 436 (1966).
3 *Moore, T.:* Vitamin A (Elsevier, Amsterdam 1957).
4 *Reitz, P.:* Experientia *29:* 168 (1973).
5 *Rodriguez, M.S. and Irwin, M.I.:* J. Nutr. *102:* 909 (1972).
6 *Sauberlich, H.E.; Hodges, R.E.; Wallace, D.L.; Kolder, H.; Canham, J.E.; Hood, J.; Raica, N., Jr., and Lowry, L.K.:* Vitams Horm. *32:* 251 (1974).
7 *Shivakumar, B. and Reddy, V.:* Br. J. Nutr. *27:* 299 (1972).
8 *Supopark, W. and Olson, James, A.:* Int. J. Vit. Nutr. Res. *45:* 113 (1975).
9 *Suthutvoravoot, S. and Olson, James A.:* Am. J. clin. Nutr. *27:* 883 (1974).
10 *Swaminathan, M.C.; Susheela, T.P., and Thimmayamma:* Am. J. clin. Nutr. *23:* 119 (1970).
11 *Underwood, B.A.; Siegel, H.; Weisel, R.C., and Dolinski, M.:* Am. J. clin. Nutr. *23:* 1037 (197).
12 *Vahlquist, A.; Rask, L.; Peterson, P.A., and Berg, T.:* Scand. J. clin. Lab. Invest. *35:* 569 (1975).
13 *Varma, R.N. and Beaton, G.H.:* Can. J. Physiol. Pharmacol. *50:* 1062 (1972).
14 *WHO:* Vitamin A deficiency and xerophthalmia: Technical Report Series, No. 590 World Health Organization, Geneva, Switzerland (1976).

Dr. *J.A. Olson,* Department of Biochemistry and Biophysics, Iowa State University, *Ames, IA 50011* (USA)

Wld Rev. Nutr. Diet., vol. 31, pp. 135–140 (Karger, Basel 1978)

Effect of Oral Contraceptive Steroids on Vitamin A Status of Women and Female Rats

Mahtab S. Bamji and Faizy Ahmed[1]
National Institute of Nutrition, Indian Council of Medical Research, Hyderabad

Use of combination type oral contraceptive (OC) containing synthetic estrogens and progestagens is associated with many clinical side effects of trivial nature as well as serious complications. The biochemical basis for the clinical manifestation is not understood, though several metabolic lesions due to the use of contraceptive steroids are known. Among these lesions are some that suggest deficiency of vitamins. Unlike most vitamins whose blood levels fall with the use of OC, plasma vitamin A levels show a significant increase (8).

Since the general vitamin status of women of low and middle income groups is poor and a large majority suffer from biochemical, if not frank clinical forms of deficiency, we decided to examine the interaction between OC and vitamin A in women of low income groups.

One study in a small group of women has been completed and another more comprehensive investigation is currently in progress. The latter is a multicentered study sponsored by the Human Reproduction Unit of the World Health Organization, Geneva.

The first study consisted of two parts. A cross-sectional investigation in which women who had been using OC for 6–12 months were compared with a matched group of women who had never received OC and a partial follow-up study in which a woman was examined initially and then at one or more points of time in the first 6 months. Thus each woman served as her own control. The women received either Ovral (ethinyl estradiol 0.05 mg and dl-norgestrel 0.5 mg) or Ovulen-50 (ethinyl estradiol 0.05 mg and ethinodiol diacetate 1.0 mg).

[1] The authors are grateful to Dr. S.G. Srikantia, Director, National Institute of Nutrition, Hyderabad, and Human Reproduction Unit, WHO, Geneva, and to the staff working on this project.

In the WHO sponsored study, three types of hormonal contraceptives are being tested for their metabolic side effects: (a) 0.05 mg ethinyl estradiol and 0.15 mg d-norgestrel, oral pill, (b) 0.03 mg ethinyl estradiol and 0.15 mg d-norgestrel, oral pill, and (c) medroxyprogesterone acetate (DMPA), 150 mg, once in 3 months injection. The two oral pills are coded as LNA and LNB trade preparations and we do not know which one is 50 μg estrogen pill and which one is 30 μg estrogen pill.

We hope to examine at least 60 women/preparation intially and at the end of one year. In addition, these women will be examined at one point (either 1st, 3rd or 6th cycle) within one year. The study is incomplete but some preliminary data will be presented.

Since starting this project the investigation on DMPA has been discontinued due to a ban on the drug, but considerable information was obtained before this ban was imposed.

Vitamin A was estimated in cyclohexane extracts of the plasma, by ultraviolet spectrophotometry before and after irradiation with UV light (6).

Tables I and II give the data on Ovulen-50 and Ovral used in the first study. It can be seen that while both the OC agents elicited a rise in plasma vitamin A, the extent of increase was greater with Ovulen-50, suggesting that the progestagen component of the pill modifies the response. The data in table II shows that the increase occurred within one month.

The results obtained in the on-going WHO study are given in table III. The 'first cycle' examination in the case of the two pill preparations, LNA and LNB, was done only 10–15 days after starting the contraceptive and within that interval plasma vitamin A levels were raised.

It was interesting to note that the magnitude of the change in plasma vitamin A was similar with LNA and LNB, indicating that there is no difference between 30 and 50 μg estrogen pills as far as the effect on plasma vitamin A is concerned.

DMPA failed to elicit a similar response. This has been observed earlier and shows that the effect on vitamin A metabolism is due to the estrogen component of the pill, though the progestagen may modify the estrogen effect.

The two pertinent questions that arise from these results are: (a) what is the biochemical basis for the observed change in plasma vitamin A and (b) what is the clinical significance of this change?

Three explanations supported by limited experimental data have been put forward to explain the rise in plasma vitamin A levels associated with OC use: (a) rise in plasma vitamin A is due to a general lipemia which is often seen in women using OC. However, no correlation seems to be apparent between triglycerides and vitamin A in our women. Similar observation was made by *Yeung and Chan* (11). Further, it has been shown that the increase in vitamin A is due to retinol rather than retinyl esters. In female rats *Supopark and Olson* (9) found

Table I. Effect of oral contraceptive (OC) on plasma vitamin A, cross-sectional study

	Control	OC treated, 6–12 months	
		Ovral	Ovulen-50
Plasma vitamin A µg/100 ml	29.8 ± 1.31[1] (43)	37.5 ± 3.25[2] (10)	45.0 ± 1.51[3, 4] (12)

[1] Mean ± S.E.
[2] $p < 0.01$ compared to control.
[3] $p < 0.001$ compared to control.
[4] $p < 0.05$ Ovral vs Ovulen-50.
Figures in parentheses indicate number of subjects.

Table II. Effect of oral contraceptives (Ovral and Ovulen-50) on plasma vitamin A, partial follow-up study

	Duration of treatment, months						Pooled SD	Between month	
	Initial	1	2	3	4	5–6		df.	F value
Plasma vitamin A µg/100 ml	31.5[1] (22)	40.7 (8)	39.7 (10)	36.7 (3)	46.1 (8)	43.3 (9)	6.2	33	9.8[2]

[1] Mean.
[2] $p < 0.001$.
Figures in parentheses indicate number of subjects.

that the ratio of free to bound retinol is not altered following the administration of OC; (b) the second explanation proposed is that OC enhances the conversion of carotene to retinol. *Horwitt et al.* (7) found inverse correlation between plasma vitamin A and carotene in OC-treated women. Several other studies, however, fail to confirm this. (c) The third explanation is that the rise in plasma vitamin A in OC users is probably secondary to an increase in retinol-binding protein (RBP). Combination type OC, but not the depoprogestagens alone, has been reported to stimulate the α_1-globulin as well as iodine-binding protein and lipid-binding protein. The results hitherto obtained in our women, however, do not show any specific changes in plasma proteins. Recently *Supopark and Olson* (9) have demonstrated a rise in rat serum RBP following the administration of Ovral.

Table III. Effect of oral contraceptives on plasma vitamin A levels

		Duration of treatment, cycles					
		Initial	1	3	6	9–12	13
Plasma vitamin A μg/100 ml	LNA	25.0[1] ± 0.70 (94)	36.8[3] ± 2.46 (16)	37.4[3] ± 2.66 (17)	34.9[3] ± 2.87 (13)	–	38.6[3] ± 2.50 (11)
	LNB	26.2 ± 0.87 (91)	31.3[2] ± 2.10 (13)	36.8[3] ± 2.16 (18)	44.8[3] ± 4.40 (5)	–	40.4[3] ± 1.84 (15)
	DMPA[4]	–	–	20.8 ± 2.57 (5)	23.5 ± 3.22 (10)	26.9 ± 4.36 (42)	–

[1] Mean ± S.E.
[2] $p < 0.05$.
[3] $p < 0.001$ compared to initial.
[4] Months of treatment.
Figures in parentheses indicate number of subjects.

Table IV. Effect of oral contraceptives on plasma and liver vitamin A of female rats[1] (24 day treatment)

	Control (8)	Ovral (8)	Ovulen-50 (8)
Plasma vitamin A μg/100 ml	24.2 ± 1.61[2]	27.7 ± 3.27	28.0 ± 2.22
Liver vitamin A μg/100 ml	407.9 ± 21.34	307.1 ± 23.12[3]	277.9 ± 22.34[4]

[1] Vitamin A – 20 IU/g.
[2] Mean ± S.E.
[3] $p < 0.01$.
[4] $p < 0.001$ compared to control.
Figures in parentheses indicate number of animals/group.

Liver vitamin A levels have been shown to fall in monkeys and rats treated with OC (1, 2, 10). The data obtained by us in adult female rats treated with one-tenth tablet of Ovral or Ovulen-50 daily is presented in table IV. Here again the fall in liver vitamin A was more marked with Ovulen-50 than with Ovral. Unlike women, female rats failed to show a rise in plasma vitamin A. However, *Supopark and Olson* (9) have shown that this rise does occur with dose of OC, 50 times the human dose on weight basis. The dose employed here was 25–30 times the human dose.

It is possible that due to an increase in circulating RBP, there is a shift of vitamin A from the liver into circulation leading to faster depletion. Faster depletion of liver vitamin A has been reported in rats treated with OC (9, 10).

The second question relates to the clinical significance of raised plasma retinol and depletion of liver stores. *Gal et al.* (4) have expressed the fear of teratogenic effects due to higher plasma vitamin A levels, should women using OC conceive soon after discontinuation of the pill. However, this fear seems unfounded, since plasma vitamin A levels never reach the toxic levels of 300 μg/100 ml.

Some workers have reported association of OC with hepatomas (3) and hence the remote possibility that higher incidence of hepatomas in pill users may be due to depletion of liver vitamin A has been suggested (5). This again seems to be an unfounded fear since no correlation has been observed between malnutrition where liver vitamin A stores are low and hepatomas.

Perhaps the only clinical consequence of concern should be hypovitaminosis A due to continuous faster depletion of liver vitamin A in OC users. This fear is particularly valid in the case of women whose initial stores may not be high and whose dietary intake is low. To investigate this possibility, a rat study was conducted in which the vitamin A intake of female rats was restricted to 4 IU/g diet. The OC treated animals on low vitamin A diet showed a significant fall not only in liver vitamin A but also plasma vitamin A in about 2 weeks. Thus, it is conceivable that prolonged use of OC may lead to biochemical hypovitaminosis A in women whose vitamin A intake is marginal.

We have examined the effects of vitamin A supplements to women using OC in a separate study. The plasma vitamin A concentration of women who received pyridoxine (10 mg) and multivitamin tablet containing 5000 IU of vitamin A along with Ovral, was similar to that of women who received Ovral and pyridoxine but not the multivitamin tablet. Thus, supplementation of women using OC with moderate doses of vitamin A may not be hazardous (as has been suggested by some workers) and may, in fact, help to maintain the liver stores.

References

1 *Ahmed, F. and Bamji, M.S.:* Ann. Rep. natn. Inst. of Nutr.; p. 100 (1975).
2 *Belvady, B.; Krishnamurthy, D.; Mohinuddin, S.M., and Udayasekhara Rao, P.:* Indian J. Exp. Biol. Med. *11:* 15 (1973).
3 *Christopherson, W.M.; Mays, E.T., and Borrows, G.H.:* Obstet. Gynec., N.Y. *46:* 221 (1975).
4 *Gal, I.; Parkinson, C., and Craft, I.:* Br. med. J. *2:* 436 (1971).
5 *Gal, I.:* Lancet *i:* 684 (1975).
6 *Gopalan, C.; Venkatachalam, P.S., and Belvady, B.:* Am. J. clin Nutr. *8:* 833 (1960).
7 *Horwitt, M.K.; Harvey, C.C., and Dahm, C.H.:* Am. J. clin. Nutr. *28:* 403 (1975).
8 *Larsson-Cohn, U.:* Am. J. Obstet. Gynec. *121:* 184 (1975).
9 *Supopark, W. and Olson, J.A.:* Int. J. Vit. Nutr. Res. *45:* 113 (1975).
10 *Yeung, D.L.:* Am. J. clin. Nutr. *27:* 125 (1974).
11 *Yeung, D.L. and Chan, P.L.:* Am. J. clin. Nutr. *28:* 125 (1975).

Dr. *M.S. Bamji,* National Institute of Nutrition, Indian Council of Medical Research, *Hyderabad 500 007* (India)

Wld. Rev. Nutr. Diet., vol. 31, pp. 141–148 (Karger, Basel 1978)

Synthetic Studies in Carotenoids

M. V. Bhatt and H.N. Venkatesh Prasad

Department of Organic Chemistry, Indian Institute of Science, Bangalore

A practical synthesis of vitamin A (I) from locally available and abundant raw material is of more than academic interest. Most of the industrially successful syntheses start from β-ionone (II) and build up the rest of the carbon atoms in installments of smaller units. Naturally formed citral (III) derived from essential oil of lemon grass – *Cymbopogon citratus* (stapf) or *Cymbopogon flexuoses* (Nees) stapf *(Gramineae)* – continues to be the widely used starting material. Much research effort has been directed to circumvent the dependence on lemon grass oil. Successful attempts have been made to obtain citral from the geographically widely distributed and cheap β-pinene. Also totally synthetic routes for β-ionone have been developed. Last year, an attractive and efficient synthesis of vitamin A starting from 2,2,6-trimethyl cyclohexanone was described (2) (fig. 1).

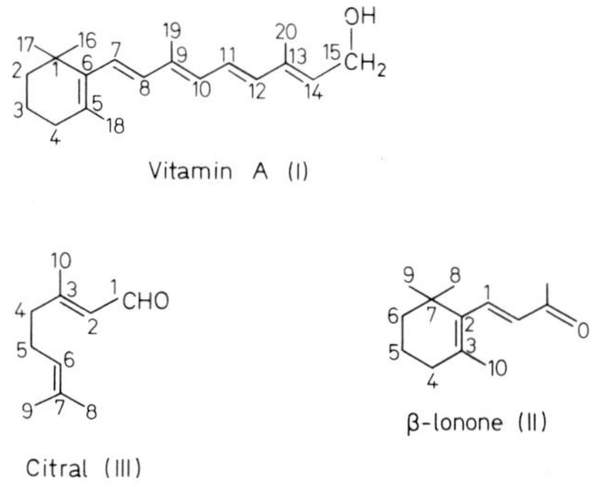

1

At the outset we decided that our synthetic approach should take a direction quite different to the direction taken by previous workers. Instead of attempting to reduce, or dispense with, dependence on natural sources, we wanted to attempt to increase the use of naturally available material. All commercial syntheses depend on natural citral for 10 out of 20 carbon atoms. We have used citral for all the 20 carbon atoms. Once the strategy was decided upon, choice of tactics became rather a simple matter. It has two crucial features, namely: (a) functionalization of C_8 position of 10-carbon unit, (b) introduction of a *trans* double bond in the 10-carbon unit to obtain an all-*trans* bifunctional derivative (fig. 2).

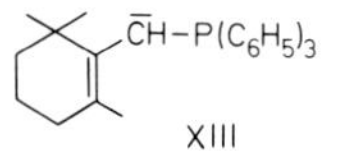

XIII

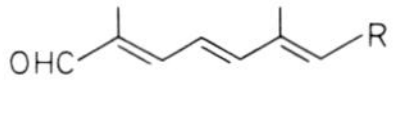

VII. R = CN
XI. R = $COOC_2H_5$

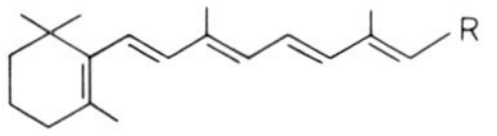

2 Retino nitrile (VIII. R = CN)
Ethyl retinoate (XII R = $COOC_2H_5$)

Selenium dioxide oxidation of allylic positions has been a fairly well studied reaction (4). It has been demonstrated that the reagent preferentially attacks the methyl group *trans* to the substituent across the double bond rather than other positions. When the reaction was carried out, a single product, the 10-carbon diene aldehyde nitrile (VI) could be isolated in 40–50% yield. The 7 and 8 methyl groups in geranonitrile (V) give poorly resolved singlets at about 1.6 δ. In the NMR spectrum of the aldehyde it is found that the signal for 8-methyl group disappears. The aldehyde proton gives a signal at 9.4 δ, the chemical shift value is consistent with a *trans* disposition of the aldehyde function. Had it been *cis*, signal would have been shifted to about 10 δ. Moreover, it has been established as a result of detailed study that the oxidation with SeO_2 takes place stereoselectively at the *trans* methyl group (4) (fig. 3).

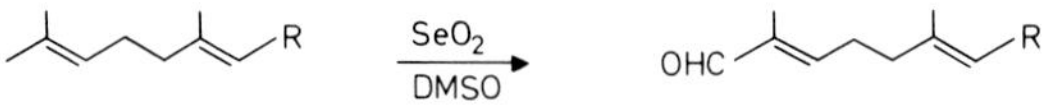

V. R = CN
IX. R = $COOC_2H_5$

VI. R = CN
X. R = $COOC_2H_5$

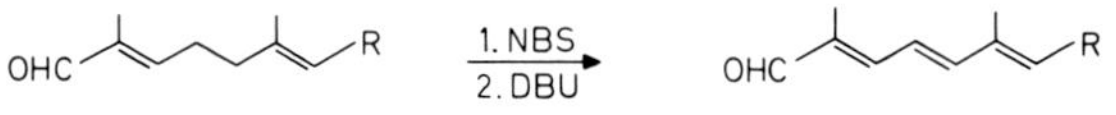

3
VI. R = CN
X. R = $COOC_2H_5$

VII. R = CN
XI. R = $COOC_2H_5$

Bromination of the aldehyde nitrile (VI) with N-bromosuccinimide (NBS) or with N,N-dibromodimethylhydantoin and dehydrobromination with 1,5-diazabicyclo (5.4.0) undec-7-ene (DBU), gave the crystalline trienealdehydonitrile with the correct all-*trans* stereochemistry (VII), m.p. 135°C.

In a similar manner, bromination with NBS and dehydrobromination with DBU of 8-oxoethylgeranate (X) yielded all *trans* trienealdehydocarboxylic ester (XI) m.p. 78°C, having the same m.p. as the compound reported in literature (3). The NMR and UV properties for this compound were consistent with the assigned structure (fig. 4).

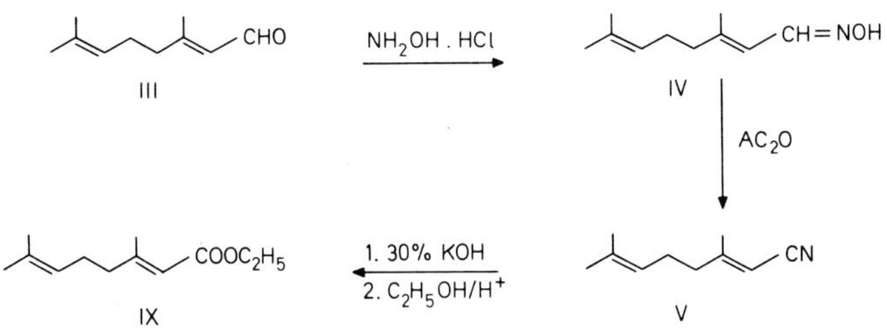

4

Considering the fact that bromination and dehydrobromination procedure gave the *trans* trienealdehyde ester, there is no reason to suppose that the reaction with the nitrile would proceed differently. The NMR data is consistent with the all-*trans* stereochemistry and different from that expected on the basis of *trans-cis-trans* stereochemistry.

In the NMR spectrum of the 2 triene aldehydes the signals for the aldehyde proton, C_7 methyl, C_6 vinyl, C_3 methyl and C_2 vinyl protons are at the positions expected for the *trans* stereochemistry. That the newly introduced double bond is also *trans* is proved by the chemical shifts for C_4 and C_5 vinyl protons which is around 6.5–6.6 δ for these two compounds, a value expected for the *trans* double bond at this position. Had the double bond been *cis* the value would have been around 6.4 δ. Thus the NMR spectrum is consistent only with all-*trans* stereochemistry of the two compounds.

Condensation of (VII) with cyclogeranyltriphenylphosphonium-ylide (XIII) gave retinonitrile (VIII). The UV and NMR spectra were consistent with the published spectroscopic data (1). All-*trans* ethyl retinoate was similarly obtained from (XI) by the Wittig reaction with (XIII) the NMR consistent only with the all-*trans* stereochemistry. The chemical shifts of the olefinic protons at the positions of C_{10}, C_{11}, C_{12} and C_{14} vinyl protons (refer to tables I and II) are informative and diagnostic regarding the stereochemistry. In the two tables the values expected for the all-*trans* and 11-*cis* compounds and the observed values are collected. There is a considerable upfield shift for C_{11} and C_{12} vinyl protons

Table I. Expected chemical shifts for olefinic protons in all *trans* and 11 *cis* isomers and observed chemical shifts (retinonitrile)

	10	11	12	14
All-*trans*	6.15	6.8	6.2	5.2
11-*cis*	6.5	6.4	5.8	5.3
Observed	6.2	6.8	6.2	5.1

Table II. Expected chemical shifts for olefinic protons in all-*trans* and 11-*cis* isomers and observed chemical shifts (ethyl retinoate)

	10	11	12	14
All-*trans*	6.13	6.99	6.27	5.79
11-*cis*	6.50	6.56	5.87	5.90
Observed	6.2	6.9	6.2	5.8

(around 0.4 δ) for the 11 *cis* compounds. While the C_{10} vinyl proton is shifted downfield to an extent of 0.4 δ in the 11-*cis* compounds, the C_{14} vinyl proton is slightly downfield (0.1 δ) in the 11-*cis* compound. From the tables it is clear that the observed chemical shifts indicate that the compounds have all-*trans* stereochemistry.

2,6-Octadienaldoxime 3,7 dimethyl (citral oxime, IV)

2,6-Octadienal 3,7 dimethyl (citral 25 g) was added to a solution of hydroxylamine hydrochloride (62 g), sodium bicarbonate (35 g) and sodium acetate (17.5 g) in 630 ml of water. 200 ml of methanol was added to dissolve the citral. The solution was stirred for 12 h and left overnight. The aqueous and the organic layer were separated and the aqueous layer extracted with 2 × 100 ml of ether. The ether layer was mixed with the organic layer and the combined layer washed with 2 × 100 ml ammonium chloride solution. The ether solution was dried over anhydrous sodium sulphate and the solvent removed to get 26.85 g of the crude oxime which was distilled in vacuum to get 24 g of the pure oxime (yield 87%). Boiling point 125–127°C (3 mm) ir ν_{max} 1660 cm^{-1}, 3400 cm^{-1}

2,6-Octadienenitrile 3,7 dimethyl (geranonitrile, V)

To 17 g of acetic anhydride at 100°C, 24 g of the corresponding oxime was added, dropwise, at such a rate that a gentle reflux was maintained. After the addition was complete, the reaction mixture was refluxed for 10 min. It was then cooled and poured into 200 ml of water. The resulting mixture was extracted with 3 X 50 ml of ether. The combined ether extract was washed with sodium carbonate solution till neutral and then again with 2 X 50 ml ammonium chloride solution. It was then dried over sodium sulphate and the solvent removed to get 23 g of crude geranonitrile. This was then distilled in vacuum to get 15 g of the pure nitrile (yield 70%). Boiling point 85°C (3 mm) ir ν_{max} 2950, 2250, 1630 cm^{-1}.

8-Oxo 2,6,octadinenitrile 3,7 dimethyl (VI)

2,6-Octadiene nitrile 3,7-dimethyl (geranonitrile, 14.5 g) and selenium dioxide (15 g) were taken in 100 ml dimethyl sulphoxide and the reaction mixture heated on a water-bath for 1.5 h and then left overnight. Afterwards the reaction mixture was filtered to remove the precipitated selenium (6.5 g). The precipitated selenium was washed with ether and water and the filtrate diluted with 300 ml water. It was then extracted with 3 X 100 ml ether and the combined ether extract washed with 2 X 100 ml saturated sodium bicarbonate solution and 2 X 100 ml saturated ammonium chloride solution. It was dried over anhydrous sodium sulphate and the solvent removed to get 14 g crude material. This was then subjected to short path distillation and the material coming out at 162°C (3 mm) was collected (8 g).

This was converted into the semicarbazone by mixing with a solution of 6 g of semicarbazide hydrochloride and 9 g of sodium acetate in 15 ml water and 10 ml methanol. About 150 ml of water was added when all the semicarbazone had precipitated out and the mixture was filtered to get 9 g of the semicarbazone of 8-oxo-2,6-octadiene nitrile 3,7-dimethyl (yield 41%) m.p. 198°C (found C–60.12; H–7.15; N–25.31; $C_{11}H_{16}N_4O$ requires C–59.98; H–7.32 and N–25.44%).

9 g of semicarbazone, 150 ml benzene and 500 ml 25% oxalic acid were mixed together and the mixture refluxed with stirring for 3 h. The benzene and the aqueous layer were separated and the aqueous layer extracted with 3 X 100 ml ether. The combined benzene and the ether layer was washed with saturated sodium bicarbonate solution till neutral and then with 2 X 100 ml of saturated ammonium chloride solution. It was then dried over sodium sulphate and the solvent removed to get 7 g of the crude aldehyde. This was sublimed (162°C; 3 mm) to get 5.6 g of the required aldehyde (yield – 84%) i.r. ν_{max} 2950, 2800, 2250, 1680 and 1630 cm^{-1} PMR ($CDCl_3$); δ 1.8 (*s*, 3H, C_7-methyl) 2.6 (*m*, 4H, methylenes) 5.2 (*s*, 1H, C–2 vinyl) 6.4 (*m*, 1H, C–6 vinyl) 9.4 (*s*, 1H, aldehyde proton).

8-Oxo 2,4,6-octatriene nitrile 3,7-dimethyl (VII)

3.2 g 8-oxo-2,6-octadienenitrile 3,7-dimethyl 1.6 g calcium oxide, 2.0 g sodium bicarbonate and 2.6 g of N-bromosuccinimide were taken in 25 ml CCl_4 and the mixture refluxed for 1 h. It was then filtered and the filtrate added drop by drop to 6 g of 1,8-diazabicyclo (5.4.0) undec-7-ene with stirring and under an atmosphere of nitrogen. After the addition was complete the resulting mixture was refluxed for 15 min. It was then poured into 50 ml 1N sulphuric acid and ice. The mixture was then extracted with 3 X 100 ml ether; the ether solution washed with 2 X 100 ml water and dried over sodium sulphate and the solvent removed to get 2.5 g of crude material. This was purified by chromatography (neutral alumina, eluted with 50:50 mixture of benzene and hexane) and crystallised to get 650 mg of all-*trans* triene aldehyde nitrile (yield – 20.3%).

λ_{max} (ethanol) 329 nm (ϵ – 48,000) and – 315 mm (ϵ – 40,000)

PMR ($CDCl_3$) [(δ 1.9 (*s*, 3H, C_7 methyl)], 2.25 (*s*, 3H, C_3 methyl), 5.5 (*s*, 1H, C_2 vinyl), 6.5–7 (m, 3H, vinyl protons) 9.5 (*s*, 1H, aldehyde proton) (found C–74.44; H–6.82; N–8.36%; $C_{10}H_{11}NO$ requires C–74.51; H–6.88; N–8.69%).

All-trans *Retinonitrile (VIII)*

280 mg of 8-oxo-2,4,6-octatrienenitrile 3,7-dimethyl, 1.2 g of β-cyclogeranyl triphenyl phosphonium bromide and 1.4 ml of 50% sodium hydroxide were stirred in 25 ml methylene chloride for 24 h in an atmosphere of nitrogen. The reaction mixture was then poured into 100 ml water and extracted with 3 X 75 ml ether. The ether solution was washed with 3 X 75 ml saturated ammonium chloride solution. The ether was removed and the residue was purified by preparative tlc (silica gel, solvent benzene) to get 120 mg of *all-trans* retinonitrile (yield – 24.5%).

i.r. ν_{max} 2920, 2210, 1580 and 965 cm^{-1}

UV λ_{max} (ethanol) 365 nm (ϵ, 43,400)

Reported λ_{max} –360 nm (ϵ, 47,000)

PMR ($CDCl_3$) δ 0 (*S*, 6H, gem dimethyl) 1.0–1.5 (*m*, 4H, methylenes), 1.7 (*s*, 3H, C_5-methyl), 2 (*s*, 3H, 3H, C_9 methyl) 2.02 (*m*, 2H, allylic methylene) 2.2 (*s*, 3H, C_{13} methyl), 5.1 (*s*, 1H, C_{14} vinyl), 6.2 (*m*, 4H, vinylic protons), 6.8 (*m*, 1H, vinylic proton).

2,6-Octadienoic acid 3,7-dimethyl ethyl ester (IX)

2,6 Octadienenitrile 3,7 dimethyl (40 g) and 400 ml 30% ethanolic potassium hydroxide were refluxed for 48 h; then neutralised with dilute hydrochloric acid and the acid extracted with ether.

The crude acid (16 g) was refluxed with 100 ml ethyl alcohol and 1 ml of concentrated sulphuric acid for 24 h; then poured into 200 ml water neutralised with sodium bicarbonate and extracted with 3 × 100 ml ether. The ether solution was washed with 3 × 100 ml saturated sodium bicarbonate solution followed by 2 × 100 ml saturated ammonium chloride solution. It was dried over sodium sulphate and the solvent removed and the residue distilled in vacuum to get 12 g of ethyl ester of 2,6-octadienoic acid 3,7-dimethyl (yield 23%).

Boiling point 120°C/3 mm

i.r. ν_{max} 2980, 1750, 1630 cm^{-1}

Ethyl 3,7-dimethyl 8-oxo-2,6-octadienoate (X)

Ethyl 3,7-dimethyl 2,6-octadienoate (10 g) was oxidised with selenium dioxide (7 g) by the usual procedure to get 2.3 g ethyl 3,7-dimethyl 8-oxo 2,6-octdienoate (yield 22.9%).

i.r. ν_{max} 2980, 1750, 1680, 1630 cm^{-1}

PMR ($CDCl_3$), δ 1.2 (*t,* 3H, ester methyl), 1.7 (*s,* 3H, 7 methyl), 2.15 (*s,* 3H, 3 methyl), 2.4 (*m,* 4H, allylic methylenes), 4.2 (*q,* 2H, ester methylene), 5.7 (*s,* 1H, 2 vinyl), 6.4 (*m,* 1H, 6 vinyl), 9.3 (*s,* 1H, aldehyde). m.p. of the semicarbozone 190°C. Analysis values for semicarbazone (found C–58.41, H–7.50 and N–16.01. $C_{13}H_{22}N_3O_3$ requires C–58.82, H–7.92, N–15.72).

Ethyl 3,7-dimethyl-8-oxo 2,4,6-octatrienoate (XI)

2 g of the preceding aldehyde was refluxed in 25 ml CCl_4, with 2 g NBS and 1 g sodium bicarbonate and 600 mg calcium oxide, for 1 h. The solution was filtered and the filtrate added drop by drop to 3 g DBU. It was then refluxed for 15 min and worked up as described previously to get 1.6 g crude material which on chromatographic purification gave 360 mg ethyl 3,7-dimethyl 8-oxo-2,4,6-octa trienoate (yield 18%). This after two recrystallizations melted at 78°C, which is identical with that reported in literature.

λ_{max} –325 nm ε–44,300

PMR ($CDCl_3$) δ 1.3 (*t*, 3H, ester methyl) 1.95 (*s*, 3H, C_7 methyl) 2.4 (*s*, 3H, C_3 methyl), 4.25 (q, 2H, ester methylene), 6.05 (*s*, 1H, 2 vinyl) 6.6–7.4 (*m*, 3H, vinyl protons), 9.6 (*s*, 1H, aldehyde).

Ethyl Retinoate (XII)

Ethyl 3,7-dimethyl-8-oxo 2,4,6-octatrienoate (100 mg) and cyclogeranyl triphenyl phosphonium bromide (315 mg) and 0.35 ml of 50% sodium hydroxide were stirred in 10 ml methylene chloride for 24 h. It was then poured into 100 ml water extracted 3 × 50 ml ether and ether solution washed with 3 × 50 ml saturated ammonium sulphate solution and dried over sodium sulphate and the solvent removed and the residue purified by chromatography to get 10 mg ethyl retinoate (yield 6.8%).

λ_{max} 348 nm Reported λ_{max} 349 nm

ϵ – 38,500 ϵ – 40,000

PMR ($CDCl_3$), δ 1 (*s*, 6H gem dimethyl), 1.3 (*t*, 3H, ester methyl), 1.55 (*m*, 4H, methylenes), 1.7 (*s*, 3H, C_5 methyl), 2 (*s*, 3H, C_9 methyl) 2.02 (*m*, 2H, allylic methylene), 2.35 (*s*, 3H, C_{13} methyl), 4.25 (q 2H, ester methylene), 5.8 (*s*, 1H, C_{14} vinyl), 6.2 (*m*, 4H, vinyl protons) 6.9 (*m*, 1H, vinyl).

Note

Melting points are uncorrected. UV spectra were determined in ethanol solution using a Unicam SP 700 spectrophotometer; i.r. spectra were determined in nujol or neat with a perkin-elmer infracord or a model 257 spectrometer; PMR spectra were recorded in $CDCl_3$ using tetramethylsilane as an internal standard using a varian associates model HA-100D spectrometer.

References

1 *Henbest, H.B.; Jones, E.R.H., and Owen, T.C.:* J. Chem. Soc. 2765 (1965).
2 *Olson, G.L.; Cheung, H.C.; Morgon, K.D.; Rene Borer, and Saucy, G.:* Helv. chim. Acta *59 (2):* 567 (1976).
3 *Schwieter, U. and Isler, O.:* In *Sebrell and Harris* The vitamins, chemistry physiology, pathology, methods; vol. I, p. 30 (Academic Press, 1967).
4 *Uday, T.; Bhale Rao, and Rapoport, H.:* J. Am. chem. Soc. *93:* 4835 (1971).

Dr. *M.V. Bhatt,* Department of Organic Chemistry, Indian Institute of Science, *Bangalore 560012* (India)

Wld Rev. Nutr. Diet., vol. 31, pp. 149–153 (Karger, Basel 1978)

Regulation of Carotenogenesis in *Blakeslea trispora*[1]

Satya Rao and V. V. Modi

Department of Microbiology, Faculty of Science, MS University of Baroda, Baroda

When plus and minus cultures of *Blakeslea trispora* are grown together, β-carotene production is enhanced by 15–20 fold. This increase is attributed to the formation of a sexual hormone called trisporic acid (TA) (12). TA regulates sexual reproduction in heterothallic mucorales (13) and conspicuously activates carotenogenesis in minus *B. trispora* but to a limited extent in the plus strain (3). *Thomas et al.* (11) have demonstrated that TA acts as a depressor of an enzyme (enzymes) in carotene pathway which is normally rate limiting. But the exact role of TA in the regulation has not been established so far.

Our main aim was to elucidate the regulation of carotene production in *B. trispora.* TA stimulates isoprenoid synthesis by derepressing the enzyme or enzymes involved in the conversion of 5-phosphomevalonate to dimethyl allyl pyrophosphate (9). Carotene pathway is repressed in single cultures. When these cultures are mated, formation of TA causes derepression resulting in a high yield of β-carotene. Attempts have been made to isolate some proteins from (+) and (–) cultures which are inhibitory to carotene synthesis and to study the significance of their presence in the mold.

The plus (NRRL 2895) and minus (NRRL 2896) strains of *B. trispora* obtained from US Department of Agriculture, Peoria, Illinois, were maintained as described by *Hesseltine and Anderson* (5) and grown in synthetic mucor medium.

Carotenoids were estimated from the wet mycelia. Mycelia were ground and carotenes were obtained in acetone:ether (1:1) mixture. Acetone was removed by washing the mixture with cold distilled water and drying over anhydrous sodium sulphate. β-Carotene was estimated by using $E_{1\,cm}^{1\,\%}$ value of 2500 at 450 nm as described by *Davies* (4).

[1] This investigation was supported by a Am-PL-480/FG-In-509 grant from the Agricultural Research Service of the USDA.

TA was extracted from potato glucose thiamine medium of 5 day-old mated cultures according to the method described by *Sutter* (10). The final TA extract was obtained in 0.1 *M* Tris-sulphate buffer, pH 7.5 and estimated by using $E_{1\ cm}^{1\ \%}$ value of 700 at 325 nm. TA extract was filter sterilised and used for the experiments.

Inhibitory proteins were isolated from cell-free extracts of single cultures and characterised by bioassay. Frozen mycelia of 4 day old single cultures were treated with chilled acetone below $-10°C$ to remove lipids. After removal of acetone, mycelia was homogenised. Cell-free extracts were obtained in 0.1 *M* Tris-HCl buffer (pH 7.5) and centrifuged at 15,000 *g* for 30 min. The supernatant was brought to 0–60, 60–80 and 80–100% saturation with solid ammonium sulphate. Precipitates, thus obtained, were dissolved in the buffer, dialysed and sterilised with (0.45 u) membrane filters. For obtaining proteins from mated cultures, cell-free extracts of mated cultures were subjected to ammonium sulphate fractionation. These proteins were estimated by biological assay. Minus cultures were grown in 50 ml of synthetic mucor medium in 250 ml Erlenmeyer flasks for 48 h. Protein fractions were added to this test system in sterile condition and incubated for 48 h further at 28°C. Carotene was estimated. Decrease of 10 μg of β-carotene/g dry wt compared to the control was taken as one unit of inhibitory protein (IP).

Inhibitory proteins were purified on Sephadex G-100 column (43.5 × 1.5) cm. Proteins were eluted with 0.05 *M* Tris-HCl buffer, pH 7.5 and 5 ml of fractions were collected. Protein from the inhibitory and stimulatory fractions were estimated by the method of *Lowry et al.* (7).

Cell-free extracts of (+) culture were subjected to $(NH_4)_2SO_4$ fractionation. When different fractions (0–60, 60–80 and 80–100%) were tested, only the 0–60% fraction was found to contain the carotene inhibitory activity. 30% Reduction in carotene formation was observed. The 0–60% fraction showed 9.8 units/mg protein of inhibitory activity. Addition of IP did not affect mycelial growth which excludes the possibility of its being some sort of metabolic inhibitor. In similar experiments with (–) culture, carotene production was inhibited by 35% on addition of 0–60% $(NH_4)_2SO_4$ precipitates. This fraction contained 12.2 units/mg protein of inhibitory activity. Results showed that single culture (+) and (–) contained some protein which was inhibitory to carotene production. In both the cultures, IP was precipitated in 0–60% $(NH_4)_2SO_4$ fraction indicating similarity between these proteins.

Inhibitory protein fraction was subjected to Sephadex G-100 column chromatography (43.5 × 1.5 cm). Fractions collected were sterilised by membrane filtration and 2 ml of each were added to the test system. Inhibition of carotene production was observed only in the case of 53rd fraction (fig. 1). Addition of all the other fractions from the column affected neither growth nor carotene synthesis. About 53% inhibition of carotene synthesis was observed.

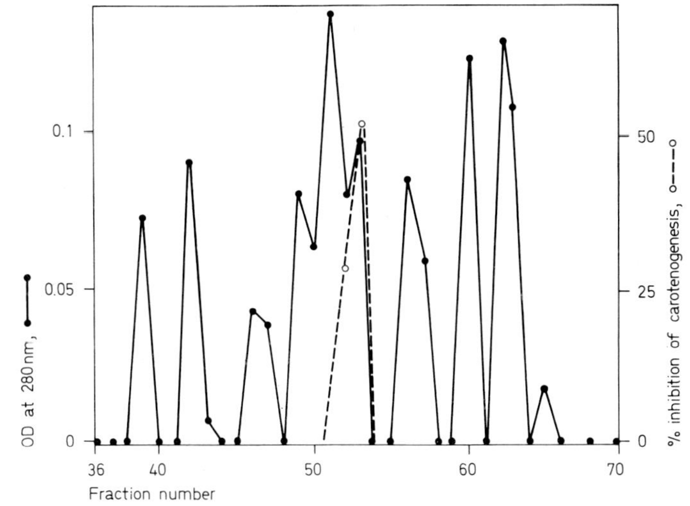

Fig. 1. Purification profile of IP on Sephadex G-100 column (43.5 × 1.5 cm).

When increasing concentrations of the purified IP fraction were added in the test system, a linear decrease in carotene synthesis was observed. About 43% inhibition of carotene production was observed on addition of 0.4 mg protein indicating the high sensitivity of carotene synthesizing system to the IP.

An attempt was also made to determine the molecular weight of IP by gel filtration (fig. 2). Data shows that the inhibitory protein has a mol wt of about 47,000. The inhibitory protein lost its inhibitory activity on the treatment with trypsin. It was inactivated when subjected to 50°C for 5 min showing that it is a heat-labile and trypsin-sensitive protein.

From the above data we could conclude that a protein inhibitory to carotene synthesis is present in single cultures of *B. trispora.* It was of interest to see what happened to the IP in the mold on treatment with TA. A 72 h old (–) culture was treated with TA for 6 and 24 h, and the IP was isolated to check its activity. Data in table I shows that (–) culture without TA treatment showed 10.58 units of IP activity but when the cultures were treated with TA for 6 h, 50% of IP activity was lost. After 24 h of TA treatment, IP was almost inactivated. Results suggest that TA was responsible for the inactivation of IP in (–) cultures.

Mated cultures consist of (+) and (–) strains together. Both the cultures contain the IP which inhibit carotenogenic pathway. TA is formed in the mated cultures which might be acting on the IP of single cultures. Cell-free extracts of mated cultures were fractionated with ammonium sulphate and were added to the testing system. It was surprising to note that there was the total absence of

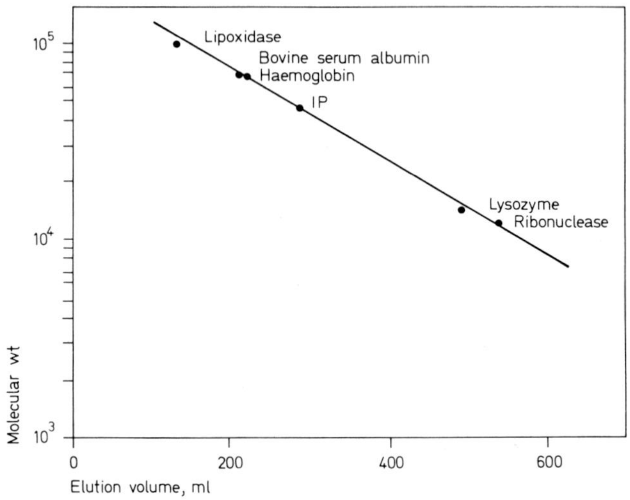

Fig. 2. Determination of Mol wt of IP fractions from *B. trispora* (–).

Table I. Effect of trisporic acid supplementation on IP fractions in *B. trispora*

Sources of IP fraction added	Carotene µg/g	Activity of IP	
		units	units/mg protein
Control	183	–	–
(–) Cultures before TA addition	128	5.5	10.58
(–) Cultures after 6 h of TA addition	139	4.4	5.95
(–) Cultures after 24 h of TA addition	175	0.8	0.73

TA (14 µg%) was added to 72 h old cultures of *B. trispora* (–) and the cultures were harvested after 6 and 24 h of incubation period for the isolation of IP fractions.

the IP in mated cultures. Instead, some proteins were isolated in 40–80% ammonium sulphate fraction which were of stimulatory nature. Addition of these proteins resulted in almost 53% stimulation of carotenogenesis compared to the control. These stimulatory proteins (SP) were isolated only from mated culture cell-free extracts. They were trypsin sensitive.

Stimulation of carotene synthesis increased with increasing concentrations of SP added (fig. 3). But a saturation level was reached after the addition of 1.8 mg protein. (+) and (–) cultures produce less carotene, but on mating, there is a rise in carotene production by 10–15 fold, which has been attributed to the formation of TA. TA is not formed in single cultures. Biosynthetic pathways of TA and β-carotene are repressed in the single cultures. When they are mated, both the pathways are derepressed. β-Carotene is the precursor of TA (2); so it is

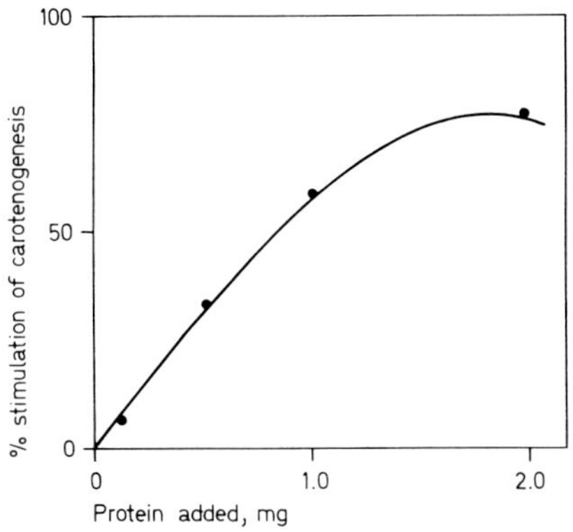

Fig. 3. Effect of SP fraction from mated cultures on carotenogenesis on *B. trispora* (—).

likely that the control of these pathways is interrelated. Presence of a repressor regulating carotene synthesis has been hypothesized, but so far no conclusive data has been obtained regarding the repressor control.

We propose that the presence of the IP in single cultures results in the repression of carotene pathway. When TA is available to the culture, it inactivates the IP along with the activation of stimulatory proteins resulting in the stimulation of carotenogenesis.

References

1 *Anderson, R.F.; Arnold, M.; Nelson, G.E.N., and Ciegler, A.:* Agricultural & Food Chemistry *6:* 543 (1958).
2 *Austin, D.J., Bu'Lock, J.D., and Goodday, G.W.:* Nature *223:* 1178 (1969).
3 *Cagliotti, L.; Cainelli, G.; Camerino, G.; Mondelli, R.; Prieto, A.; Quilico, A.; Salvalori, T., and Selva, A.:* Chem. Ind. (Milan) *46:* 1 (1964).
4 *Davies, B.H.:* Analysis of carotenoid pigments; in *Goodwin* Chemistry & biochemistry of plant pigments, pp. 489–532 (A.P., London 1965).
5 *Hesseltine, C.W. and Anderson, R.F.:* Mycologia *49:* 449 (1957).
6 *Hesseltine, C.W.:* US Dept. Agr. Tech. Null. *1245:* 33 (1961).
7 *Lowry, O.H.; Rosenbrough, N.J.; Farr, A.L., and Randall, R.J.:* J. biol. Chem. *193:* 265 (1951).
8 *Murillo, F.J. and Corda-Olmedo, E.:* Xth IEBS Meeting, Paris, July 1975.
9 *Satya Rao and Modi, V.V.:* Experientia *33:* 31 (1977).
10 *Sutter, R.P.:* Science N.Y. *168:* 1590 (1970).
11 *Thomas, D.M.; Harris, R.C.; Kirk, J.T.O., and Goodwin, T.W.:* Phytochemistry *6:* 361 (1967).
12 *Van den Ende, H.:* Nature *215:* 211 (1967).
13 *Van den Ende, H. and Stegwee, D.:* Bot. Rev. *37:* 22 (1971).

Dr. *S. Rao,* Department of Microbiology, Faculty of Science, MS University of Baroda, *Baroda 390 002* (India)

Wld Rev. Nutr. Diet., vol. 31, pp. 154–158 (Karger, Basel 1978)

Carotenoids in Fruits and Flowers

Pro-Vitamin A-Rich Tomatoes

B.R. Premachandra, V.N. Vasantharajan and H.R. Cama*

Department of Biochemistry, Indian Institute of Science, Bangalore, and
*Microbiology & Cell Biology Laboratories, Indian Institute of Science, Bangalore

Carotenoids play a vital role in human as well as animal nutrition as those with the right structure and configuration give rise, on consumption, to vitamin A in the body.

Detailed investigations on the carotenoid composition of several fruits and flowers for their pro-vitamin A content have been carried out in our laboratory for some years (1, 2, 3, 6, 7, 8, 9). Among the various flower petals analysed, those of GulMohr *(Delonix regia)* were found to be very rich in β-carotene (2). Among the thirty different carotenoids identified in these flower petals, about 35% of the total carotenoid content was found to be β-carotene. This observation prompted us to employ them as an economical substitute for the rather costly, synthetic vitamin A which is normally supplemented in the poultry feed.

Dried, dehydrated GulMohr petal powder was supplemented in the poultry feed at 1,5 and 10% (by wt) over 8 weeks in laying hens. The appearance, vitamin A, and carotene contents of the egg yolk of 10 birds placed in each group are in table I. As is evident from the data, supplementation at 5 and 10% levels could significantly improve the colour and quality of the yolk. For all practical purposes it is recommended that synthetic vitamin A in the poultry feed could be substituted by 5% (by wt) of dried dehydrated GulMohr flower petal powder.

Mangoes, papaya and oranges are the most commonly cultivated fruit in the country. The carotenoid composition of these fruit suggested that they serve as a good source of the pro-vitamins A, namely, β-carotene and cryptoxanthin (1, 3, 8,9). These fruits, however, are beyond the common man's economy for daily consumption.

Vitamin A deficiency is widely prevalent (with 15,000–20,000 people going permanently blind in India every year); a cheaper and easily available pro-vitamin A-rich source is always welcome in a country like ours where the majority of people are vegetarians. This directed our attention to tomatoes, a widely

Table I. The effect of supplementation of dehydrated GulMohr flower petals in the poultry feed on carotenoid composition, vitamin A content and quality of egg-yolk

Diet composition	Colour of egg-yolk	β-Carotene, μg/g	Xanthophyll	Vitamin A, IU/g
White maize (synth. Vitamin A)	white	traces	traces	5.0
Yellow maize (synth. Vitamin A)	pale	traces	18.0	6.3
Yellow maize + 1% petals	bright yellow	2.0	19.2	11.3
Yellow maize + 5% petals	orange	6.3	23.6	12.6
Yellow maize + 10% petals	deep orange red	13.5	36.0	14.0

10 birds have been placed in each group on the various diet compositions indicated in the first column. The figures represent the mean values obtained for the group.

cultivated and consumed crop in our country. They are unique in that they can serve both as vegetable and fruit.

Commonly cultivated, 38 different varieties of tomatoes were analysed for their carotenoid composition (7). The analysis revealed that β-carotene is present in very small amounts constituting only about 5% (1–5 μg/g fresh wt) whereas the bulk of the pigment is accounted for by lycopene, which is not a precursor of vitamin A. It would be of immense nutritive value if the red pigment lycopene in the tomatoes is replaced by β-carotene. During the course of their classical work aimed at the study of carotenoid biosynthesis in tomatoes, *Lincoln and Porter* (5), and *Tomes et al.* (11) had shown that mutants with high amounts of β-carotene in their fruit could be developed. We obtained samples of seeds of such 'High-β' tomatoes from the US, UK and Poland to assess how they propagate under our climatic conditions. The carotene compositions of these alien strains are compared with that of the local variety 'Pusa Ruby' (table II).

In the local Pusa Ruby, the bulk of the pigment is accounted for by lycopene whereas in OF(US) and 'H-β' Poland, β-carotene is found in large amounts. In ORF(US) and Int.β(UK), intermediate amounts of β-carotene and lycopene were realised. Even though all the alien strains were rich in β-carotene, yet they were all poorly pigmented (ranging from pale yellow to orange in colour) due to lack of sufficient lycopene and lower total carotene contents. Hence, it was decided to cross them with the local Pusa Ruby in order to develop a new hybrid

Table II. Carotene composition: parent strains and their F_1 hybrids (μg/g fresh wt)

Strain/cross	β-Carotene	Lycopene
Pusa Ruby (Local)	4.5 (4.7)	90.5 (94.2)
Orange flesh (USA)	25.9 (82.1)	3.7 (11.1)
Orange red flesh (USA)	24.2 (58.6)	16.1 (36.3)
Intermediate-β (UK)	28.9 (56.8)	19.6 (38.5)
Pol-H-β (Poland)	25.4 (61.3)	14.3 (32.9)
Pusa x OF (USA)	25.1 (40.4)	34.5 (53.5)
OF (USA) x Pusa	25.7 (42.1)	33.1 (52.0)
Pusa x Pol-H-β (Poland)	28.4 (41.3)	37.1 (53.6)
Pol-H-β (Poland) x Pusa	28.0 (40.3)	39.0 (54.2)
Pusa x ORF (USA)	22.8 (32.0)	45.9 (63.9)
ORF (USA) x Pusa	23.4 (36.1)	40.4 (58.6)
Pusa x Int-β (UK)	21.1 (36.0)	37.9 (59.3)
Int-β (UK) x Pusa	20.1 (35.0)	35.8 (60.8)

Figures in parentheses are % of total carotenes (β-carotene + γ-carotene + lycopene).

with adequate amount of β-carotene for nutrition and sufficient amount of lycopene for the colour appeal, as well as to study their genetic make up.

All possible twentyfive different types of matings were made among the strains given in table II. Carotene composition of the off-spring of only eight select matings is quoted in the above table. It can be observed from this table that intermediate levels of β-carotene and lycopene were observed among all the F_1-hybrids. It should also be noted that lycopene is present in slightly predominent amounts in the F_1-hybrids of (PUSA × ORF) and (PUSA × Int.β) compared with (PUSA × OF) and (PUSA × Pol). A daily intake of 50–100 g (1–2 fruits) of such hybrids would adequately meet the requirements of vitamin A. These hybrids ranged in color from deep orange-red to red-orange hue that might better promote their market acceptibility. Apart from these eight crosses, the progenies of the inbred parent strains indicated that they breed true to their carotenoid composition presented in table II. The study of the progenies of the remaining twelve matings made among the alien 'High-β' strains showed that they yielded fruits ranging from orange to orange-red in colour with intermediate levels of β-carotene and lycopene as given in table II. Since progenies of reciprocal matings have yielded similar results, any cytoplasmic factor or maternal inheritance involved in carotene biosynthesis can be ruled out.

The progenies of four crosses, namely (PUSA × OF)F_1, (OF × PUSA)F_1, (PUSA × Pol)F_1 and (Pol × PUSA)F_1 were studied for segregation in F_2 generation. The data for (PUSA × OF)F_1 and (OF × PUSA)F_1, F_2 segregates are given in table III. The F_2 population was classified into Reds (that resembled Pusa

Table III. Carotene composition of tomatoes of F_2 generation ($\mu g/g$ fresh wt)

Type	Pusa x OF (USA)				OF (USA) x Pusa			
	β-carotene		lycopene		β-carotene		lycopene	
Reds	5.2	(6.3)	80.1	(92.6)	7.2	(9.4)	72.4	(89.0)
Red Oranges	29.0	(33.5)	54.5	(62.5)	31.6	(37.7)	50.3	(58.6)
Orange Reds	25.9	(50.6)	22.0	(44.1)	23.4	(46.9)	24.8	(48.7)
Oranges	37.9	(78.2)	7.0	(13.9)	40.9	(77.1)	8.7	(16.7)
Entire 'High-β'	30.9	(54.1)	27.8	(40.1)	31.9	(53.9)	27.9	(41.3)

Values in parentheses are % of total carotenes (β-carotene + γ-carotene + lycopene).

Ruby), Red Oranges (those with 25 μg β-carotene and about 45% of total carotene content as lycopene), Oranges (those with 75% and above of total carotene content as β-carotene) and the rest as Orange Reds (with intermediate levels of β-carotene and lycopene). The Red Oranges constitute the 'hybrids of choice' with adequate amounts of β-carotene for nutrition and sufficient amount of lycopene for its attractive red orange colour. As is evident from table III, the reciprocal matings have yielded similar results, even among their F_2 segregates, again indicating the nuclear origin of the genes responsible for carotene biosynthesis. Since the original parent selection of Pol-H-β had significantly higher lycopene content (35% of total carotene content) compared to OF selection (about 10% of total carotene content), the identical results obtained in case of (PUSA X Pol) and (PUSA X OF) matings both at F_1 and F_2 were attributed to the independent segregation of the modifier locus of gene B.

Finally, it was necessary to confirm by bioassay trials the pro-vitamin A potency of the pigment identified as β-carotene in these genetic mutants, since the chances of other carotenoids with the same adsorption and absorption characteristics (but biologically inactive) must be ruled out. The liver storages of vitamin A in vitamin A-deficient rats fed on 'High-β' hybrids were nearly four times compared with the Pusa Ruby-fed ones. Further, it was also evident from these experiments that the presence of lycopene does not affect the intestinal conversion of β-carotene to vitamin A.

Thus, a tomato strain, like the Red Orange phenotype described in the above studies, with adequate amounts of β-carotene for nutrition and sufficient amounts of lycopene for colour appeal, would form an ideal fruit and vegetable source of vitamin A. In view of the extensive vitamin A deficiency in our country, introduction of such a novel strain of tomatoes to the market would form one of the vital measures to tackle the problem of vitamin A deficiency.

Acknowledgements

The authors thank Prof. T.W. Goodwin, FRS, CBS, Liverpool, UK, Prof. *J.W. Porter,* Madison, USA, and Prof. Stan Berger, Poland, for their generous gifts of the samples of seeds of 'High-β' strains of tomatoes. The technical assistance rendered by Miss R.V. Jayamma is gratefully acknowledged.

References

1 *Jacob, John; Subbarayan, C., and Cama, H.R.:* J. Fed. Sci. *35:* 262 (1970).
2 *Jungalwala, F.B. and Cama, H.R.:* Biochem. J. *85:* 1 (1962).
3 *Jungalwala, F.B. and Cama, H.R.:* Indian J. Biochem. *1:* 36 (1963).
4 *Kargle, T.E.; Quackenbush, F.W., and Tomes, M.L.:* Proc. Am. Soc. Hort. Sci. *75:* 574 (1960).
5 *Lincoln, R.E. and Porter, J.W.:* Genetics N.Y. *35:* 206 (1950).
6 *Premachandra, B.R.; Jacob John, and Cama, H.R.:* Indian J. Nutr. Dietet. *11:* 28 (1974).
7 *Premachandra, B.R.; Vasantharajan, V.N., and Cama, H.R.:* Curr. Sci. *45:* 56 (1976).
8 *Subbarayan, C. and Cama, H.R.:* Indian J. Chem. *2:* 451 (1964).
9 *Subbarayan, C. and Cama, H.R.:* Indian J. Chem. *3:* 463 (1965).
10 *Subbarayan, C.; Jungalwala, F.B., and Cama, H.R.:* Ann. Biochem. *12:* 275 (1965).
11 *Tomes, M.L.; Quackenbush, F.W., and Kargle, T.E.:* Botanical Gaz. *119:* 250 (1958).

Dr. *B.R. Premachandra,* Department of Biochemistry, Indian Institute of Science, *Bangalore 560 012* (India)

Wld Rev. Nutr. Diet., vol. 31, pp. 159–161 (Karger, Basel 1978)

Biological Utilization of β-Carotene from Amaranth and Leaf Protein in Preschool Children

Rajammal P. Devadas and Nirmala K. Murthy
Sri Avinashilingam Home Science College for Women, Coimbatore

It is one of those anomalies of nature and man that the countries with the highest rates of xerophthalmia are among the perennially greenest of the world, but the nutritious green leaves do not find their way into the mouth of the small child (3). If only they had had enough of vitamin A or its precursor, β-carotene, in their food, this tragedy could have been averted.

Foods containing preformed vitamin A are expensive and beyond the reach of the poor (6). Hence, carotene derived from plant foods needs to be the chief source of vitamin A (2, 5). These carotenes are not fully absorbed by human subjects and the absorption has been found to vary over a wide range. However, studies relating to the utilization of carotenes from different vegetable food stuffs by Indian children who are sub-clinically malnourished are limited. This study was designed to estimate the biological utilization of β-carotene, from two rich sources, in preschool children: namely, amaranth and leaf protein as compared with standard β-carotene.

The study was conducted on 15 preschool children of 3–5 years of age selected from Sri Avinashilingam Balwadi (Preschool). The study consisted of four phases. As a preliminary step, a food weighment survey was done to formulate the Balwadi supplement for the children. In order to formulate the dietary supplement, the β-carotene content of amaranth and leaf protein were analysed. During the first phase, the Balwadi supplement alone was given to the children along with their home diet for a period of one month. This period was considered as the basal period of the study. During the second, third and fourth phases, each of one month's duration, three different sources of β-carotene, namely, 40 g of amaranth, 8 g of leaf protein and 1 ml of standard β-carotene solution, respectively, were given to the children. These amounts carried 1200 μg of β-carotene. During the terminal three days of each phase, faeces were collected to estimate the excretion of β-carotene, and hence the utilization from the three sources.

Table I. Comparison of percentage utilization of β-carotene from three different sources in 15 children

Source of β-carotene	Percentage of β-carotene utilized		
	mean	range	SD
Amaranth	61.4	41.2–78.3	± 9.35
Leaf protein	76.7	58.3–90.0	± 7.48
Standard β-carotene	85.4	82.1–90.5	± 6.143

Table II. Mean serum vitamin A levels of the 15 children before and after supplementation of 1200 μg of β-carotene for a period of 3 months

Dietary intake of β-carotene	Serum vitamin A level, μg/100 ml
272 μg	20.5 ± 4.39
1200 μg (from leaf protein)	29.2 ± 2.09

Table III. Mean serum protein and albumin levels of the children before and after the 3 month study period

Dietary intake of protein, g	Total serum protein, g/100 ml	Albumin level g/100 ml
Before 20	5.9 ± 1.4	3.2 ± 1.7
After 35	6.7 ± 0.68	3.5 ± 0.35

The initial and final levels of serum vitamin A, total serum proteins, albumins, globulins and blood haemoglobin, which were analysed, served as indices of evaluation.

The mean β-carotene content of amaranth was 3000 μg/100 g, and that of leaf protein was 14,000 μg/100 g. About 20–25% of β-carotene was lost from amaranth, and about 10% was lost from leaf protein, during cooking.

During the terminal days of the first phase, faeces were collected and analysed. The mean excretion of β-carotene during the basal period was 23.2 ± 13.6 μg/ /day. During the subsequent phases, the amount of β-carotene excreted was determined. The mean value of β-carotene excreted in the basal period was subtracted from the amount of β-carotene excreted in faeces after feeding the different sources of β-carotene (7). The utilization of β-carotene was determined by determining the difference between the intake and excretion. The percentage utilization of β-carotene from various sources of β-carotene are presented in table I.

When the Balwadi diet was supplemented with amaranth 40 g/day/child, supplying about 1200 μg of β-carotene, the absorption of β-carotene was 61.4%.

When amaranth was substituted by 8 g of leaf protein supplying an equivalent amount of 1200 μg of β-carotene/day/child, the β-carotene absorption was 76.7%. This increase in absorption of β-carotene from leaf protein was significantly higher than that from amaranth.

When the leaf protein was substituted by 1 ml standard β-carotene solution providing 1200 μg of β-carotene/day/child, the absorption was 85.4%. The absorption of standard β-carotene was significantly higher than that from amaranth or leaf protein.

The mean serum vitamin A values of the children before and after the three month study are given in table II.

The result showed that there was a significant increase in serum vitamin A levels after feeding the different sources of β-carotene. A similar observation has been reported by *Pereira and Begum* (4) and by *Vinodini and Lala* (7).

The mean total protein and albumin levels of the children before and after supplementation are given in table III.

Statistical analysis was done for estimating the correlation between plasma levels of vitamin A and proteins among the children. Vitamin A and albumin showed a significant positive correlation at the 0.1% level of significance. On the other hand, there was no significant correlation between vitamin A and globulin.

The children also showed an increment in the haemoglobin levels from 8.4 ± 1.4–12 ± 0.9 g/100 ml which was considered to be due to the increase in intake of iron, folic acid and other nutrients provided by the supplements.

References

1 *Devadas, R.P.; Joseph, A.; Murthy, N.K., and Saroja, S.:* Indian J. Nutr. & Dietet. *10:* 65 (1972).
2 *Devadas, R.P. and Murthy, N.K.:* X Internat. Congr. Nutr., Kyoto, Japan. Symposia and free communication, p. 114 (1975).
3 *Oomen, H.A.P.C.:* Nutr. Rev. *32:* 161 (1974).
4 *Pereira, S.H. and Begum, A.:* Indian J. Med. Res. *56:* 362 (1968).
5 *Rao, N.C. and Rao, N.B.S.:* Absorption of dietary carotenes in human subjects. Am. J. clin. Nutr. *23:* 105–109 (1970).
6 *Srikantia, S.G.:* Wld. rev. nutr. diet., vol. 20, p. 184 (Karger, Basel 1975).
7 *Vinodini, R. and Lala, V.R.:* Am. J. clin. Nutr. *23:* 110 (1970).

Dr. *R.P. Devadas,* Sri Avinashilingam Home Science College for Women, *Coimbatore 641 011* (India)

Wld Rev. Nutr. Diet., vol. 31, pp. 162–167 (Karger, Basel 1978)

Studies on Carotene and Vitamin A with Regard to Nutritional Status, Utilization and Requirements

R. Rajalakshmi and C. V. Ramakrishnan
Biochemistry Department, MS University of Baroda, Baroda

Our interest in vitamin A nutrition began in 1964 when we undertook the responsibility for the Applied Nutrition Programme in Gujarat State. We had to identify existing dietary intakes and the prevalence of nutritional deficiencies in different age groups, and suggest means for the prevention and alleviation of malnutrition. In rural areas around Baroda we found the typical pattern in developing countries of a deficiency of food energy, protein and vitamin A and, to some extent, other nutrients such as calcium and riboflavin (19). Our approach to this problem was to use locally available or producible foods (19–22).

In Gujarat, practically all the vitamin A needed has to be derived from carotenoids, as the daily consumption of other foodstuffs that contain vitamin A is negligible. β-Carotene derived from vegetables would amount to about 450 μg, after allowing for cooking losses (3, 25, 28), and even less among the rural poor, the Bhils in Gujarat and in coastal Kerala.

Carotene intakes do not vary to the same extent as calorie intakes. Consequently, the degree of inadequacy varies in different age groups. The intake, as carotene, is about 400–500 μg in most age groups, although requirements, as retinol, vary from about 150 μg at the age of 1 year, to 750 μg in the adult and are greater in the pregnant or lactating woman. Thus, the very young children in Gujarat show less evidence of vitamin A deficiency. The incidence of corneal and conjunctival xerosis was 60% among school boys as against 34% in preschool children. Bitot spots were found occasionally in school boys but seldom in young children. Serum vitamin A levels were higher in young children (about 20–25 μg/100 ml) than in older school boys (10–15 μg). They were comparatively less in young children studied in Calicut (12 μg/100 ml). In tribal Gujarat adult men also showed a high incidence of xerophthalmia. Yellow maize, formerly the staple food in tribal Gujarat, has been replaced by white maize hybrid strains; an unfortunate change, as yellow maize may be a better source for carotenoids. We found liver·vitamin A to be 21 μg/g in rats fed yellow maize supplemented with amino acids, as against none in those fed a diet comparative nutritively but containing no carotene or vitamin A. Total vitamin A in the liver was 42% of intake in the former. The major carotenoids in maize are reported to be cryptoxanthin, but analyses in this laboratory showed an appreciable amount of β-carotene (132 μg/100 g) (3). Cryptoxanthin has also vitamin A activity (13).

The comparative availability of carotene in selected sources was investigated in a series of experiments. The general procedure was to use a basal diet devoid of carotenoids and vitamin A and add to this a known amount of carotene in the form of the test source and monitor growth as well as the vitamin A content of liver and serum. Additional studies were also carried out on the effects of variation in protein and fat content on the utilization of carotene. The results of these experiments are summarized in tables I and II. They suggest the generally good availability of carotene in leafy vegetables. Spinach, fenugreek, mustard greens, yellow pumpkin, coriander leaves and radish tops appear to be particularly good sources (table I). These studies showed that about 4 μg of β-carotene or less may yield at least 1 μg of vitamin A under physiological conditions. Similar conclusions are to be derived from other reports (9).

In the case of spinach, procedures such as cooking, mashing and/or addition of oil were not found to result in appreciable increase in availability, perhaps because of the already excellent availability of carotene in the same.

The addition of oil to a diet composed of wheat, Bengal gram and the test source of carotene had no effect on the availability (table II), perhaps because the basal diet provided small amounts of fat indigenously present in wheat (1–2%) and bengal gram (5–6%). In any case, several reports do not suggest a beneficial effect of fat (7, 30).

Contrary to expectation, no differences were apparent between animals fed low and high protein diets with regard to the utilization of carotene as judged by liver stores. This may be because of a decrease in utilization as well as requirements (table II). On the other hand, total liver vitamin A concentration was increased from 37–50 μg when the protein quality of a maize diet was improved by the addition of lysine. In the former experiment, the protein deficiency was not so severe as to result in growth arrest as the weight gain was of the order of 5 g/week as against 3 g with a maize diet.

Carotene in oil was not found to be better utilized than that in vegetables (table II). Similar observations have been made earlier (8, 30). A lower availability of vegetable carotene has been reported (7) using a much larger dose of carotene (1 mg/100 g) as dehydrated alfalfa, which is not a typical vegetable. Similarly, *De* (4) found the availability of carotene in amaranth to be poorer (45%) than that of carotene in red palm oil (65%). Here again, the vegetable chosen is one which is found to have relatively low availability. It is reassuring that Mrs. *Pirie* is inclined to agree with us in this regard (16).

Table I. Comparative availability of β-carotene of leafy vegetables to rats (26)

Vegetable source[1]	% availability[2]
Amaranth leaves	16
Colocasia leaves	17
Drumstick leaves	30
Fenugreek leaves	19–40
Spinach leaves	50
Kankoda	15
Yellow pumpkin	19
Coriander leaves	19
Radish tops	21
Mint leaves	9
Khol-Khol greens	13
Portulace	14
Mustard greens	18
β-carotene in oil	13
Vitamin A acetate	50–60

[1] Vitamin A or carotene source was added to contain 150–300 μg/100 g diet.
[2] % of vitamin A or carotene intake during 6 or 8 weeks of the experiment that is stored as vitamin A in liver at the end of 6 or 8 weeks.

Table II. Effects of variations of dietary protein and fat contents on the utilization of carotene and vitamin A in rats (26)

Dietary regimen	Availability (%)[1]		
	vitamin A acetate	β-carotene	fenugreek leaves
5% casein[2]	14	17	24
20% casein[2]	37	17	22
2.5 g groundnut oil[3]	–	–	15
5 g groundnut oil	–	–	18
10 g groundnut oil	–	–	18
None	–	–	16

[1] As explained for table I; experimental period 8 weeks.
[2] 100 μg of vitamin A or 300 μgs of carotene was provided in the diet.
[3] Diet contained wheat 60 g, bengal gram 15 g, sugar 22.5 g, salt 2 g, freeze-dried fenugreek leaves 3 g and providing 330 μg of β-carotene.

Because of the reported effects of protein status on vitamin A utilization (2), we expected vitamin A deficiency to be induced more rapidly in low protein-fed animals. We found the reverse; the concentration of liver vitamin A being 60 μg in low protein-fed animals as against 34 μg in animals fed on a high protein, a result not surprising in retrospect in view of the higher plane of metabolism in high protein-fed animals. We discovered subsequently that similar observations have been made by *McLaren* (12). These results are supported by recent observations on the serum levels of holo-RBP in animals fed low and high protein diets, subjected to vitamin A deficiency (15).

In protein deficiency in humans, the utilization, transport, storage and retrieval of vitamin A are all said to be affected (17, 29). However, vitamin A deficiency does not appear to be an invariable concommitant of severe protein deficiency in children. Kwashiorkor children exhibit symptoms such as severe corneal xerosis and keratomalacia in Madurai, whereas they seldom do in Trivandrum. A similar difference between children in the coastal areas and the interior was noticed several decades ago in Japan by Mori as early as 1904 (*McCollum,* 11). Such differences cannot be attributed to those in intestinal parasite infestation as it is heavy in both regions. It is possible that differences in the liver stores of vitamin A acquired before the onset of severe protein deficiency are responsible for this anomaly. A lack of association between kwashiorkor and vitamin A deficiency is also reported in African regions where red palm oil is used (Prof. E.M. Widdowson, personal discussion).

Contrary to popular impression, we found a greater incidence of xerosis of the eye in pregnant women (82%) than in lactating women (26%) belonging to the urban poor socio-economic group. We found this confirmed in longitudinal studies on 18 women, 9 of whom showed eye symptoms during pregnancy as against 3 in lactation (22). Disappearance of night-blindness after delivery has been reported by *Dixit* (5) and *Mandal et al.* (10). This is consistent with the fall in serum vitamin A during pregnancy which contrasts with the rise in vitamin E (14).

Since placental transfer of vitamin A during pregnancy is limited, fetal deficiency of vitamin A should be neither expected nor found, but congenital blindness apparently resulting from vitamin A deficiency is sometimes found (Dr. J.K. Patel, personal discussion). Both the weight and protein concentration of the placenta are seriously reduced in some malnourished women (23), and the possibility of this influencing placental transport cannot be ruled out.

This raises questions regarding the relative requirements of vitamin A during pregnancy and lactation and also, perhaps, during growth. The requirements of carotene in relation to vitamin A need clarification. The FAO Committee's equation of 6 μg of carotene with 1 μg of retinol appears to underestimate the potency of carotene in most vegetables. In our experience, 30 g of leafy vegetables providing 1200–1300 μg of carotene are found to be adequate to maintain normal vitamin A status in young children. About 50 g appear to achieve a similar result in older children. These would provide after-cooking losses of about 800–1400 μg of carotene, as against recommended 200–600 μg. In adult men, the response of serum vitamin A to 50 g of leafy vegetables appears to compare well with that of 600 μg of vitamin A as palmitate (24). Similar observations with regard to young children have been made by other investigators at Vellore and Madurai (18).

In view of the wide prevalence of vitamin A deficiency in young children, prophylactic measures such as administration of massive doses have been considered. This procedure is perhaps not without some disadvantages, since at least a small proportion of the children show symptoms of toxicity. Since carotene is well utilized by children, it may be worthwhile to explore the feasibility of giving a suitable mixture of carotene and vitamin A, or vitaminised oil when the distribution of leafy vegetables poses problems. We found groundnut oil fortified with vitamin A (150 μg/teaspoon) given twice daily along with food to be effective (27).

Another problem that needs a satisfactory answer is the fate of absorbed carotene in species such as man. Recent studies suggest its partial excretion via the bile and its catabolism to steroids. Volunteers subjected to deprivation showed first a fall in serum carotene levels (6), raising the question of whether the carotene stored in the body is utilized, perhaps after rerouting to the intestine, under conditions of vitamin A deprivation. Unfortunately, most of the studies on carotene appear to have been done in species such as the rat which does not usually store carotene.

Finally, the determination of vitamin A requirements poses problems in determining the absorption, utilization, normal levels of storage and the rate of depletion and criteria for deficiency and adequacy. Pragmatic efforts to eradicate deficiency will have to be made without waiting for unequivocal answers to the above questions.

References

1 *Arroyave, G.; Wilson, D.; Castellanos, and Scrimshaw, N.S.:* Fed. Proc. Fed. Am. Socs exp. Biol. *20:* 372 (1961).
2 *Berger, S.; Rechcigl, M.; Loosli, J.K., and Williams, H.H.:* J. Nutr. *77:* 174 (1962).
3 *Chari, K.V.:* MS (food and nutrition) dissertation, MS University, Baroda (1967).
4 *De, N.K.:* Indian J. med. Res. *25:* 11 (1937).
5 *Dixit, D.T.:* Indian J. med. Res. *54:* 791 (1966).
6 *Mitchell, H.H.:* Comparative nutrition of man and domestic animals, vol. II (Academic Press, New York 1964).
7 *Kemmerer, A.R. and Fraps, G.S.:* J. Nutr. *16:* 309 (1938).
8 *Kemmerer, A.R. and Fraps, G.S.:* Archs. Biochem. *8:* 197 (1945).
9 *Koehn, C.J.:* Archs. Biochem. *17:* 337 (1948).

10 *Mandal, G.S.; Nanda, K.N., and Bose, J.:* J. Obstet. Gynaec. India *19:* 453 (1969).
11 *McCollum, E.V.:* History of nutrition (Haughton Miflin Company, Boston 1956).
12 *McLaren, D.S.:* Br. J. Opthal. *29:* 893 (1959). See 14 below (1970).
13 *Moore, T.:* Vitamin A; chap. 14; p. 159 (Elsevier, Amsterdam 1957).
14 *Moore, T.:* The biochemistry of vitamin A in the general system; in *Morton* Fat soluble vitamins, vol. 9, chap. 7 (Pergamon Press, New York 1970).
15 *Muhilal, H. and Glover, J.:* Br. J. Nutr. *32:* 549 (1974).
16 *Pirie, A.:* Baroda J. Nutr. *2:* 79 (1975).
17 *Pereira, S.M.; Begum, A.; Issac, T., and Dumm, M.E.:* Am. J. clin. Nutr *20:* 297 (1967).
18 *Pereira, S.M. and Begum, A.:* Indian J. med. Res. *56:* 362 (1968).
19 *Rajalakshmi, R. and Ramakrishnan, C.V.:* in *Cremer* Nutrition under various geographic and climatic conditions, Proc. VIIth Int. Congr. Nutr., Hamburg 1966, vol. III, symposium VI, p. 95 (Pergamon Press, Oxford 1967).
20 *Rajalakshmi, R. and Ramakrishnan. C.V.:* Pl. Fds. Hum. Nutr. *1:* 79 (1969).
21 *Rajalakshmi, R. and Ramakrishnan, C.V.:* Pl. Fds. Hum. Nutr. *1:* 163 (1969).
22 *Rajalakshmi, R. and Ramakrishnan, C.V.:* Terminal Report of PL-480 Research Project No. FG-IN-224, Biochemistry Department, MS University, Baroda.
23 *Rajalakshmi, R.; Subbulakshmi, G.; Parekh, B.S.; Bhat, R.V., and Joshi, S.K.:* in *Rajalakshmi* Perspectives in nutrition (Baroda University, Baroda 1972).
24 *Rajalakshmi, R.; Sail, S.S., and Ramachandran, K.:* Baroda J. Nutr. *1:* 29 (1974).
25 *Rajalakshmi, R.; Subbulakshmi, G., and Kothari, B.:* Baroda J. Nutr. *1:* 117 (1974).
26 *Rajalakshmi, R.; Chari, K.V.; Advani, M.; Chary, T.M.; Patel, M.A.; Mutalik, A.M.; Bhat, T.K., and Vyas, A.D.:* Baroda J. Nutr. *2:* 103 (1975).
27 *Rajalakshmi, R. and Ramakrishnan, C.V.:* Wld. Rev. Nutr. Diet. *27:* 34–104 (Karger, Basel 1977).
28 *Sail, S.S.:* Doctoral thesis, MS University of Baroda, Baroda.
29 *Trowell, H.C.; Davies, J.N.P., and Dean, R.F.A.:* Kwashiorkor (Arnold, London 1954) *Munro and Allison*, Vol. II, Chapter 23 (Academic Press, New York/London 1964).
30 *Wilson, H.E.C.; Ahmed, B., and Majumdar, B.N.:* Indian J. med. Res. *24:* 399 (1936).

Dr. *R. Rajalakshmi,* Biochemistry Department, MS University of Baroda, *Baroda* (India)

Wld Rev. Nutr. Diet., vol. 31, pp. 168–172 (Karger, Basel 1978)

The Metabolism and Function of Vitamin D

D.R. Fraser

Dunn Nutritional Laboratory, University of Cambridge and Medical Research Council, Cambridge

During the past ten years much interest has been shown by biochemists and physiologists in the molecule of vitamin D because the nature of its metabolism and mechanism by which it acts indicate that it has an endocrine function in calcium homoeostasis. The metabolic feature of interest is the conversion of vitamin D to a dihydroxylated derivative, and the hormonal role of this metabolite in the target tissues is very similar to that of classical steroid hormones. Hence, vitamin D has come to be regarded as a hormone precursor – a noticeably different function from those suggested for other isoprenoid-derived vitamins.

The physiology of vitamin D is, however, not just concerned with its conversion to a regulatory factor for calcium metabolism. Another equally important aspect is the acquisition of vitamin D from the environment. Consideration of the relationship between the aspects of functional metabolism and the supply of the basic molecule gives rise to doubt as to whether a dietary source of vitamin D is, indeed, physiological.

The metabolism of vitamin D to a functional form ought, with hindsight, to have been predicted before this metabolism was discovered. Earlier studies had indicated that vitamin D acted, like the steroid hormones, by inducing the synthesis of mRNA (5, 14, 15, 18) which coded for proteins mediating the effect of the vitamin. All the steroid hormones characteristically have oxygen functions at the extremities of the long axis of the molecule e.g., cortisol, corticosterone and aldosterone each have 3-keto- and 21-hydroxy- groups. This polar oxygenation enables the steroids to interact, with high affinity, with specific receptor proteins in the target cells. The specificity of the interaction is enhanced by the presence of functional groups deployed elsewhere on the steroid structure e.g., 11β-hydroxy- and 20-keto- groups on corticosterone.

Unlike these hormonal steroids, vitamin D has only one oxygen function – a hydroxyl group on C-3. Thus, in the functional form, 1,25-dihydroxyvitamin

D, (1,25$(OH)_2$D), the polar oxygens are provided by hydroxy- groups on C-3 and C-25 and the group giving the functional specificity is the hydroxyl on C-1.

Conversion of vitamin D to this active form takes place in two steps which differ, both in their significance for vitamin D economy, and also in the anatomical site of the enzyme. 25-Hydroxylation takes place in the endoplasmic reticulum of liver cells (2, 16) and 25-hydroxy-vitamin D (25(OH)D) is 1-hydroxylated in the mitochondria of kidney cells (8). The 1,25$(OH)_2$D is secreted by the kidney into blood from which it is taken up by the target cells of the intestinal mucosa, bone and, possibly, the kidney itself. By action in these sites, it maintains calcium homoeostasis.

In order to act as a regulatory factor, its synthesis must itself be controlled according to the needs of calcium metabolism. Thus, during rapid growth or in pregnancy and lactation, the formation of 1,25$(OH)_2$D is increased. Similarly, in vitamin D deficiency the activity of the 1-hydroxylase system is stimulated. In growing chickens, for example, the concentration of 1,25$(OH)_2$D in the intestinal mucosa is about 0.4 ng/g (6) while when vitamin D-deficient chickens are repleted with vitamin D, the level rises to about 3 ng/g (13).

Regulation of 25(OH)D-1-hydroxylase is mediated mainly by a trophic action of parathyroid hormone on the kidney (9, 10, 17). The output of 1,25$(OH)_2$D by the kidney cannot, however, be increased by supplying more vitamin D or 25(OH)D to an animal.

Most studies on vitamin D metabolism have been done with animals which are vitamin D-deficient and hence have a stimulated 1-hydroxylase system. Some information about the metabolism of vitamin D under more normal conditions can be obtained by giving chickens sufficient radioactively-labelled cholecalciferol to enable normal growth (6). In the plasma of such chickens the concentration of 1,25$(OH)_2D_3$ is no more than 20 pg/ml while the concentration of the precursor, 25,$(OH)D_3$, is about 10 ng/ml. This 500-fold difference emphasises the quantitative dissimilarity between the two steps in the metabolism of vitamin D. While the formation of 1,25$(OH)_2$D is under homoeostatic control, the formation of 25(OH)D is essentially unregulated. The more vitamin D enters the liver, the more 25(OH)D is produced and passes into the circulation. This can be demonstrated experimentally by giving chickens cholecalciferol in doses from 0.5 to 5000 μg. After 36 h the plasma concentrations of 25$(OH)D_3$ ranged from 1.5 ng/ml at the lowest dose, to 117.6 ng/ml at the highest dose (6).

Since the concentration of 25(OH)D in blood plasma is 5–10 times higher than in any other tissue and since the concentration of vitamin D itself is low in all tissues ($<$0.5 ng/g), the plasma can, therefore, be regarded as the body store of substrate for the production of the hormonal form, 1,25$(OH)_2$D. Traditionally, the liver has been considered as a storage site for vitamin D, partly because the liver contains vitamin D, as measured by biological assay, and partly by analogy with this role for the other fat-soluble vitamins. In fact, the metabolism of vitamin D by the liver appears to be non-conservative and most of that which is not converted to 25(OH)D is metabolically inactivated and excreted in bile (1).

Vitamin D, like vitamin A, is toxic when consumed in quantities greatly in excess of requirements. For vitamin A, the liver acts as a regulating store and accumulates the vitamin, esterfied with long chain fatty acids. The esterified vitamin A is hydrolysed and released into the circulation in a controlled fashion, thus preventing toxic levels from reaching the peripheral tissues.

Although fatty acid esters of vitamin D can be found in liver, they do not represent either an effective protection against excess vitamin D, nor are they quantitatively a major storage form of the vitamin. Hence, the destruction of vitamin D by liver appears to be a protective mechanism against toxicity. Since in states of hypervitaminosis D very high levels of 25(OH)D (>500 ng/g) can be found in plasma (3, 12), it is likely that this form of the vitamin produces the toxic effects.

The metabolism of vitamin D by the liver is, therefore, characterised firstly by the production of 25(OH)D in quantities related to the uptake of the parent molecule and, secondly, by the inactivation and excretion of the remainder. Massive input of vitamin D into the liver may, however, give rise to toxic levels of 25(OH)D in the circulation.

Two sources of vitamin D are described to supply the needs of animals and man. One is preformed vitamin D obtained nutritionally from eggs, milk and fish, while the other is the formation of vitamin D in skin by the photochemical action of ultraviolet light on the pro-vitamin, 7-dehydrocholesterol. The way in which vitamin D is handled in the body differs markedly according to its mode of entry.

Dietary vitamin D, like the other fat-soluble vitamins, is absorbed in association with dietary fat and is transported in chylomicrons via the intestinal lymph into blood. A large proportion of chylomicron fat is taken up rapidly by liver so that shortly after absorption, dietary vitamin D is quantitatively presented to the 25-hydroxylase and inactivating enzymes of the liver. Thus, dietary intake of vitamin D is soon followed by hepatic secretion of 25(OH)D into the circulation.

Vitamin D formed in skin, diffuses into blood probably via the cutaneous capillaries. There it complexes with a circulating vitamin D-specific binding protein. This protein also transports 25(OH)D for which the binding capacity in man is approximately 600–700 ng/ml of plasma (11). With the normal 25(OH)D concentrations of 10–50 ng/ml this protein is less than 10% saturated. It is postulated that the very large reserve of specific binding sites act, in the manner of a buffer, to regulate the uptake of vitamin D by the liver. Thus, vitamin D produced in the skin diffuses slowly into blood and is only gradually removed from the circulating binding protein by the liver. In this situation, hepatic secretion of 25(OH)D is not rapidly elevated, but the availability of vitamin D for 25-hydroxylation is maintained for considerably longer than if the same amount of vitamin had been obtained from the diet. It is concluded that vitamin D, absorbed from the intestine, avoids this protective mechanism which prevents excess 25(OH)D production.

Throughout nature, the metabolism of vitamin D is noted for its avoidance of over-production of 25(OH)D despite the lack of regulation of the 25-hydroxylase enzyme. An example can be seen in the supply of vitamin D for the developing chick embryo. The yolk of one egg contains the equivalent of 1–2 μg of vitamin D biological activity which is a much higher concentration than that in the plasma of the domestic hen producing the egg. Moreover, the form of the vitamin D is almost entirely as the unchanged molecule whereas the plasma of the laying hen contains mainly 25(OH)D (7). Thus, a mechanism exists which enables low concentrations of vitamin D from plasma to be specifically accumulated in egg yolk. This mechanism depends on a second binding protein in plasma which has a high affinity for unmetabolized cholecalciferol (4). This protein associates with the yolk protein, phosvitin, through the intermediary linking action of divalent calcium ions. The quaternary complex of vitamin D, its binding protein (Ca^{2+}) and phosvitin is then transferred from blood into yolk during egg formation (7).

By this means a depot of vitamin D is provided for the developing chick embryo. The embryonic liver then produces 25(OH)D as the vitamin D is slowly made available during yolk resorption. If 10 μg 25(OH)D are injected into the yolk during embryogenesis, embryo mortality is very high thus indicating the toxicity of excess 25(OH)D and the need to control its supply.

The classification of vitamin D as a vitamin occurred mainly because it was identified during the same era as most of the nutritional vitamin factors. Nevertheless, the significance of vitamin D as a nutritional factor has been difficult to evaluate, partly because of the scarcity of the molecule in most diets, and also because solar irradiation provides an alternative source. With the discovery of an endocrine role for metabolites of vitamin D, this molecule has lost its functional analogy with other classes of vitamins. From the physiological analysis presented here, it is suggested that vitamin D should lose its status as a nutritional factor altogether and be considered as an environmental molecule to be derived only from ultraviolet irradiation of skin.

References

1 *Bell, P.A. and Kodicek, E.:* Biochem. J. *115:* 663 (1969).
2 *Bhattacharyya, M.H. and DeLuca, H.F.:* Archs Biochem. Biophys. *160:* 58 (1974).
3 *Counts, S.J.; Baylink, D.J.; Shen, F.H.; Sherrard, D.J., and Hickman R.O.:* Ann. intern. Med. *82:* 196 (1975).
4 *Edelstein, S.; Lawson, D.E.M., and Kodicek, E.:* Biochem. J. *135:* 417 (1973).
5 *Eisenstein, R. and Passavoy, M.:* Proc. Soc. exp. Biol. Med. *117:* 77 (1964).

6 *Fraser, D.R.:* Proc. Nutr. Soc. *34:* 139 (1975).
7 *Fraser, D.R. and Emtage, J.S.:* Biochem. J. *160:* 671 (1976).
8 *Fraser, D.R. and Kodicek, E.:* Nature, Lond. *228:* 764 (1970).
9 *Fraser, D.R. and Kodicek, E.:* Nature new Biol. *241:* 163 (1973).
10 *Garabedian, M.; Holick, M.F.; DeLuca, H.F., and Boyle, I.T.:* Proc. natn. Acad. Sci. USA *69:* 1673 (1972).
11 *Haddad, J.G.; Hillman, L., and Rojanasathit, S.:* J. clin. Endocr. Metab. *43:* 86 (1976).
12 *Hughes, M.R.; Baylink, D.J.; Jones, P.G., and Haussler, M.R.:* J. clin. Invest. *58:* 61 (1976).
13 *Lawson, D.E.M.:* Proc. Nutr. Soc. *30:* 47 (1971).
14 *Norman, A.W.:* Science *149:* 184 (1965).
15 *Norman, A.W.:* Biochem. biophys. Res. Commun. *23:* 335 (1966).
16 *Ponchon, G.; Kennan, A.L., and DeLuca, H.F.:* J. clin. Invest. *48:* 2032 (1969).
17 *Rasmussen, H.; Wong, M.; Bikle, D., and Goodman, D.B.P.:* J. clin. Invest. *51:* 2502 (1972).
18 *Zull, J.E.; Czarnowska-Misztal, E., and DeLuca, H.F.:* Science *149:* 182 (1965).

Dr. *D.R. Fraser,* Dunn Nutritional Laboratory, University of Cambridge and Medical Research Council, *Cambridge CB4 1XJ* (England)

Wld Rev. Nutr. Diet., vol. 31, pp. 173–177 (Karger, Basel 1978)

Avitaminosis E in Relation to Kidney Abnormalities in the Rat

T. Moore and I.M. Sharman [1]

Strangeways Research Laboratory, Cambridge, and Dunn Nutritional Laboratory, University of Cambridge and Medical Research Council, Cambridge

Martin and Moore (6) reported that histological sections from the kidneys of rats that had been subjected to prolonged deficiency of vitamin E showed severe cortical degeneration. Structure was lost in many of the cells of the convoluted tubules, leaving only the basement membrane intact. *Emmel* (2, 3) confirmed the appearance of the abnormalities but established that they were a *post mortem* effect, avoidable by the fixation of the tissues immediately after the rat had been killed. Moreover, dietary fat was essential for the production of the abnormality, with highly unsaturated fat, such as linseed oil, having the greatest autolytic effect. *Moore et al.* (8) agreed that both dietary unsaturated fat and a period for autolysis were necessary to cause the loss of structure. Even in promptly fixed kidneys, however, vitamin E deficiency seemed to be associated with the presence of unusually large numbers of brown granules, or concretions, in or near the tubular cells. In view of the claims of *Dam et al.* (1) that many 'redox' substances, including methylene blue, can partially replace vitamin E, this dye-stuff was tested for the prevention of kidney autolysis, and found to be effective (7). The incidence of the kidney abnormality was so predictably dependent on the vitamin E history, provided the diet contained fat, that it was used successfully by *Moore et al.* (9) as a criterion for the destruction of the vitamin in trials on various flour improvers.

The purpose of the present work was: (a) to examine the effect of incubating kidneys in various media *in vitro* rather than in the rat's carcase; (b) to compare the kidneys with other organs as sites for autolysis, and (c) to explore the possibility of inducing changes, similar to those in autolysis, in the living animal.

[1] Dr. T. Moore thanks the Commonwealth Foundation for the travel grant which enabled him to accept Professor Homi Cama's kind invitation to attend the symposium.

The dietary preparation of rats, and the cutting and staining of histological sections followed the procedures of *Moore et al.* (8), who published an illustration showing arbitrary gradings for the severity of 'histolysis'. This term was then preferred to 'autolysis' on an editorial suggestion that the latter word usually refers to biochemical, rather than to histological changes. Although the same workers tried the effect of various changes in the fat content of the diet, their standard basal diet (vitamin-free casein 25, sucrose 50, lard 10, dried brewers' yeast 10, and minerals 5%) was uniformly employed throughout this work. The rats, mostly females, received this diet for periods of about 9–12 months. They reached a severe state of avitaminosis E, as evidenced by brown discolouration of the uterus, paralysis, emaciation, etc. Control rats, dosed with dl-α-tocopheryl acetate (Roche) remained free from these abnormalities.

Autolysis in vitro

The kidneys were promptly dissected out after the rats had been killed, and were incubated for 3 h in either Ringer's solution or normal saline, with or without various additions. In general, autolysis *in vitro* ran parallel to that observed after delayed dissection. The rate of autolysis seemed to be reduced by cold (1°C) and increased by warmth (37°C). Adjustments of pH over the range 2.6–11.7 gave no clear indication of an optimum value for autolysis. At the extremes of this range, however, cellular injuries, not related to the vitamin E status, particularly pyknosis, complicated the histological picture. Additions of sodium cyanide, sodium fluoride or ascorbic acid, all as 0.1% of the incubation medium, all failed to prevent autolysis. Neither was autolysis retarded by the replacement of NaCl in the incubation fluid by equimolecular KCl.

The Particular Liability of the Kidney to Autolysis

The kidney of a rat that had been kept for about 9 months on the deficient diet showed severe PMRA, with a marking of 2.5 (max 3.0). No comparable histological changes were observed in liver, lung, heart, adrenal, pancreas or spleen taken from the same rat.

Kidney Degeneration in vivo *in the Vitamin E-Deficient Rat*

This part of our work was made possible by the kind cooperation and operative skill of our colleague, Dr. *David Fraser.* Rats of both sexes, prepared as for the experiments already described, were submitted under anaesthesia to unilateral ligature of the kidney blood vessels. They all recovered from this operation, but were killed exactly 3 h after the ligatures had been tied. The kidneys were then quickly removed and promptly fixed.

A typical result is shown in figure 1. As expected, no autolysis occurred in the non-ligated kidneys from either the vitamin E-deficient or the control rat. The ligated kidney from the control rat was abnormal in showing changes, particularly pyknosis, which can presumably be ascribed to congestion, but changes typical of autolysis were absent. In contrast, the ligated kidney from the deficient rat showed much the same changes as could have been produced by delayed fixation. PMRA, therefore, was successfully simulated in the living animal.

Discussion

As already stated PMRA occurs with such regularity in rats deprived of vitamin E, but not unsaturated fat, that it can be used as an indication of the vitamin E content of the diet. It cannot be claimed, however, that estimations based on this abnormality could ever be made either rapid or convenient. Prolonged dietary treatment is required to induce PMRA. The histological examination of the kidney, while by no means difficult, involves laborious section-cutting, staining and microscopic examination. Once induced, moreover, PMRA is eliminated only by weeks or months of dosing with vitamin E. Unlike the well known haemolysis test (*György and Rose* (5)), therefore, PMRA reflects the longterm history in regard to the vitamin E intake, rather than the current vitamin E status.

For these reasons PMRA, in itself, could well be regarded merely as a nutritional, or histological curiosity. Perhaps it merits more interest, however, as an outward sign of the complicated interplay in the tissues between readily oxidisable lipoids, typified by PUFA, and anti-oxidants, typified by the tocopherols. The phenomenon may gain in practical importance, moreover, from our findings on the effect of kidney ligature, which transferred observations from the dead to the living animal. Thus failure to balance dietary PUFA with adequate vitamin E caused degeneration of the kidney tubules during life, when the rat was subjected not only to dietary, but also to vascular stress.

More realistic appreciation of the importance, if any, of an 'autolytic diathesis' must obviously await the results of further research, both in the rat and in other species. Possibly the peculiar liability of the kidney tubules to autolysis may have wide general significance and be complementary to their recently discovered powers in lipoid metabolism, as evidenced by their unique ability to introduce additional hydroxyl groups into the D vitamins (*Fraser and Kodicek* (4)).

Rat 1 (Control) Rat 2 (Deficient)

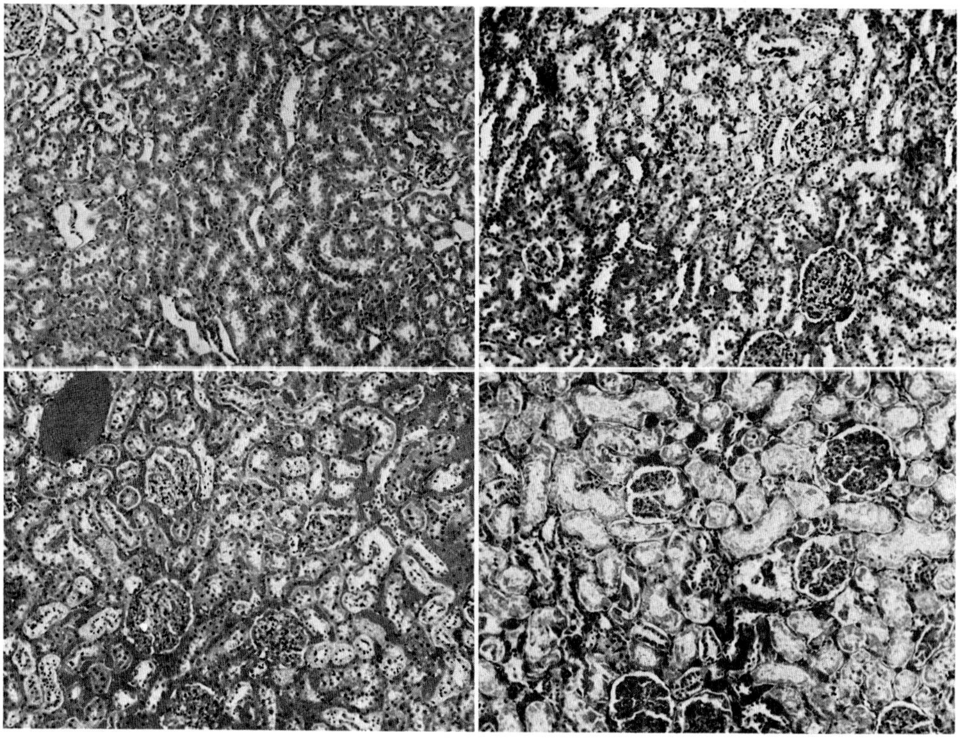

Fig. 1. Kidney autolysis in the living rat. Sections from the kidneys of rats removed 3 h after unilateral ligature of the renal artery and vein. Rat 1 had received adequate doses of dl-α-tocopheryl acetate, but rat 2 was in an advanced state of avitaminosis E. The kidneys were fixed promptly after dissection, so as to avoid autolysis *post mortem.*

Non-ligated kidneys (above): No autolysis can be seen in either kidney. The brown concretions which are prominent in the tubules of the deficient rat, when seen in colour, are difficult to distinguish in monochrome.

Ligated kidneys (below): Extensive degeneration can be seen in the tubules of the kidney from the deficient rat. The picture is very similar to that seen in *post mortem* autolysis, except that much blood has accumulated between the tubules.

The kidney of the rat dosed with tocopherol is certainly not normal but the changes differ from those in autolysis. Again there are massive accumulations of blood between the tubules. In the tubules the cell nuclei are pyknotic, but have not completely disappeared, as in the kidney of the deficient rat.

Even at our present state of knowledge, however, it seems unwise that recommendations for an increased dietary PUFA intake, as a precaution against heart disease, should not be made without full assurance that the vitamin E intake is correspondingly high. Danger of heart disease must not be replaced by danger of kidney disease.

References

1 *Dam, H.; Kruse, I.; Prange, I., and Søndergaard, E.:* Acta physiol. scand. *22:* 299 (1951).
2 *Emmel, V.M.:* Anat. Rec. *124:* 399 (1956).
3 *Emmel, V.M.:* J. Nutr. *61:* 51 (1957).
4 *Fraser, D.R. and Kodicek, E.:* Nature, Lond. *228:* 764 (1970).
5 *György, P. and Rose, C.S.:* Trans. N.Y. Acad. Sci. *52:* 231 (1949).
6 *Martin, A.J.P. and Moore, T.:* J. Hyg. Camb. *39:* 643 (1939).
7 *Moore, T.; Sharman, I.M., and Ward, R.J.:* Soc. of biol. Chem., India: Souvenir, p. 71 (1955).
8 *Moore, T.; Sharman, I.M., and Symonds, K.R.:* J. Nutr. *65:* 183 (1958).
9 *Moore, T.; Sharman, I.M., and Ward, R.J.:* Br. J. Nutr. *12:* 215 (1958).

Dr. *I.M. Sharman,* Dunn Nutritional Laboratory, Milton Road, *Cambridge CB4 1XJ* (England)

Wld Rev. Nutr. Diet., vol. 31, pp. 178–183 (Karger, Basel 1978)

The Biological Function of Vitamin E and the Nature of the Interaction of the Vitamin with Selenium

A. T. Diplock

Department of Biochemistry and Chemistry, Guy's Hospital Medical School, University of London, London

The understanding of the mode of action of vitamin E has been largely due to three early observations: (a) the nutritional antagonism between vitamin E and dietary polyunsaturated fatty acids (PUFA) (28); (b) vitamin E-like activity of certain unphysiological antioxidants, and (c) that selenium is an essential trace element, the function of which is intimately linked with vitamin E (36).

Selenium, Vitamin E and Tissue Peroxidation

The Antioxidant Hypothesis

The hypothesis advanced by *Tappel* (37) some 15 years ago has been widely discussed by several workers and most recently by the present author (10). *Green and Bunyan* (14) found that antioxidant hypothesis untenable because, in their view, it failed to satisfy two fundamental premises. First, that it should be possible to demonstrate the existence of lipid peroxides in tissues; their amount should increase as vitamin E and/or selenium deficiency proceeds and as the level of dietary PUFA is increased and, conversely, that the amount of tissue peroxide should be decreased by vitamin E administration. Secondly, damage to oxidizable components of intracellular structures, such as lysosomes or substrates, such as tocopherol itself, should increase in vitamin E and/or selenium deficiency and the destruction should be exacerbated by increased dietary PUFA.

Evidence for Lipid Peroxidation

The test most frequently used for lipid peroxides is the malondialdehyde (MDA) test. MDA is formed *in vitro* as a breakdown product of peroxidized PUFA (7) and the extent of peroxidation is quantitatively related to the amount of MDA produced. If precautions to exclude oxygen are good, MDA values in vitamin E-deficient or normal tissues are usually indistinguishable from zero and are not correlated with the development of vitamin E deficiency disease (1, 2).

The direct measurement of true lipid peroxides in tissues is very difficult. When special precautions were taken to exclude oxygen, tissues of rats were shown to contain only 10–40 μEq. of peroxide per gram of tissue (5); these values were unaltered by substantial increases in the dietary lipid unsaturation and by deprivation of vitamin E.

Damage to Lysosomes

According to *Tappel*'s hypothesis (37), free radicals generated during the peroxidation processes *in vivo*, are predicted to have damaging consequences for subcellular structures. Thus, damage to lysosomes would cause release of lysosomal enzymes resulting in widespread hydrolysis damage which, *Tappel* considered, would account for all the various manifestations of vitamin E deficiency disease. Although, it is possible to demonstrate elevated levels of free lysosomal enzymes in tissues of vitamin E-deficient animals (41), time sequence studies failed to show a relationship between the appearance of free lysosomal enzyme activity and the onset of disease (3, 4). There is, furthermore, no evidence that free hydrolase activity is causally related to lipid peroxidation and, in muscular dystrophy in chicks, there is clear evidence that it is not (1).

Metabolism of Tocopherol

Peroxidation *in vitro* proceeds at a finite rate in the presence of inhibitors and *Witting* (39) has stated that the oxidation of the fatty acid is accompanied by oxidation of the inhibitor. Since the antioxidant theory predicts that the processes that occur *in vivo* should be accelerated by the addition of the diet of more unsaturated fat and consequently the rate of oxidative destruction of tocopherol should increase. A series of experiments by the present author and his colleagues, on the rate of destruction of (^{14}C)-labelled tocopherol in many of the nutritional situations known to lead to vitamin E and/or selenium deficiency, failed to support the concept that vitamin E and selenium deficiency diseases are accompanied by an increased destruction of tocopherol that is causally related to lipid peroxidation in the tissues (11, 15, 16).

Thus, the antioxidant hypothesis in its original form appears to fail. However, at the present time many aspects of the hypothesis may be seen to be valid in the light of recent observations and it is vital that in drawing attention to the flaws in the hypothesis, the opposite extreme of repudiating entirely all aspects of the theory is avoided.

Selenium and Glutathione Peroxidase

The importance of the discovery (18, 35) that glutathione peroxidase contains selenium cannot be overemphasised. In studies on the susceptibility to haemolysis of erythrocytes derived from selenium-deficient and vitamin E-deficient animals it was found (34) that dietary selenium decreased both autohaemolysis and ascorbic acid-induced haemolysis of rat erythrocytes *in vitro* provided that glucose was present in the incubation medium; in the absence of glucose, no protective effect of selenium was found. The ascorbic acid-induced oxidation of haemoglobin and the formation of Heinz bodies was also inhibited by dietary selenium in the presence of glucose. Dietary vitamin E, in contrast to selenium, decreased haemolysis whether or not glucose was present, but was without effect on haemoglobin oxidation and Heinz body formation. The membrane and the haemoglobin of the erythrocytes of adequately fed rats were both protected in the presence of glucose, but glucose was without effect when selenium was withdrawn from the diet. The maintenance of GSH levels by glucose is important in maintaining erythrocyte integrity and it was found that, in selenium-deficient rat erythrocytes, the levels of GSH were in fact higher than normal rather than being depressed as might have been expected. These findings were correctly interpreted as meaning that the enzyme involved in GSH utilisation, namely glutathione peroxidase, was affected in selenium deficiency. Since glutathione peroxidase had been shown to be a major means of removing hydrogen peroxide from erythrocytes (6), and that the enzyme could also utilise lipid peroxides as substrates (23), involvement of selenium in peroxidase would explain both the haemolytic phenomenon and the destruction of haemoglobin in selenium-deficient erythrocytes. Shortly afterwards (35) it was shown that, following daily administration of $Na_2{}^{72}SeO_{3-}$ for a period, most of the ^{75}Se of the erythrocytes was associated with glutathione peroxidase and remained associated with it during purification. Subsequently, it was confirmed that the ovine enzyme (31) and the bovine enzyme (13) contain selenium in the constant proportion of 4 g atoms of selenium per mole of enzyme. These observations give rise to a key question: does glutathione peroxidase function under physiological conditions *in vivo* to remove lipid peroxides which may arise in sensitive membrane structures as a result of spontaneous interaction of the polyunsaturated fatty acyl moieties of membrane phospholipids with oxygen? No complete answer can be given at the present time, but this question is central to the debate concerning the physiological function of selenium and its relationship to that of vitamin E.

Vitamin E and Membrane Physiology

Much circumstantial evidence exists that vitamin E may play a structural role in biological membranes. Following the classic observation that vitamin E functions specifically to prevent the dialuric acid or hydrogen peroxide-induced haemolysis of erythrocytes (33), it was found that haemolysis by retinol of rabbit erythrocytes was also prevented by the addition *in vitro* of vitamin E (26). More pertinent, however, was the discovery (26) that 6-0-acetyl tocopherol, squalene, phytol, phylloquinone and ubiquinone-30 also inhibited the haemolysis, whereas classical antioxidants did not. The liquid-like properties of the hydrocarbon chain of α-tocopherol might play an important part in the stabilization of biological membranes in general, in a manner unrelated to the antioxidant properties of the tocopherol (24).

Biological phenomena that indicate that vitamin E may play a role in the stabilization of biological membranes have been observed by many workers. (a) Both vitamin E and selenium were shown (22) to cause a stimulation of the transport of Rb^+ from the medium into liver slices and there was no correlation with peroxidative changes; (b) electron microscopy of human jejunum of patients with a β-lipoproteinaemia (29) suggested that the underlying vitamin E deficiency in these patients caused a loss of contrast in membranes; treatment with α-tocopherol resulted in a rapid restoration of normal ultrastructure. Similar phenomena were observed in the jejunal epithelium of vitamin E-deficient Peking ducklings (30) and these ultrastructural changes were interpreted and subsequently confirmed (38) as being due to specific loss of PUFA from the membranes. Membrane associated enzymes may be either increased or decreased in vitamin E deficiency by changes in the membrane architecture (20, 21, 27).

From the results of model building experiments, we proposed (12, 25) that the observed effects of vitamin E on biological membranes might be due to specific physico-chemical interactions between the phytyl chain of tocopherol and membrane phospholipids with PUFA in the 2-position of their glyceryl moiety.

The consequences of vitamin E deficiency would, according to our hypothesis, be expected to be as follows: (a) the packing of hydrocarbon regions of membranes would be disordered, which would facilitate in a limited manner the oxidative destruction by free-radical chain reactions of membrane PUFA *in vivo*; (b) increase in membrane permeability to cations and solutes such as that described in the mitochondrial membranes of the liver of rats deprived of vitamin E and selenium (40); (c) an increase in the degradation of membrane phospholipids *in vivo* by endogenous phospholipases which might be expected to become activated by the less compact structure of the membrane in the absence of vitamin E; (d) alterations in the activity of membrane-associated enzymes, as their active sites become either more or less accessible to their substrates because of changes in the membrane architecture.

Selenium-Tocopherol Interaction

Catalase is largely located in peroxisomes in liver (9) so that localisation of glutathione peroxidase in the cytosol and within the mitochondria would imply that it exists, either to destroy peroxisomal hydrogen peroxide or for some other purpose. The principle role of glutathione peroxidase (and, by derivation, of selenium) in liver and other tissues may be to catalyse the destruction of lipid peroxides, as many lipid peroxides can serve as substrates for the enzyme (17, 23). Thus, if lipid peroxide radicals are formed *in vivo,* two mechanisms appear theoretically to be available for their immediate discharges, namely, either interaction with tocopherol, or conversion of the hydroperoxide to a hydroxy acid by glutathione peroxidase. If animals are adequately nourished with selenium, then the failure (5) to demonstrate lipid peroxides in the tissues of rats deprived of vitamin E and given adequate or high levels of dietary PUFA, can be simply explained by supposing that the peroxides were discharged, as soon as they were formed, by glutathione peroxidase.

In vitamin E-deficient animals it might be thought that the reason that (^{14}C)-α-tocopherol was not destroyed more rapidly in the presence of dietary PUFA than in its absence was because peroxides were destroyed as they were formed, by glutathione peroxidase. But the key experiments would seem to be those undertaken with vitamin E and selenium-deficient animals (11, 16); no accelerated destruction of (^{14}C)-tocopherol was seen in rats and chicks, which presumably had depressed levels of glutathione peroxidase as well as deficiency of vitamin E. It is not necessary, however, to invoke lipid peroxidation kinetics at all if one accepts our physico-chemical hypothesis (12, 25). Under these circumstances, although the metabolic consequences of increased dietary PUFA might prove to be fatal no accelerated destruction of α-tocopherol would necessarily be expected to occur even with absence as well of dietary selenium. In this context it is of particular interest to note that, using the ethane evolution technique (32), it has been possible to demonstrate lipid peroxidation *in vivo* in rats shortly before their death from liver necrosis (19). One can deduce from this finding that substantial amounts of lipid peroxide only accumulate when an animal is *in extremis* and it seems highly probable that it is the peroxide which causes the death of the animal.

References

1 *Bunyan, J.; Diplock, A.T.; Edwin, E.E., and Green, J.:* Br. J. Nutr. *16:* 519 (1962).
2 *Bunyan, J.; Green, J., and Diplock, A.T.:* Br. J. Nutr. *17* (1963).
3 *Bunyan, J.; Green, J.; Diplock, A.T., and Robinson, D.:* Br. J. Nutr. *21:* 127 (1967).
4 *Bunyan, J.; Green, J.; Diplock, A.T., and Robinson, D.:* Br. J. Nutr. *21:* 137 (1967).
5 *Bunyan, J.; Murrell, E.A.; Green, J., and Diplock, A.T.:* Br. J. Nutr. *21:* 175 (1967).
6 *Cohen, G. and Hochstein, P.:* Biochemistry *2:* 1420 (1963).
7 *Dahle, L.K.; Hill, E.G., and Holman, R.J.:* Archs Biochem. Biophys. *98:* 253 (1962).
8 *Desai, I.D.; Calvert, C.C., and Scott, M.L.:* Archs Biochem. Biophys. *108:* 60 (1964).
9 *De Duve, C. and Baudhuin, P.:* Physiol. Rev. *46:* 323 (1966).
10 *Diplock, A.T.:* CRC critical rev. Toxicol. *4:* 271 (1976).
11 *Diplock, A.T.; Bunyan, J.; McHale, D., and Green, J.:* Br. J. Nutr. *21:* 103 (1967).
12 *Diplock, A.T. and Lucy, J.A.:* FEBS Lett. *29:* 205 (1973).
13 *Flohe, L.; Gunzler, W.A., and Schock, H.H.:* FEBS Lett. *32:* 132 (1973).
14 *Green, J. and Bunyan, J.:* Nutr. Abstr. Rev. *39:* 321 (1969).

15 *Green, J.; Diplock, A.T.; Bunyan, J.; McHale, D., and Muthy, I.R.:* Br. J. Nutr. *21:* 69 (1967).
16 *Green, J.; Diplock, A.T.; Bunyan, J.; Muthy, I.R., and McHale, D.:* Br. J. Nutr. *21:* 497 (1967).
17 *Gunzler, W.A.; Vergin, H.; Muller, I., and Flohe, L.:* Hoppe-Seyler's Z. physiol. Chem. *353:* 1001 (1972).
18 *Hoekstra, W.G.:* Trace element metabolism in animals; vol. 2, p. 61 (University Park Press, Baltimore 1974).
19 *Hoekstra, W.G.:* Personal communication.
20 *Hulstaert, C.E.; Gijzel, W.D.; Hardonk, M.J.; Froon, A.M., and Molenaar, I.:* Lab. Invest. (in press, 1976).
21 *Kawai, K.; Nakao, M.; Nakao, J., and Katsui, G.:* Am. J. clin. Nutr. *27:* 987 (1974).
22 *Levander, O.A. and Morris, V.C.:* J. Nutr. *101:* 1013 (1971).
23 *Little, C. and O'Brien, P.J.:* Biochem. biophys. Res. Commun. *31:* 145 (1968).
24 *Lucy, J.A.:* Biochem. J. *99:* 579 (1966).
25 *Lucy, J.A.:* Proc. natn. Acad. Sci. USA *203:* 4 (1972).
26 *Lucy, J.A. and Dingle, J.T.:* Nature, Lond. *304:* 156 (1964).
27 *Machado, E.A.; Porta, E.A.; Hartroft, W.S., and Hamilton, F.:* Lab. Invest. *24:* 13 (1971).
28 *Mattill, H.A. and Golumbic, C.:* J. Nutr. *23:* 625 (1942).
29 *Molenaar, I.; Hommes, F.A.; Braams, W.G., and Holman, H.A.:* Proc. natn. Acad. Sci. USA *61:* 982 (1968).
30 *Molenaar, I.; Vos, J.; Jaeger, F.C., and Hommes, F.A.:* Nutr. Metabol. *12:* 358 (1970).
31 *Oh, S.-H.; Canther, H.E., and Hoekstra, W.G.:* Biochemistry *13:* 1825 (1974).
32 *Riely, C.A.; Cohen, G., and Lieberman, M.:* Science *183:* 208 (1974).
33 *Rose, C.S. and György, P.:* Blood *5:* 1062 (1950).
34 *Rotruck, J.T.; Pope, A.L.; Ganther, H.E., and Hoekstra, W.G.:* J. Nutr. *102:* 689 (1972).
35 *Rotruck, J.T.; Pope, A.L.; Ganther, H.E.; Swanson, A.B.; Hafeman, D.G., and Hoekstra, W.G.:* Science *179:* 588 (1973).
36 *Schwarz, K.:* Proc. Soc. exp. Biol. Med. *78:* 852 (1951).
37 *Tappel, A.L.:* Vitams Horm. *20:* 493 (1962).
38 *Vos, J.; Molenaar, I.; Searle van-Leuwen, M., and Hommes, F.A.:* Ann. N.Y. Acad. Sci. *203:* 74 (1972).
39 *Witting, L.A.:* Fed. Proc. Fed. Am. Socs. exp. Biol. *24:* 912 (1965).
40 *Yeh, Y. and Johnson, R.M.:* Archs Biochem. Biophys. *159:* 821 (1973).
41 *Zalkin, H.; Tappel, A.L.; Caldwell, K.A.; Shibko, S.; Desai, I.D., and Holliday, T.A.:* J. biol. Chem. *237:* 2678 (1962).

Prof. *A.T. Diplock,* Department of Biochemistry, Guy's Hospital Medical School, *London* (England)

Wld Rev. Nutr. Diet., vol. 31, pp. 184–189 (Karger, Basel 1978)

Structural Interactions between Vitamin E and Polyunsaturated Lipids

Jack A. Lucy

Department of Biochemistry and Chemistry, Royal Free Hospital School of Medicine, University of London, London

Molecular interactions of synthetic phospholipid molecules with α-tocopherol and derivatives of α-tocopherol have been investigated in monolayers of phospholipids at the air-water interface. Of the tocopherols studied, the naturally occurring α-tocopherol exhibited the maximum interaction with polyunsaturated phospholipids in monolayers. Furthermore, all of the tocopherols penetrated into monolayers more readily as unsaturation in the phospholipids increased. α-Tocopherol is thus likely to be closely associated with polyunsaturated phospholipids in membranes and this may aid the inhibition of lipid peroxidation by an antioxidant mechanism. Our observations are also consistent, however, with the hypothesis that α-tocopherol facilitates molecular packing of polyunsaturated phospholipid molecules and hence may stabilize membranes containing high proportions of polyunsaturated phospholipid molecules.

In the preceding paper, Dr. *Diplock* has referred to the fact that the rate of destruction of trace quantities of α-(^{14}C) tocopherol in the tissues of vitamin E-deficient animals is not increased by dietary polyunsaturated fatty acids (3), as would be expected according to the antioxidant hypothesis (8, 9). This indicates that the nutritional interaction between α-tocopherol and unsaturated lipids cannot be ascribed solely to an antioxidant mechanism. We have therefore proposed, on the basis of molecular-model building, that α-tocopherol may physically stabilize biological membranes that are rich in polyunsaturated phospholipids. As Dr. *Diplock* has explained, this stabilization might arise from interactions between the phytyl side chain of α-tocopherol and the polyunsaturated fatty acyl residues of phospholipid molecules in the hydrophobic regions of biological membranes (1, 4).

This paper is concerned with experiments on lipid monolayers that were undertaken in collaboration with Dr. *Diplock* and with Dr. *Bruno Maggio* (British Council Fellow from the National University of Cordoba, Argentina). The work was designed to see whether or not physical interactions occurred between α-tocopherol and polyunsaturated phospholipids in a model system *in vitro* and to characterize any interactions that might be observed. Surface monolayers at the air-water interface provide a very suitable experimental system with which to investigate molecular interactions occurring in an oriented molecular array (2). The techniques that we have used and the equipment employed have been described earlier (5, 6). A more detailed account of the experiments reported in the present paper is also available (7).

Mixed Monolayers of Phospholipids and Tocopherols

In one type of experiment, monolayers of synthetic phospholipids with differing composition in their fatty acyl chains, monolayers of synthetic α-tocopherols with different lengths of phytyl chain and mixed monolayers of phospholipids with tocopherols were investigated at a surface pressure of 5 $mN \cdot m^{-1}$. From the experimental data obtained, the areas per molecule were calculated for phospholipid alone and for tocopherol alone. Mean molecular areas per molecule were also obtained for the mixed films of phospholipid and tocopherol and these values were plotted as functions of the molar composition of the mixed monolayers.

It was found that mixed monolayers of tocopherol with distearoylglycerylphosphorylcholine followed the additivity rule with respect to mean molecular areas. In other words, the different molecular species mixed ideally in the monolayer and, therefore, showed no evidence of any molecular interactions.

By contrast, all four of the tocopherols studied in this type of experiment, which had two, three (α-tocopherol), four and seven isopentane units in the side chain, exhibited negative deviations in plots of mean molecular area against molar composition in mixed films with dioleoylglycerylphosphorylcholine and also, in particular with diarachidonylglycerylphosphorylcholine. This latter finding showed that α-tocopherol and the polyunsaturated phospholipids are packed more closely together than in an ideally mixed film, indicating the existence of a molecular interaction between the two components of the monolayer. Thus, these experiments on mixed monolayers of tocopherols and phospholipids support the hypothesis that α-tocopherol and diarachidonylglycerylphosphorylcholine interact physically in a way that is not available to mixtures of α-tocopherol and distearoylglycerylphosphorylcholine.

Penetration of Phospholipid Films by Tocopherol Components

In a second type of experiment, we measured the increase in surface pressure that occurred at constant area when a tocopherol was injected into the subphase below a monolayer of phospholipid, which was spread at a surface pressure that was greater than the collapse pressure of the tocopherol. Tocopherol, dissolved in ethanol, was injected below the compressed phospholipid monolayer while the aqueous subphase was briefly stirred with a magnetic stirrer. Subsequent changes in the surface pressure of the monolayer were measured. Penetration of the tocopherols into monolayers of phospholipid was very rapid and equilibrium values of surface pressure were usually reached within 1 or 2 min. Final readings were taken after 5 min. Ethanol injected into the subphase did not produce any variation in the surface properties studied.

Initial experiments were undertaken to test the ability of α-tocopherol to penetrate and increase the surface pressure (at constant area) of diarachidonylglycerylphosphorylcholine spread in a monolayer at an initial pressure of 30 $mN \cdot m^{-1}$. The extent of penetration, as measured by the increase in surface pressure of the monolayer, was approximately constant for values of molar ratio of 0.5–2.0 (mol of α-tocopherol/mol of phospholipid). Penetration was greatly decreased only when the quantity of α-tocopherol present was less than 0.3 mol/mol of diarachidonylglycerylphosphorylcholine. In all of the remaining experiments on the penetration of phospholipid monolayers by tocopherols that are described in this paper, equimolar ratios of phospholipid and penetrating molecule were used.

Next, the abilities of a number of tocopherols to penetrate and increase the surface pressure of dioleoylglycerylphosphorylcholine were investigated, at differing initial surface pressures in the phospholipid monolayer. It was found that tocopherols with 2, 3 (α-tocopherol) and 4 isopentane units in the side chain appeared to penetrate the phospholipid monolayers at high surface pressures more effectively, as judged by the measured increase in surface pressure occurring on penetration, than the higher molecular weight tocopherols (with 5–9 isopentane units in the side chain). However, this finding was due, at least in part, to the relatively high collapse pressures of the shorter chain tocopherols which enabled them to penetrate the phospholipid monolayer with greater ease. Nevertheless, it is interesting to note that α-tocopherol penetrated the phospholipid film more effectively than analogues with shorter or with longer side chains.

In subsequent experiments, in order to obtain more comparable measures of penetration, we studied the ability of tocopherols to penetrate phospholipid monolayers that were spread at initial surface pressures that were higher, by known increments, than the collapse pressures of the individual tocopherols. When the penetration experiments were done in this way, the ability of 'tocopherols' with no side chain at all (tocols), or with 2 isopentane units in the chain, was less marked than previously. It was also interesting to observe that in both types of experiments, α-tocopherol (with the naturally occurring length of side chain) penetrated dioleoylglycerylphosphorylcholine most effectively and gave the largest increases in surface pressure.

Effect of Unsaturation in Phospholipid Molecules

Of particular interest, in relation to possible mechanisms of action of α-tocopherol at the molecular level in biological membranes, is the effect of unsaturation in the fatty acyl chains of phospholipid molecules on the interaction of phospholipids with α-tocopherol. Experiments were, therefore, made on the interaction with tocopherols of phospholipids containing increasing numbers of double bonds in their fatty acyl chains. In these and subsequent experiments, the initial surface pressures of the phospholipid monolayers were 15 $mN \cdot m^{-1}$ higher than the collapse pressure of the individual tocopherol under study. We observed that the capacity of α-tocopherol to penetrate monolayers of phospholipid increased with increasing unsaturation of the acyl chains up to 2 double bonds/chain (dilinoleoylglycerylphosphorylcholine) but remained almost constant thereafter. This finding is consistent with our proposal that α-tocopherol may interact physically with polyunsaturated phospholipids in membranes. It was also interesting to note that for each monolayer of phospholipid studied, there was a sharp increase in the ability of tocopherols to penetrate the monolayer on increasing the length of the isopentane chain to 3 isopentane units (α-tocopherol). With 4 isopentane units in the chain, penetration was slightly less than, or comparable with, that found with α-tocopherol itself. Higher molecular weight tocopherol derivatives penetrated less effectively.

In naturally occurring biological membranes, both saturated and unsaturated phospholipids are present in differing proportions. It is, therefore, important to know how tocopherols interact with phospholipid monolayers that contain both saturated and unsaturated phospholipids. To this end, we studied the interaction of tocopherols with a mixed monolayer of diarachidonyl- and distearoylglycerylphosphorylcholine in a 1:1 molar ratio. Interestingly, the behaviour of this mixed monolayer much more closely resembled that of the unsaturated phospholipid component, i.e., more extensive penetration by the tocopherols than that of the distearoylglycerylphosphorylcholine. Increases in surface pressure that were practically equal to those found with monolayers of the unsaturated phospholipid alone were obtained with mixed monolayers containing only about 20% of the unsaturated component. It was thus apparent that penetration by α-tocopherol is greatly facilitated by the presence of relatively small quantities of unsaturated phospholipid in the monolayer.

Unlike their behaviour with phospholipids, the tocopherols exhibited very little penetration of a monolayer of cholesterol which was spread at a surface pressure that was initially 15 $mN \cdot m^{-1}$ higher than the collapse pressure of the individual tocopherols. Furthermore, increases in surface pressure produced by the penetration of the tocopherols into mixed monolayers of dioleoylglycerylphosphorylcholine/cholesterol (1:1 molar ratio) were intermediate between those observed for monolayers of the components.

Changes in surface pressure observed on the penetration of derivatives of α-tocopherol into monolayers of dipalmitoyl- and dioleoyl-glycerylphosphoryl-ethanolamine were very similar to those obtained with monolayers of phosphatidylcholines possessing corresponding fatty acyl chains. This finding indicates that the ability of α-tocopherol and its analogues to penetrate monolayers of phospholipids is regulated more by the hydrophobic chains of the phospholipid and by the length of the phytyl chain of the tocopherol, than by the polar head group of the phospholipid.

Some caution is necessary in attempting to relate the observations made on the model system used in this paper to the behaviour of α-tocopherol *in vivo.* Furthermore, it should not be overlooked that the phospholipids of biological membranes normally have one unsaturated and one saturated fatty chain. Phospholipids of this type, having a polyunsaturated 2-acyl chain were not available for our studies.

Despite these necessary reservations, it is nevertheless important to consider what bearing our observations may have on the biochemical functions of α-tocopherol *in vivo.* If α-tocopherol is involved in the protection of the polyunsaturated phospholipids of biological membranes against destructive peroxidation, in accordance with the antioxidant hypothesis, it would seem from our investigations that α-tocopherol is likely to be located in close association with the polyunsaturated phospholipid molecules that are at risk. Vitamin E may, therefore, be in an optimum position to inhibit lipid peroxidation. Equally, however, our observations are also consistent with the hypothesis that α-tocopherol may facilitate the molecular packing with biological membranes of polyunsaturated phospholipid molecules and hence the vitamin may stabilize biological membranes containing high proportions of polyunsaturated phospholipid molecules. This latter possible function of α-tocopherol may thus be additional to the antioxidant behaviour of the vitamin.

Acknowledgement

The work reported in this paper was supported by the award of a British Council Fellowship to Dr. *Bruno Maggio.*

References

1 *Diplock, A.T. and Lucy, J.A.:* FEBS Lett. *29:* 205 (1973).

2 *Gaines, G.L.:* Interscience monographs on physical chemistry; Insoluble monolayers at liquid-gas interfaces (Interscience, New York 1966).

3 *Green, J.; Diplock, A.T.; Bunyan, J.; McHale, D., and Muthy, I.R.:* Br. J. Nutr. *21:* 69 (1967).

4 *Lucy, J.A.:* Ann. N.Y. Acad. Sci. *203:* 4 (1972).
5 *Maggio, B. and Lucy, J.A.:* Biochem. J. *149:* 597 (1975).
6 *Maggio, B. and Lucy, J.A.:* Biochem. J. *155:* 353 (1976).
7 *Maggio, B.; Diplock, A.T., and Lucy, J.A.:* Biochem. J. *161:* 111 (1977).
8 *Tappel, A.L.:* Vitams Horm. *20:* 493 (1962).
9 *Tappel, A.L.:* Ann. N.Y. Acad. Sci. *203:* 12 (1972).

Dr. *J.A. Lucy,* Department of Biochemistry and Chemistry, Royal Free Hospital, School of Medicine, University of London, 8 Hunter Street, *London WC1N 1BP* (England)

Wld Rev. Nutr. Diet., vol. 31, pp. 190–195 (Karger, Basel 1978)

Role of Vitamin E in Cellular Processes

A.S. Pappu, P. Fatterpaker and A. Sreenivasan

Biochemistry & Food Technology Division, Bhabha Atomic Research Centre, Trombay, Bombay

The nonspecific role of vitamin E or α-tocopherol as a lipid soluble antioxidant is well documented. Evidence has now accumulated implicating this vitamin in the maintenance of structural and functional integrity of cell membranes, but this is not understood clearly. In the present investigation an attempt has been made to define vitamin E functions in terms of specific biochemical reactions, namely (i) regulation of membrane-bound phospholipase activity and (ii) involvement in vitamin B_{12} metabolism.

Regulation of Membrane-Bound Phospholipase Activity

Our interest in vitamin E stemmed from our recent observations on a specific lipoprotein in the intestinal mucosa, serum and liver cytosol of rats that bind vitamin E and help in its absorption, transport and subcellular distribution. Much of the cellular vitamin E is present in the cell sap and 80% of this exists in the lipoprotein-bound form.

As a first step to an understanding of vitamin E function, vis-à-vis this lipoprotein carrier, a detailed study of the effects of vitamin E-deficiency in the rat in terms of membrane lipids was undertaken. It was observed that there was a significant increase in the lyso-lecithin levels of the subcellular membranes. Lysolecithin which accounted for 0.5% total phospholipid in mitochondria of control animals, increased to 3.2% in vitamin E-deficient animals. It varied from 1.3 to 1.6% in rough microsomes, smooth microsomes and lysosomes in control animals but increased to 2.5–2.8% in E-deficient rats. Also in CNS myelin, lysolecithin increased from 0.5 to 2.3% in vitamin E-deficient animals.

Lysolecithin, a highly lytic natural surfactant is one of the least prevalent phospholipids in the tissues and body fluids with the exception of blood plasma, constituting less than 2% of the total tissue phospholipids under normal physiological condition (19). However, elevated levels of lysolecithin are reported in atherosclerosis (17), some nutritional (18) and genetic (11) muscular disorders.

Table I. Lecithin cholesterol acyl transferase (LCAT) activity in vitamin E deficiency

Group	LCAT activity	
	plasma[1]	cell sap[2]
Control	2.33 ± 0.21	1.08 ± 0.17
Vitamin E-deficient	0.61 ± 0.27	0.51 ± 0.04
% reduction	81.1	30.0

LCAT activity was measured following the radioactivity incorporated in cholesterol esters from (^{14}C)-cholesterol. Aliquots of plasma and/or cell sap were incubated in (^{14}C)-cholesterol (0.5 μCi) in suitable buffer system at 37°C for 3 h according to the procedure of *Akiyama et al.* (1). Cholesterol and its esters were separated by thin layer chromatography on silica gel G, using petroleum ether:ether:acetic acid (82:18:1, v/v/v) as developing solvent (23). The counting of radioactivity (5) was carried out in a Beckman LS 100 Liquid Scintillation Spectrometer with an efficiency of 94% for ^{14}C. The results are mean of five different experiments ± SEM.

1 $\frac{\text{cpm in esterified cholesterol}}{\text{cpm in added cholesterol}} \times 100$ per ml plasma

2 $\frac{\text{cpm in esterified cholesterol}}{\text{cpm in added cholesterol}} \times 100$ per g liver

Lysolecithin is known to promote lysis of red cells (10) and fusion of cellular membranes (16). The increased lysolecithin levels of cellular membranes can perhaps give rise to several structural and functional abnormalities observed in vitamin E deficiency condition. It was, therefore, of interest to know whether vitamin E exerts a regulatory role, direct or indirect, on lysolecithin metabolism. A study of enzymes responsible for lysolecithin production, lecithin cholesterol acyl transferase (LCAT) of plasma and liver cell sap, and phospholipase A_2 of liver mitochondria and utilization, acylating enzyme complex of liver mitochondria and microsomes, in vitamin E deficiency, was studied. Effect *in vitro* of bound and free vitamin E on phospholipase A_2 activity was also ascertained.

There is a decrease in LCAT activity of plasma and cell sap (table I) to the extent, respectively, of 80 and 30% of the normal values. This reduction in enzyme activity could not be due either to possible elevation of lipid peroxides or to any polyunsaturated fatty acids (PUFA) destruction because neither intravenous administration of peroxides nor essential fatty acids (EFA) deficiency could inactivate the enzyme (24, 25). There is on the contrary stimulation of LCAT activity in EFA deficiency.

The phospholipase A_2 activity of rat liver mitochondria showed a two-fold increase in vitamin E deficiency (table II). Incubation of mitochondria with control cell sap reduced the enzyme activity almost to control values, suggesting the presence of a factor in control cell sap that can inhibit mitochondrial phos-

Table II. Phospholipase A_2 activity in vitamin E deficiency

Group	Phospholipase A_2 activity $\frac{\text{cpm in lysolecithin}}{\text{cpm in added lecithin}}$ × 100/mg protein		
	mitochondria, Mt	Mt + cell sap, control	Mt + cell sap, deficient
Control	7.50 ± 1.12	8.00 ± 1.14	6.80 ± 0.74
Vitamin E-deficient	16.50 ± 0.83	6.00 ± 0.75	17.00 ± 0.67

Phospholipase A_2 activity was measured by following the radioactivity in (^{32}P)-lysolecithin formed from (^{32}P)-lecithin, according to the procedure of *Waite and Sission* (26). Cell sap was obtained from a 50% liver homogenate in 0.25 *M* sucrose containing 0.01 *M* Tris-HCl pH 7.4 and 0.001 *M* EDTA (21). Mitochondrial suspension equivalent to 2–3 mg protein was preincubated with cell sap, either from control or deficient rats, in a total volume of 0.5 ml (6–7 mg of protein) at 37°C for 15 min. The results are averages ± SEM of five independent experiments.

Table III. Activity of lysolecithin acylating enzyme complex in vitamin E deficiency

Group	Lysolecithin acylating activity mmol (^{14}C)-palmitic acid incorporated/mg protein/2 h	
	mitochondria	microsomes
Control	0.230 ± 0.016	2.260 ± 0.435
Vitamin E-deficient	0.056 ± 0.014	0.520 ± 0.089
% reduction	78.4	78.0

The enzyme activity was determined by measuring the radioactivity incorporated in (^{14}C)-lecithin formed from (^{14}C)-palmitic acid and lysolecithin (20). 0.5 μCi of (^{14}C)-palmitic acid (5 mCi/mmol) was included in the reaction mixture. Results are averages of five independent experiments ± SEM.

pholipase A_2. This inhibitor appears to be absent in the deficient cell sap (table II). In further experiments it was found that vitamin E in the free form, or in lipoprotein-bound form, prepared according to *Rajaram et al.* (21) inhibits the enzyme activity in the E-deficient mitochondria, lipoprotein-bound vitamin being much more effective. These observations are consistent with *Lucy*'s hypothesis (12) that vitamin E *in vivo* may function by inhibiting membrane-bound phospholipases.

The acylating enzyme activity of liver mitochondria and microsomes exhibits a 78% reduction in vitamin E deficiency (table III). From these results it would seem that vitamin E has a direct role in controlling lysolecithin levels in membranes.

Involvement of Vitamin E in Vitamin B_{12} Metabolism

Increased urinary excretion of methyl malonic acid is known to be associated with deficiencies of both vitamin E (2, 15) and vitamin B_{12} (3, 8, 22). This symptom is reversed by vitamin E therapy (15).

We have observed that excretion of methyl malonic acid in E-deficient rats during a 24 h period is about four times (41.2 ± 5.5 μmoles) of that found in the control animal (10.6 ± 1.02 μmoles). Preliminary experiments have indicated that the conversion *in vivo* of intraperitoneally administered 1-(^{14}C) propionate into 1-(^{14}C) methyl malonic acid was much higher in the livers of vitamin E-deficient rats which is subsequently reflected in an increased excretion of this metabolite in the urine.

In vitamin B_{12} deficiency, the increased excretion of methyl malonic acid has been traced to an impairment in the methyl malonyl CoA mutase, requiring B_{12} coenzyme (dimethyl benzimidazol cobamide coenzyme – DMBC) (8). The observed disturbance in methyl malonic acid metabolism could therefore result from a secondary deficiency of vitamin B_{12} in vitamin E deficiency condition. An interdependence of these two vitamins was indeed postulated by *Hove and Hardin* (9). However, we did not find any significant change in vitamin B_{12} levels in serum and liver in E-deficient animals. This suggests that vitamin E deficiency does not interfere with the absorption transport or storage of vitamin B_{12} in the rat. These results fail to provide information regarding interference if any, by lack of vitamin E, in the utilization of vitamin B_{12} in cellular processes. The formation *in vitro* of methyl malonic acid from propionate and its subsequent conversion to succinic acid by liver enzymes of vitamin E-deficient rats were next investigated.

It was observed that the extent of conversion *in vitro* of 1-(^{14}C) propionate to methyl malonic acid by the propionyl CoA carboxylase of homogenate and mitochondria was unaffected in E deficiency. However, further isomerization of methyl malonic acid to succinic acid regulated by the B_{12} requiring methyl malonyl CoA mutase seems to be impaired to the extent of 45% in the homogenate and 31% in mitochondria (table IV). Addition of DMBC to the reaction mixture almost completely restored the values in the deficient group to normal levels. The conversion of propionate to succinic acid in presence of DMBC increased to some extent in the control group, also. This may be due to the known fact that the apoenzyme of the methyl malonyl CoA mutase is not fully saturated even in the normal animals (3).

The results of these experiments thus indicated that the defective conversion of methyl malonate to succinic acid in vitamin E deficiency is not due to a secondary deficiency of vitamin B_{12}, but to an impairment in methyl malonyl CoA mutase activity because of vitamin B_{12} coenzyme being limiting. Involvement of vitamin E in the utilization of vitamin B_{12} to its coenzyme function is thus indicated.

Table IV. Effect of E deficiency on conversion of 1-(^{14}C) propionate via methyl 1-(^{14}C) malonic acid to 1-(^{14}C) succinic acid *in vitro* by rat liver enzymes

	Radioactivity, cpm/mg protein of acetone powder				% efficiency of conversion to succinic acid		% decrease
	methyl malonic acid		succinic acid				
	control	vitamin E-deficient	control	vitamin E-deficient	control	vitamin E-deficient	
Homogenate	3.6×10^3	3.9×10^3	3.15×10^3	1.5×10^3	96.0	53.0	44.6
Mitochondria	3.1×10^4	3.4×10^4	3.2×10^4	2.1×10^4	94.4	67.8	30.8

The method used is essentially according to *Flavin and Ochoa* (7). The incubation mixture contained 100 m*M* Tris-HCl buffer, pH 8.5, 4 m*M* $MgCl_2$, 4 m*M* ATP, 5 m*M* GSH, 15 m*M* $KHCO_3$, 1 m*M* CoA, 10 m*M* propionate, 0.5 μCi (9.5×10^5) 1-(^{14}C) propionate and enzyme suspension from homogenate and mitochondria equivalent to 5 mg or 2.5 mg of protein, respectively. 20 m*M* malonate was added to inhibit conversion to succinic acid wherever necessary (6). The dicarboxylic acids were extracted by ether and separated by descending paper chromatography using butanol:acetic acid:water (100:22:50) as developing solvent (13). The results are typical of four independent experiments.

Our observations can explain some of the functional defects observed in vitamin E deficiency. The reported alterations in the structure and function of cellular membranes in vitamin E deficiency may be partly due to incorporation of branched chain fatty acids derived from methyl malonyl CoA precursors. It is reported (4) that succinyl CoA formed from methyl malonyl CoA is preferentially utilized for heme synthesis. The reduced formation of succinate could explain, partly at least, the reduction in heme synthesis in vitamin E deficiency (14).

References

1 *Akiyama, M.; Minari, O., and Sakagami, T.:* Biochim. biophys. Acta *137:* 525 (1967).
2 *Barness, L.A.:* Am. J. clin. Nutr. *20:* 573 (1967).
3 *Barker, H.A.:* Ann. Rev. Biochem. *41:* 55 (1972).
4 *Cavender, F.L.:* Biochem. Med. *5:* 515 (1971).
5 *Chase, C.D. and Rabinowitz, J.C.:* Principles in radioisotope methodology; p. 203 (Burger Publishing, Minneapolis 1962).
6 *Flavin, M.; Ortiz, P.J., and Ochoa, S.:* Nature *176:* 823 (1955).
7 *Flavin, M. and Ochoa, S.:* J. biol. Chem. *229:* 96 (1957).
8 *Gurnani, S.; Mistry, S.P., and Johnson, B.C.:* Biochim. biophys. Acta *38:* 187 (1960).
9 *Hove, E.L. and Hardin, J.O.:* Fed. Proc. Fed. Am. Socs exp. Biol. *10:* 385 (1951).
10 *Inoue, K. and Kitakawa, T.:* Biochim. biophys. Acta *363:* 361 (1974).
11 *Iyer, S.L.; Katyare, S.S., and Howland, J.L.:* Neuroscience Lett. *2:* 103 (1976).
12 *Lucy, J.A.:* Ann. N.Y. Acad. Sci. *203:* 5 (1972).
13 *Macek, K.:* in *Hais and Macek* Paper chromatography; p. 344 (Academic Press, New York & London 1963).
14 *Nair, P.P.:* Ann. N.Y. Acad. Sci. *203:* 53 (1972).
15 *Oski, F.A.; Myerson, R.; Barness, L.A., and Williams, W.J.:* Am. J. clin. Nutr. *18:* 307 (1966).
16 *Poole, A.R.; Howell, J.I., and Lucy, J.A.:* Nature *227:* 815 (1970).
17 *Portman, O.W. and Alexander, M.:* J. Lipid Res. *10:* 158 (1969).
18 *Portman, O.W.; Soltys, P.; Alexander, M., and Osuga, T.:* J. Lipid Res. *11:* 596 (1970).
19 *Portman, O.W. and Illingworth, D.R.:* J. Lipid Res. *326:* 34 (1973).
20 *Rajaram, O.V.; Fatterpaker, P., and Sreenivasan, A.:* Biochem. biophys. Res. Commun. *52:* 459 (1973).
21 *Rajaram, O.V.; Fatterpaker, P., and Sreenivasan, A.:* Biochem. J. *140:* 509 (1974).
22 *Reed, E.B. and Tarver, H.:* Br. J. Nutr. *23:* 343 (1970).
23 *Schlierf, G. and Wood, P.:* J. Lipid Res. *6:* 317 (1961).
24 *Sugano, M. and Portman, O.W.:* Archs Biochem. Biophys. *109:* 302 (1965).
25 *Takatori, T. and Privette, O.S.:* Lipids *9:* 1018 (1974).
26 *Waite, M. and Sission, P.:* Biochemistry *12:* 2377 (1971).

Dr. *A.S. Pappu,* Biochemistry and Food Technology Division, Bhabha Atomic Research Centre, Trombay, *Bombay 400 085* (India)

Wld Rev. Nutr. Diet., vol. 31, pp. 196–201 (Karger, Basel 1978)

The Vitamin K-Dependent Carboxylation of Glutamyl Residues in a Prothrombin Precursor

J. W. Suttie

Department of Biochemistry, College of Agricultural and Life Sciences, University of Wisconsin-Madison, Madison, Wisc.

Although vitamin K was discovered by Dam in the mid-1930's, little progress in our understanding of the role of the vitamin was made until the mid-1960's. It was clear from early investigations that the vitamin was involved in the biosynthesis of prothrombin (Factor II) and clotting Factors VII, IX and X. Evidence gradually accumulated to support the hypothesis that this vitamin functioned to convert a liver precursor protein to an active prothrombin molecule and this has been recently reviewed (26, 27).

Direct evidence for the presence of a liver precursor was obtained when *Shah and Suttie* (20) demonstrated that the prothrombin produced when hypoprothrombinemic rats were given vitamin K and cycloheximide did not contain radioactive amino acids if they were administered at the same time as the vitamin. The liver precursor hypothesis was strengthened by observations (7, 12) that the plasma of man or animals treated with coumarin anticoagulants contained a protein which was antigeneically similar to prothrombin, but which lacked biological activity. A similar protein was first demonstrated in bovine plasma by *Stenflo* (22). *Carlisle et al.* (1) found little evidence of such a protein in rat plasma but did detect some abnormal prothrombin in the plasma of anticoagulant-treated chicks. They reported that this protein was absent in plasma from anticoagulant-treated mice, hamsters, guinea pigs, rabbits and dogs. The initial studies of this protein indicated that it had the same molecular weight and amino acid composition as normal prothrombin. It did not adsorb to insoluble barium salts as did normal prothrombin and showed a difference in calcium-binding properties (15). The observation (16) that the abnormal prothrombin would yield thrombin when treated with trypsin or snake venoms, indicated that this portion of the molecule was normal and that the critical difference in the two proteins was the inability of the abnormal protein to bind to calcium ions needed for a phospholipid association. This difference has subsequently been directly demonstrated (2). *Nelsestuen and Suttie* (17) isolated an acidic peptide

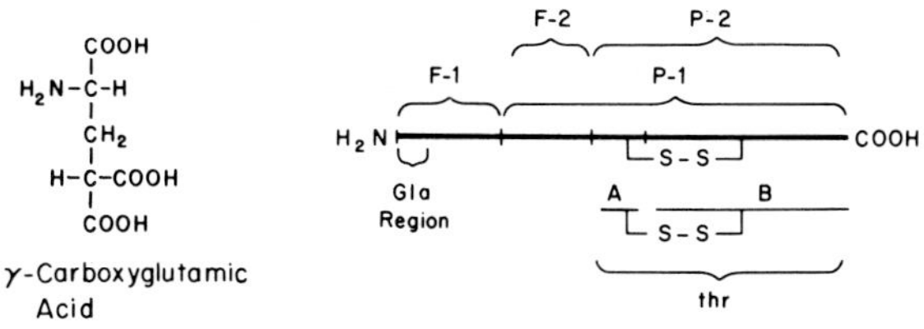

Ala-Asn-Lys-Gly-Phe-Leu-Gla-Gla-Val-Arg-Lys-Gly-Asn-Leu-Gla-Arg-Gla-Cys-Leu-

Gla-Gla-Pro-Cys-Ser-Arg-Gla-Gla-Ala-Phe-Gla-Ala-Leu-Gla-Ser-Leu-

Fig. 1. Structure of γ-carboxyglutamic acid and diagram of prothrombin structure. Prothrombin can be degraded by specific proteases to yield nonthrombin-containing fragments 1 and 2 (F-1, F-2) and thrombin-containing peptides prethrombin 1 and 2 (P-1, P-2). During normal activation of prothrombin, P-2, is cleaved to yield two-chain thrombin. The Gla residues are located in the first 33 residues of the F-1 peptide (14).

from a tryptic digest of normal bovine prothrombin which would adsorb to insoluble barium salts and which bound calcium ions in solution. *Stenflo* (23) later isolated two acidic peptides from prothrombin by different methods. These peptides could not be obtained when similar isolation procedures were applied to preparations of abnormal prothrombin and both groups postulated the existence of some unkown acidic nonpeptide prosthetic group attached to prothrombin in the molecule.

Stenflo et al. (24) succeeded in isolating a tetrapeptide, residues 6–9 of prothrombin which had an apparent sequence of Leu-Glu-Glu-Val and demonstrated that the glutamic acid residues of this peptide were modified as γ-carboxyglutamic acid. (3-amino-1,1,3-propanetricarboxylic acid) residues (fig. 1). Independently, *Nelsestuen et al.* (18), characterized γ-carboxyglutamic acid from a dipeptide (residues 33 and 34 of prothrombin) which appeared originally to be Glu-Ser. These findings have been confirmed by *Magnusson et al.* (14) who have shown that the ten Glu-residues nearest the amino terminal end prothrombin have been modified in this fashion.

Isolation of Liver Precursor Proteins

Early studies suggested that there is an appreciable pool of the precursor in the liver of hypoprothrombinemic animals and *Suttie* (25) demonstrated that when microsomes were isolated from vitamin K-deficient or anticoagulant-treated rats, solubilized with detergent and the extract treated with *Echis carinatus* venom, thrombin activity was generated. Two proteins have subsequently been isolated (3, 8, 9) from the livers of warfarin-treated rats which have the properties predicted for the prothrombin precursor. The first was a glycoprotein immunochemically similar to the prothrombin with a molecular weight (85,000) indistinguishable from rat prothrombin. Electrophoretic and isofocussing analyses indicated that the precursor was less negatively charged (pI – 5.8) than prothrombin (pI – 5.0) and specific proteolysis of the precursor yielded fragments indistinguishable from those formed by similar proteolysis of prothrombin. This protein did not adsorb to $BaSO_4$ and its rate of activiation to thrombin by Factor Xa and Ca^{++} was not stimulated by the addition of phospholipid. The protein isolated appears to differ from rat prothrombin only in that it lacks γ-carboxyglutamic acid residues and the sialic acid residues which are present in plasma prothrombin. More recently, a second protein has been isolated (8) from the same source which has similar properties but which has a pI of 7.2. The charge differences in these two proteins is a property of the F-1 region of the molecule, but the chemical nature of the change has not been determined.

Vitamin K-Dependent Carboxylase

The first vitamin K-dependent *in vitro* system which produced prothrombin was a postmitochondrial supernate preparation described by *Shah and Suttie* (21). Prothrombin production was dependent on an energy supply and was inhibited by antagonists of vitamin K but not by cycloheximide. After the vitamin K-dependent step in prothrombin synthesis was shown to be the formation of γ-carboxyglutamic acid residues, *Esmon et al.* (4), demonstrated that the same postmitochondrial supernatant would catalyze a vitamin K-dependent carboxylation of the endogenous microsomal precursor. Radioactive prothrombin was isolated from this system following incubation and it was shown that essentially all of the radioactivity was present as γ-carboxyglutamic acid residues in the amino-terminal region of prothrombin. The vitamin K-dependent carboxylase has been studied by *Sadowski et al* (19) in washed microsomes where the activity requires the presence of microsomal precursor, O_2, vitamin K, and HCO_3^- and is stimulated by an energy source and factor(s) present in the postmicrosomal supernatant. A major factor in the supernatant is a protein(s) acting as a NAD^+ ($NADP^+$) reductase. That this requirement can be replaced with the addition of NAD(P)H to the system and systems has now been shown (19) to be largely a requirement for the reduced form of vitamin K. The carboxylase activity in this microsomal preparation can be inhibited by warfarin and this inhibition can be overcome by high concentrations of vitamin K.

The carboxylase activity has now been solubilized (5) and the solubilized preparation retains many of the properties of the membrane associated system. The solubilized system still requires O_2, but not ATP and although it is not

Table I. Properties of the vitamin K-dependent carboxylase

A *Absolute requirements*	B *Known inhibitors*
Vitamin K and NAD(P)H	Chloro-K
or vitamin KH_2	Warfarin[1]
O_2	*p*-Hydroxymercuribenzoate
$HCO_3^-(CO_2)$	Spin-trapping agents
Presence of a CO_2 acceptor	Anaerobic conditions
C *Noninhibitory conditions*	D *Stimulatory conditions*
ATP analog AMPP(NH)P[2]	Dithiothritol
Avidin	Additional substrate (peptide)
Cyt. P_{450} inhibitors	
EDTA	

There is not complete agreement in the published literature on all points; the properties assigned represent the authors' evaluation of the consensus of the published literature (4, 5, 6, 10, 11, 13, 19) and unpublished data.
[1] Only when intact microsomes are present.
[2] Some inhibition when intact microsomes are present.

inhibited by warfarin, it is still sensitive to a direct vitamin K antagonist such as 2-chloro-3-phytyl-1,4-naphthoquinone. Other workers (6, 10, 11, 13) have adopted this basic *in vitro* system and have obtained data that is in general consistent with that obtained in our laboratory. The available data (table I) suggest that the energy to drive the carboxylation comes from the reoxidation of the reduced vitamin in the system, but the mechanism remains unclear. There is no evidence to indicate that either biotin or the coenzyme A esters of the glutamyl residues are involved in this carboxylase and it is usually assumed that the vitamin must function either to 'activate' or transfer the HCO_3^- (CO_2) or to labilize the hydrogen on the γ-methylene group of a glutamyl residue.

Carboxylation of Low Molecular Weight Substrates

To study the mechanism of the vitamin K-dependent carboxylase we have developed a series of low molecular weight peptides which would serve as substrates for this enzyme. The first such peptide tested, Phe.Leu.Glu.Glu.Val, which would be analogous to residues 5–9 of the postulated bovine precursor, was shown to be a substrate for the carboxylase (28). The requirements for carboxylation in this system have been studied and they have been found (table II) to be very similar to those observed for carboxylation of the endogenous

Table II. Requirements and inhibitors of peptide carboxylation

Alteration of basic system	Peptide carboxylation % of control system
Complete system	100
— Vitamin K	<10
N_2 atmosphere	15
+ AMPP (NH)P (2 m*M*)	100
— NADH	<10
— Dithiothreitol (DTT)	60
+ Warfarin (40 μg/ml)	95
+ Chloro-K (20 μg/ml)	<10
+ *p*-Hydroxymercuribenzoate (1 m*M*)	<10

The complete system consisted of solubilized microsome from vitamin K-deficient rats incubated with 0.5 *M* peptide, 10 μg/ml vitamin K_1, 1 m*M* DTT, and 1 mg/ml NADH. The data presented have been combined from a number of different experiments.

Table III. Activity of precursor sequence analogs as substrates for the vitamin K-dependent carboxylase and as inhibitors of endogenous precursor carboxylation

Peptide added	Net carboxylation, DPM/ml	
	peptide	protein
None	0	12,700
Phe·Leu·Glu·Glu·Ile	36,800	13,100
Phe·Leu·Glu·Glu·Leu	31,700	13,500
Phe·Glu·Leu·Glu·Leu	0	11,500
Phe·Gly·Glu·Glu·Leu	1,080	11,700
Phe·Glu·Ala·Leu·Glu·Ser·Leu	780	11,600

All peptides were added at 1 m*M*. Previously unpublished peptides were synthesized by Lehrman and D.H. Rich.

precursor. The relative effectiveness of a number of recently synthesized peptides is shown in table III. Six of the ten γ-carboxyglutamic acid residues in prothrombin occur in pairs (fig. 1), and it can be seen that peptides with Glu. Glu. sequences are the best substrates. The various peptides which have been used as substrates do not appreciably influence the carboxylation of the endogenous protein precursors.

Acknowledgement

Previously unpublished data reported here was supported by the College of Agricultural and Life Sciences, University of Wisconsin-Madison, and in part by Grant #AM-14881 from the National Institute of Health.

References

1 *Carlisle, T.L.; Shah, D.V.; Schlegel, R., and Suttie, J.W.:* Proc. Soc. exp. Biol. Med. *148:* 140 (1975).
2 *Esmon, C.T.; Jackson, C.M., and Suttie, J.W.:* J. biol. Chem. *250:* 4095 (1975).
3 *Esmon, C.T.; Grant, G.A., and Suttie, J.W.:* Biochem. *14:* 1595 (1975).
4 *Esmon, C.T.; Sadowski, J.A., and Suttie, J.W.:* J. biol. Chem. *250:* 4744 (1975).
5 *Esmon, C.T. and Suttie, J.W.:* J. biol. Chem. *251:* 6238 (1976).
6 *Friedman, P.A. and Shia, M.:* Biochem. biophys. Res. Commun. *70:* 647 (1976).
7 *Ganrot, P.O. and Nilehn, J.E.:* Scand. J. clin. Lab. Invest. *22:* 23 (1968).
8 *Grant, G.A. and Suttie, J.W.:* Biochem. *15:* 5387 (1976).
9 *Grant, G.A. and Suttie, J.W.:* Archs Biochem. Biophys. *176:* 650 (1976).
10 *Giradot, J.-M.; Mack, D.O.; Floyd, R.A., and Johnson, B.C.:* Biochem. biophys. Res. Commun. *70:* 655 (1976).
11 *Jones, J.P.; Fausto, A.; Houser, R.M.; Gardner, E.J., and Olson, R.E.:* Biochem. biophys. Res. Commun. *72:* 589 (1976).
12 *Josso, F., Lavergne, J.M.; Goualut, M.; Prou-Wartelle, O., and Soulier, J.P.:* Thromb. Diath. haemorrh. *20:* 88 (1968).
13 *Mack, D.O.; Suen, E.T.; Girardot, J.-M.; Miller, J.A.; Delaney, R., and Johnson, B.C.:* J. biol. Chem. *251:* 3269 (1976).
14 *Magnusson, S.; Sottrup-Jensen, L.; Petersen, T.E.; Morries, H.R., and Dell, A.:* FEBS Lett. *44:* 189 (1974).
15 *Neisestuen, G.L. and Suttie, J.W.:* Biochem. *11:* 4961 (1972).
16 *Nelsestuen, G.L. and Suttie, J.W.:* J. biol. Chem. *247:* 8176 (1972).
17 *Nelsestuen, G.L. and Suttie, J.W.:* Proc. natn. Acad. Sci. USA *70:* 3366, 4095 (1973).
18 *Nelsestuen, G.L.; Zytkovicz, T.H., and Howard, J.B.:* J. biol. Chem. *249:* 6347 (1974).
19 *Sadowski, J.A.; Esmon, C.T., and Suttie, J.W.:* J. biol. Chem. *251:* 2770 (1976).
20 *Shah, D.V. and Suttie, J.W.:* Proc. natn. Acad. Sci. USA *68:* 1653 (1951).
21 *Shah, D.V. and Suttie, J.W.:* Biochem. biophys. Res. Commun. *60:* 1397 (1974).
22 *Stenflo, J.:* Acta chem. scand. *24:* 3762 (1970).
23 *Stenflo, J.:* J. biol. Chem. *249:* 5527 (1974).
24 *Stenflo, J.; Fernlund, P.; Egan, W., and Ropestorff, P.:* Proc. natn. Acad. Sci. USA *71:* 2730 (1974).
25 *Suttie, J.W.:* Science *179:* 192 (1973).
26 *Suttie, J.W.:* Vitams Horm. *32:* 463 (1973).
27 *Suttie, J.W. and Jackson, C.M.:* Physiol. Rev. *57:* 1 (1977).
28 *Suttie, J.W.; Hageman, J.M.; Lehrman, S.R., and Rich, D.H.:* J. biol. Chem. *251:* 5827 (1976).

Dr. *J.W. Suttie,* Department of Biochemistry, College of Agricultural and Life Sciences, University of Wisconsin-Madison, *Madison, WI 53706* (USA)

Wld Rev. Nutr. Diet., vol. 31, pp. 202–209 (Karger, Basel 1978)

Biological Role of Vitamin K at the Molecular Level

B. Connor Johnson, Jean Marie Girardot, Eric T. Suen, Donald O. Mack, Robert A. Floyd and Robert Delaney

Vitamin and Nutrition Research Laboratory, Oklahoma Medical Research Foundation, and Department of Biochemistry and Molecular Biology, University of Oklahoma Health Sciences Center, Oklahoma City, Okla.

Vitamin K was shown to be required for prothrombin synthesis in the rat (22, 23) and the site of action of vitamin K was shown to be post-transcriptional (13) and post-translational (1, 14). Finally, the controversy was solved by the discovery of prothrombin carboxylation (9) and the concurrent discovery that the structural difference between normal bovine prothrombin and prothrombin made in the presence of warfarin, was γ-carboxylation of glutamyl residues (20, 28). It was shown by *Magnusson et al.* (17) that 10 glutamyl residues of the pro-piece of prothrombin were carboxylated in this vitamin K-dependent 'completion' step.

The *in vitro* 'finalization' of prothrombin by post-mitochondrial supernatants from vitamin K-deficient rat liver (26) provided the lead for the development of a vitamin K-dependent microsomal carboxylation system (4, 16). It was found that this *in vitro* carboxylation of glutamyl residues of prothrombin (and certain other proteins) did not require the microsomal supernatant, nor the addition of ATP but required vitamin K-deficient liver microsomes, vitamin K, NAD(P)H, bicarbonate and oxygen and was further stimulated by the addition of dithiothreitol (16). Later, the hydroquinone of vitamin K_1 was prepared and found to completely replace the requirements for vitamin K_1 and NADH, and to very greatly reduce the oxygen requirement (8, 10, 24). It was suggested that the semiquinone of vitamin K may be functional, since the carboxylation reaction was blocked by spin-trapping agents (10). Kidney microsomes will also carry out the vitamin K-dependent carboxylation (12) and among the vitamin K forms tested for *in vitro* activity, the 2-methyl-2-fanesyl-1,4-naphthoquinone (MK3) was the most active. However, other reports indicate no significant difference *in vitro* activity between various vitamin K homologues (15).

In this report, I will discuss only our recent unpublished work on the *in vitro* carboxylation system. These studies involve the activity of some forms of vitamin K, the requirement for the β–γ double bond of the phytyl side chain of vitamin K_1, the comparison of the microsomal and solubilized systems, the effect of the hydroquinone on the need for DTT and SH requirement, the lack of involvement of the methyl group of vitamin K, the non-replaceability of the oxygen requirement, the potential function of the semiquinone, evidence against a double-bond derivative of the glutamyl residues as a precursor of di-γ-carboxyl glutamyl groups, and the role of ATP and related compounds.

Preparation of vitamin K-deficient rats, liver microsomal fractions, solubilization of the system, incubation conditions and assay of carboxylation reaction has been described (10, 11, 16).

In the *in vitro* prothrombin carboxylation reaction in the DOC-solubilized vitamin K-deficient rat liver microsomal system, vitamin K_1 quinone (plus NAD(P)H) showed 100% activity while vitamin K_1 hydroquinone showed 160% activity. In this solubilized system, the epoxide, the chromanol, the chromanol phosphate and menadione are without activity. The inactivity *in vitro* of menadione in the absence of dithiothreitol is in agreement with other reports (8, 15, 24). Vitamin K_1, β, γ-dihydride hydroquinone was inactive showing the essentiality of unsaturation in the β,γ position of the phytyl side-chain. This is unexpected in view of the inactivity of the chromanol, and must indicate either ring closure in some other manner or an enzyme binding function for this position. This inactivity of the saturated side-chain compound is in agreement with the reported inactivity of the unnatural β–γ–*cis* configuration (8). The *in vitro* inactivity in carboxylation of demethyl vitamin K has been reported (8), in agreement with its inactivity *in vivo* (6).

The soluble incubation system (solubilized with either Triton X-100 or DOC) is compared to the intact microsome incubation system in table I. Three notable differences are seen. Vitamin K_1 epoxide, while inactive in the soluble system, is highly active in the microsomal system, indicating that the enzyme required for its reconversion to vitamin K_1 has been lost during the solubilization. This appears to finally settle the controversy as to a direct role of the epoxide in vitamin K-dependent carboxylation (30). It appears that the epoxide cannot function without reduction to the vitamin.

The interpretation of the non-effectiveness of warfarin in blocking both K and KH_2-induced carboxylation in the soluble system, while blocking the microsomal system, is less clear. However, in the soluble system, at levels up to 20 μg/ml, inhibition was uniformly about 50%.

On the other hand, while trichloropyridinol inhibited both systems, the inhibition was greater at lower levels in the soluble system. For example, at 0.6 μg/ml, 55% inhibition was obtained in DOC-solubilized system, while the microsomal system gave only 31% inhibition at 5 μg/ml TCP. Does the TCP act as a direct analog inhibitor, or does it act by promoting reoxidation of KH_2 to K, as do similar compounds (chloranil and DDQ)?

Table I. Composition of soluble and microsomal system

Soluble system	Microsomal system
KH_2 active	KH_2 active
K + NAD(P)H active	K + NAD(P)H active
KO inactive	KO active
Less KH_2 required to induce carboxylation with added DTT	KH_2 induced carboxylation does increase with added DTT
With K_1 NADH not completely replaceable	With K_1 DTT can completely replace NADH
Warfarin does not block K or KH_2	Warfarin blocks K or KH_2
TCP inhibits K_1 or KH_2	TCP inhibits
pCMP blocks K_1 or KH_2	pCMP blocks

Table II. Relationship between K and KH_2 and NADH and DTT and SH requirement

Additions	Relative carboxylation activity, %	
	soluble system	microsomal system
K_1 + NADH + DTT	100	100
K_1 + DTT	6	100
K_1 + NADH	77	90
K_1	7	7
K_1 + NADH + PHMB	0	0
K_1H_2	190	
K_1H_2 + NADH	190	
K_1H_2 + DTT	190	
K_1H_2 + NADH + DTT	164	
K_1H_2 + PHMB	6	

Vitamin K_1 and vitamin K_1 hydroquinone (K_1H_2), 20 μg/ml; NADH and DTT, 2 m*M*; PHMB, 1.6 m*M*.

Finally, in the microsomal system, DTT can completely replace NADH in K_1H_2. It will not completely replace the NADH requirement with K_1, even though the SH requirement seems intact in both systems, as evidenced by the complete block brought about by pCMB.

The results for the soluble system are given in table II. They show clearly the inability of DTT to replace NADH under these conditions. However, in the microsomal system, while NADH cannot completely replace DTT, DTT can completely replace NADH. Apparently, some reduction system has been lost by the solubilization.

A number of other reducing agents have been tried in place of NADH and DTT. Reduced glutathione and β-mercaptoethanol in the microsomal system gave 10% of the activity of NADH and DTT, while ascorbic acid, benzhydroquinone, sodium bisulfite and sodium dithionite, had no activity.

In view of the proposal by *Vilkas and Lederer* (29) that the 2-methyl of vitamin K_1 might form an active methine acceptor of a phosphate (and thus, perhaps, of a phosphocarbonate), a number of experiments were carried out to determine whether there was a replaceable hydrogen formed in the vitamin K molecule during the carboxylation reactions. When the incubation was carried out in $[^3H]H_2O$, no incorporation of $[^3H]$ into the vitamin K_1 molecule in any position was found. Similarly, *Sadowski and Suttie* (25) carried out incubations in D_2O and found no deuterium incorporation into vitamin K_1.

While these data indicate that the methyl group cannot be the carrier of the carboxyl group, the essentiality of the 2-methyl group for vitamin K activity, is well established *in vivo* and *in vitro.* The 2-ethyl compound is completely inactive *in vivo* (6), while the 2-methoxy derivative is a vitamin K antagonist (19) and the 2-demethyl vitamin K_1 has been shown to be inactive, both *in vivo* (6) and *in vitro* in carboxylation (8), although it occurs in bacteria (3).

One of the problems in understanding the carboxylation reaction is the oxygen requirement. While it was shown that the use of the hydroquinone of vitamin K_1 greatly decreased the oxygen requirement as compared to the use of vitamin K_1 quinone plus NADH and DTT (10), it was found that even with K_1H_2, there remained a residual O_2 requirement (5). In the soluble system with vitamin K_1 hydroquinone, we observed 100% activity in the presence of oxygen and only 1.8% in its absence. This oxygen requirement is not replaceable by other physiological electron withdrawing agents, such as FAD and vitamin K_1 quinone. A possible role of oxygen was the formation of the semiquinone of vitamin K_1 from K_1H_2; however, FAD should also bring about this reaction. In addition, we also found recently that the semiquinone still requires O_2 to function. $^{18}O_2$ has been shown to be incorporated into vitamin K epoxide (25).

The suggestion was made earlier (10) that the semiquinone of vitamin K may be functional in the carboxylation reaction. By means of electron spin resonance (ESR), it has been established that the partial oxidation product of the hydroquinone in $NaBH_4$ solution is the semiquinone, rather than the quinhydrone. The ESR spectra we obtained for vitamin K_1 semiquinone prepared from vitamin K_1 hydroquinone, is in close agreement with the ESR spectra for the semiquinone free radical of vitamin K_1 (2). The free radical is assigned to the hydroxyl adjacent to the 2-methyl position on the basis of the spectra. When vitamin K_1 quinone was hydrogenated with W_1 Raney Nickel catalyst in metha-

Table III. Inhibition of vitamin K-dependent carboxylation by three spin-trapping agents (vitamin K_1 quinone is used as an initiator of carboxylation)

	Vitamin K_1 quinone[1]				Vitamin K_1 hydroquinone[2]			
	phenyl N-tert -butyl-nitrone							
Amount of spin-trap agent m*M*	0	10.0	50.0	100.0	0	9.0	18.0	36.0
% Activity	100	91	·37	6	100	81	81	83
	5,5-dimethyl-1-pyrroline-N-oxide							
Amount of spin-trap agent m*M*	0	15.0	31.0	92.0	0	18.0	36.0	72.0
% Activity	100	55	41	23	100	54	40	23
	2-methyl-2-nitroso-propane							
Amount of spin-rate agent m*M*	0	10.0	50.0	100.0	Not Done			
% Activity	100	92	56	59				

[1] Complete deoxycholate-solubilized microsomal system. 100% = 5,500 cpm/ml.
[2] Complete deoxycholate-solubilized microsomal system, without added NADH or dithiothreitol. 100% = 8,000 cpm/ml.

nol, two atoms of hydrogen were taken up per molecule of vitamin K. However, the rate of uptake of the first atom was considerably faster than that for the second atom. This result further emphasises the difference between the two carbonyls of the vitamin K_1 quinone.

Further suggestion of the semiquinone function is given by the spin-trapping data shown in table III. A double reciprocal plot of the inhibition of the vitamin K_1 quinone catalysed carboxylation by phenyl-N-tert-butyl-nitrone appeared to indicate competitive inhibition as would be expected if the reagent is trapping an obligatory free radical, may be the semiquinone, may be $\dot{CO}_2$ or $OH^{\cdot}$.

The vitamin K-dependent prothrombin carboxylation reaction must involve at least activation and transfer of a carboxyl group (e.g., a vitamin K carboxyl transfer complex) and activation and removal of hydrogen from the γ-position of the appropriate glutamyl residues of the acceptor protein. If the latter reaction proceeds via oxidation (cf. molecular O_2 requirement) and dehydration, the resultant β–γ unsaturated glutamyl residue would be expected to accept a proton from the medium along with the carboxyl group. Results of a number of experiments in which the reaction was carried out in $[^3H]H_2O$ media, showed no vitamin K-dependent tritiation of protein. Fractionation of the protein by

Table IV. Effects of NADH and dithiothreitol in the carboxylation (menadione versus vitamin K_1)

Additives to the system	Concentration µg/ml	^{14}C cpm NADH	DTT	NADH + DTT
None		53 ± 5	63 ± 6	110 ± 3
Vitamin K_1	10	375 ± 16	55 ± 6	1451 ± 5
	25	695 ± 47	70 ± 1	2943 ± 20
Menadione	10	142 ± 8	1475 ± 88	2092 ± 102
	25	142 ± 8	1806 ± 16	2594 ± 169

[1] The soluble system was prepared as follows: 0.1 ml of vitamin K-deficient microsomes (0.25 g of liver), 0.05 ml 7% Triton X-100, 800 m*M* NaCl, 8 m*M* benzamidine HCl.
The carboxylation assay was conducted as follows: after centrifugation, 0.05 ml of 0.025 *M* imidazole buffer, pH 7.2, containing 5 µCi of ^{14}C sodium bicarbonate, are added to 0.15 ml of supernatant. NADH was 1 m*M* and DTT was 2 m*M* in a final volume of 0.2 ml.

blue dextran affinity chromatography failed to show more tritiation of the vitamin K-dependent proteins. Hence, it appears that the vitamin K-dependent carboxylation must involve some type of direct displacement.

While there is no disagreement as to the lack of biotin participation (11), the question of a role of ATP in the carboxylation has been somewhat less clear. ATP was required in the *in vitro* prothrombin formation system using post-mitochondrial supernatant (26), and more recently the reaction has been shown to be inhibited by the ATP analog AMP-P(NH)P (24). However, no dependence of vitamin K-dependent carboxylation on exogenous ATP can usually be shown (10, 18). We have found that carboxylation was blocked by the addition of apyrase (sigma, impure ATPase). ATP did have a protective effect if included in a preincubation period, and this protection was equally provided by a number of adenine-containing compounds including ATP, ADP, AMP and by NAD and NADP, but not by cyclic AMP. The protective effect of NAD may prove helpful in stabilizing the enzyme system during purification.

Finally, *Fieser and Turner* (7) showed that menadione adds to certain mercaptans and *Nickerson et al.* (21) have shown that glutathione reacts with menadione by nucleophilic substitution to form a thiol addition compound with a UV absorption at 420 nm. *Stadtman* (27) reported that *C. sticklandii* enzyme requires menadione thio ether as a cofactor. In table IV, are given the results of experiments in which the effects of DTT and of NADH on the activity of menadione were studied. These data clearly show that menadione plus DTT is active in vitamin K-dependent carboxylation.

Acknowledgements

This work was supported in part by NIH grants HL 16515 and HL 17619. We also wish to acknowledge the contributions of Dr. Arthur Patchett and his group at Merck, Sharp and Dohme Laboratories, Rahway, New Jersey, for the synthesis of the vitamin K_1 chromanol and chromanol phosphate. Additional acknowledgement is given to Dr. *John Matschiner,* Department of Biochemistry, University of Nebraska Medical Center, Omaha, Nebraska, for vitamin K_1 epoxide.

References

1 *Babior, B.M.:* Biochim. biophys. Acta *123:* 606 (1966).
2 *Blois, M.S., Jr. and Maling, J.E.:* Biochem. biophys. Res. Commun. *3:* 132 (1960).
3 *Dolin, M.I. and Baum, R.H.:* Biochem. biophys. Res. Commun. *18:* 202 (1965).
4 *Esmon, C.T.; Sadowski, J.A., and Suttie, J.W.:* J. biol. Chem. *250:* 4744 (1975).
5 *Esmon, C.T. and Suttie, J.W.:* J. biol. Chem. *251:* 6238 (1976).
6 *Fieser, L.F.; Tishler, M., and Sampson, W.L.:* J. biol. Chem. *137:* 659 (1941).
7 *Fieser, L.F. and Turner, R.:* J. Am. chem. Soc. *69:* 2335 (1947).
8 *Friedman, P.A. and Shia, M.:* Biochem. biophys. Res. Commun. *70:* 647 (1976).
9 *Girardot, J.M.; Delaney, R., and Johnson, B.C.:* Biochem. biophys. Res. Commun. *59:* 11 (1974).
10 *Girardot, J.M.; Mack, D.O.; Floyd, R.A., and Johnson, B.C.:* Biochem. biophys. Res. Commun. *70:* 655 (1976).
11 *Girardot, J.M.; Mack, D.O.; Suen, E.; Delaney, R., and Johnson, B.C.:* J. biol. Chem. (submitted for publication)
12 *Hauschka, P.V.; Friedman, P.A.; Traverso, H.P., and Gallop, P.M.:* Biochem. biophys. Res. Commun. *71:* 1207 (1976).
13 *Hill, R.B.; Gaetani, S.; Paolucci, A.M.; Rama Rao, P.B.; Alden, R.; Ranhotra, G.S.; Shah, D.V.; Shah, V.K., and Johnson, B.C.:* J. biol. Chem. *243:* 3930 (1968).
14 *Johnson, B.C.; Hill, R.B.; Alden, R., and Ranhotra, G.S.:* Life Sci. *5:* 385 (1966).
15 *Jones, J.P.; Fausto, A.; Houser, R.M.; Gardner, E.J., and Olson, R.E.:* Biochem. biophys. Res. Commun. *72:* 1207 (1976).
16 *Mack, D.O.; Suen, E.T.; Girardot, J.M.; Miller, J.A.; Delaney, R., and Johnson, B.C.:* J. biol. Chem. *251:* 3269 (1976).
17 *Magnusson, S.; Sottrup-Jensen, L., and Petersen, T.E.:* FEBS Lett. *44:* 189 (1974).
18 *Metta, V.C.; Nash, L., and Johnson, B.C.:* J. Nutr. *74:* 473 (1961).
19 *Molho, D.; Moraux, J., and Meunier, P.:* Bull. Soc. Chim. biol. Paris *30:* 637 (1948).
20 *Nelsestuen, G.L.; Zytkovicz, T., and Howard, J.B.:* J. biol. Chem. *249:* 6347 (1974).
21 *Nickerson, W.J.; Falconi, G., and Strauss, G.:* Biochemistry *2:* 537 (1963).
22 *Olson, R.E.:* Science *145:* 926 (1964).
23 *Olson, R.E.:* Adv. Enzyme Reg. *7:* 83 (1969).
24 *Sadowski, J.A.; Esmon, C.T., and Suttie, J.W.:* J. biol. Chem. *251:* 2770 (1976).
25 *Sadowski, J.A. and Suttie, J.W.:* Fed. Proc. Fed. Am. Socs exp. Biol. *35:* Abstr. 2517; 662 (1976).
26 *Shah, D.V. and Suttie, J.W.:* Biochem. biophys. Res. Commun. *60:* 1397 (1974).
27 *Stadtman, T.C.:* J. biol. Chem. *234:* 636 (1959).

28 *Stenflo, J.; Fernlund, P.; Egan, W., and Roepstorff, P.:* Proc. natn. Acad. Sci. USA *71:* 2730 (1974).
29 *Vilkas, M. and Lederer, E.:* Experientia *18:* 546 (1962).
30 *Willingham, A.K.; Laliberte, R.E.; Bell, R.G., and Matschiner, J.T.:* Biochem. Pharm. *25:* 1063 (1976).

Dr. *B.C. Johnson,* Department of Biochemistry and Molecular Biology, University of Oklahoma Health Sciences Center, *Oklahoma City, Okla.* (USA)

Wld Rev. Nutr. Diet., vol. 31, pp. 210–215 (Karger, Basel 1978)

Role of Vitamin K in Oxidative Phosphorylation in Mycobacteria[1]

P. Suryanarayana Murthy

Department of Biochemistry, University College of Medical Sciences, New Delhi

Naphthoquinones are present in many species of mycobacteria (4). *Brodie* and co-workers have carried out extensive studies on the role of vitamin K in bioenergetics of *Mycobacterium phlei* (4, 11). Vitamin K is essential not only for electron transport but also for phosphorylation coupled to the oxidation of NAD and $NADP^+$-linked substrates and for the oxidation of malate via the malate vitamin K reductase pathway. Investigations on the metabolism of mycobacteria by several groups of workers have revealed that *M. phlei* is not a true representative of mycobacteria. There are only limited studies on the electron transport mechanisms in other mycobacteria. The NADH oxidase of *Mycobacterium tuberculosis* $H_{37}R_a$ requires vitamin K_2 [45] (9).

Studies on the reconstitution of oxidative phosphorylation in irradiated electron transport particles (ETP) of *M. phlei* with naphthoquinones have indicated that a methyl group at the C-2 position and at least one isoprene unit in the C-3 side chain are required for restoring both oxidation and phosphorylation (3). Maximum restoration of phosphorylation is observed only with vitamin K_2 [10] and K_2 [15]. There appears to be some specificity with regard to the geometric arrangement of the side chain of the naphthoquinone as well (6). *DiMari et al.* (5) and *Schnyder and Rapoport* (14) have contradicted the above findings of *Gutnick and Brodie* (7). Therefore, studies on the mechanism of electron transport and coupled phosphorylation with various substrates have been undertaken using two species of mycobacteria, namely *Mycobacterium smegmatis,* a fast grower, and *M. tuberculosis* $H_{37}R_v$, the slow growing human pathogen. For comparison *M. phlei* has been used.

The strains of mycobacteria used, preparation of coupled electron transport particles, methods of estimation of dehydrogenases and measurements of oxidative phosphorylation have been described earlier (12).

[1] This work was carried out in the Department of Biochemistry, V.P. Chest Institute, University of Delhi, Delhi, in association with *T.L.P. Reddy* and *T.A.V. Subramanian.*

Table I. Localization and activity[1] of some dehydrogenases in mycobacteria

	Cofactor or electron acceptor	*M. smegmatis*		*M. phlei*		*M. tuberculosis* $H_{37}R_V$	
		ETP	S	ETP	S	ETP	S
Malate dehydrogenase	NAD^+	ND	0.4	ND	170.0	ND	338.0
Malic enzyme	$NADP^+$	ND	15.0	ND	13.0	ND	ND
Malate-vitamin K reductase	FAD-MTT	156.0	23.0	112.0	84.0	1.6	1.8

ETP = Electron transport particle; S = supernatant fraction; ND = not detectable.
[1] Enzyme activity is expressed as nmoles of cofactor or dye reduced/min/mg protein.

Localization and Role of Malate Vitamin K Reductase in Mycobacteria

Flavin-dependent malate dehydrogenase requiring vitamin K (malate vitamin K reductase) takes part in the oxidation and phosphorylation of malate in *M. phlei* (1, 15). The activity of this enzyme was tested in the two mycobacteria. The enzyme was present in the two fast growers *M. smegmatis* and *M. phlei* (table I). It is also clear from table I that malate vitamin K reductase was the only malate dehydrogenase present in *M. smegmatis,* the usual NAD^+-dependent malate dehydrogenase being absent. On the other hand, in the slow grower *M. tuberculosis* $H_{37}R_V$ malate vitamin K reductase was present only in negligible amounts and the organism possessed NAD^+-dependent malate dehydrogenase. The significance of malate vitamin K reductase in the generation of ATP is clear when it is realised that in both *M. smegmatis* and *M. tuberculosis* $H_{37}R_V$, malate was the preferred substrate for oxidation. Malate oxidation was associated with phosphorylation. Since the ETP of *M. smegmatis* were capable of oxidising malate without supplementation by supernatant fraction or any exogenous cofactors, it appeared that the ETP possessed all the cofactors necessary for malate vitamin K reductase activity. As stated earlier, malate vitamin K reductase requires FAD, vitamin K_1 or the natural naphthoquinone, a phospholipid and Mg^{++} ions (1, 15). The enzyme was sensitive to heat treatment. Heating at 55°C for 15 min, as done by *Bogin et al.* (2), for unmasking the ETP of *M. phlei* with respect to succinate and NADH oxidation, resulted in almost complete loss of malate oxidation in *M. smegmatis.*

Participation of Vitamin K in the Respiratory Chain of Mycobacteria

To understand the possible role of vitamin K in the respiratory chains of mycobacteria, it is necessary to establish the sequence of the respiratory components. By following the reduction of endogenous cytochromes and by using inhibitors of oxidative phosphorylation with various systems the respiratory chains of *M. smegmatis* and *M. tuberculosis* have been established (12). Cytochromes *b, c,* $(a+a_3)$ and *o* are functional in *M. smegmatis* while cytochrome *o* is absent in *M. tuberculosis* $H_{37}R_v$ (unpublished observations). Irradiation of ETP with UV light (360 nm) to destroy the natural naphthoquinone, and solvent extraction to remove selectively the lipid quinones have been used as tools in *M. phlei* to demonstrate the role of vitamin K in oxidative phosphorylation. Irradiation of ETP prepared from *M. smegmatis* for 10 min resulted in about 50% loss of oxidation as well as phosphorylation with malate, succinate and NADH. When such preparations were supplemented with vitamin K_1, only malate and NADH oxidations were partially restored. However, irradiation for 30 min or more resulted in total loss of phosphorylation while a very low rate of oxidation indicating that phosphorylation was more sensitive to UV irradiation than oxidation. The loss in oxidation and phosphorylation could not be reversed by vitamin K when the ETP were exposed to UV light for 30 min or more. These results point to the possible existence of a second light sensitive component in malate (FAD) and NAD^+-pathways, besides vitamin K, in *M. smegmatis.* Loss of succinate oxidation by the ETP when irradiated for even 10 min could not be restored by vitamin K_1. This observation rules out the participation of vitamin K in the succinate pathway of *M. smegmatis.* The results of the present investigation on irradiation studies are in contrast to the observations of *Brodie and Ballantine* (3).

High protein concentrations of the crude extracts protected the light-sensitive component of *M. phlei* from destruction (16). Vitamin K_1 could almost completely restore malate oxidase activity when crude extracts of *M. smegmatis* irradiated for 30 min, whereas with ETP alone there was irreversible loss of activity. However, after 30 min of irradiation, the crude extracts also were inactive even after supplementation with vitamin K_1. These results suggest that high protein concentration of supernatant protects the second light sensitive component in *M. smegmatis*, at least up to 30 min. Isooctane extraction of *M. smegmatis* ETP resulted in complete loss of malate oxidation which, however, could be restored by adding vitamin K_1. This implied that isooctane probably extracted the natural naphthoquinone but not the second light-sensitive component.

These studies show that as in *M. phlei, M. smegmatis* also possesses three respiratory chain pathways, namely: NAD^+-pathway for NAD^+ and $NADP^+$-linked substrates, malate-FAD pathway for malate oxidation and succinate pathway.

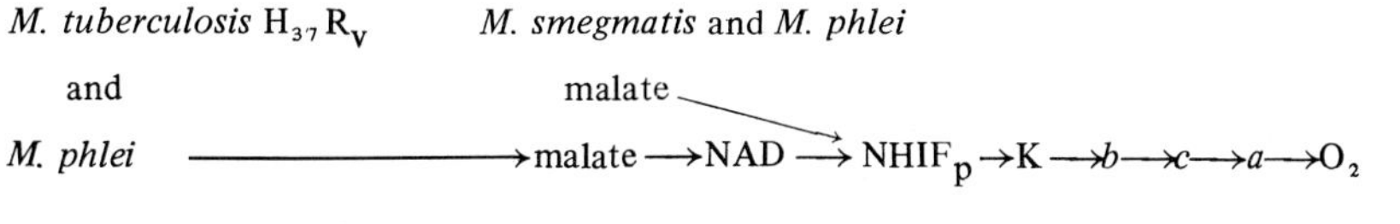

Fig. 1. Pathways of malate oxidation in mycobacteria.

Vitamin K takes part in the NAD^+-pathway and malate FAD pathway but not in the succinate pathway.

Cell-free extracts of *M. tuberculosis* $H_{37}R_V$ lost malate oxidase activity on irradiation, which could be restored by addition of vitamin K_1. This observation and the sensitivity of malate oxidase to dicumarol, suggest for the participation of vitamin K in malate oxidation in this bacterium. Thus, in *M. tuberculosis* also there are NAD^+ and succinate pathways but no malate FAD pathway since malate vitamin K reductase is absent.

Role of Vitamin K in the Three Enzyme Systems for Malate Oxidation in Mycobacteria

It is clear from the above studies that vitamin K is essential for the oxidation of malate as well as for coupled phosphorylation. However, the three species of mycobacteria investigated represent the three different systems known for malate oxidation and the differences appear to be in the dehydrogenases which initiate malate oxidation (12). These are shown in fig. 1.

Location of Vitamin K and Non-Heme Iron in the Malate FAD Pathway in M. smegmatis

According to *Kurup and Brodie* (8) non-heme iron acts at a site between vitamin K_1 and the artificial electron acceptor MTT tetrazolium insoluble malate vitamin K reductase of *M. pheli.* These authors have not investigated the sequence in the electron transport particles. *M. smegmatis* is suited for a study of this type because, unlike *M. phlei*, it possesses only malate vitamin K reductase. Therefore, experiments were conducted on the FAD-cytochrome *b* segment of malate FAD pathway in the particulate malate vitamin K reductase. A combination of phenazine methosulphate (PMS) and dichlorophenol indophenol (DCPIP) as well as (MTT) tetrazolium were used as electron acceptors since these are known to tap the electrons at flavin and cytochrome *b* levels, respectively (8). The lower activity (one third) of malate vitamin K reductase assayed with the electron acceptor MTT when compared with PMS-DCPIP may indicate that some

Table II. Effect of o-phenanthroline and irradiation on particulate malate – vitamin K reductase of *M. smegmatis*

System	Malate – vitamin K reductase activity, nmoles of the dye reduced/min/mg protein	
	PMS – DCPIP	MTT
ETP	89.0	26.0
ETP + *o*-phenanthroline (5 m*M*)	33.5	9.3
ETP + *o*-phenanthroline (10 m*M*)	3.6	1.5
Irradiated ETP	10.0	2 0

component of the respiratory chain between the flavin and cytochrome may be rate limiting.

The malate vitamin K reductase activity in the irradiated ETP (table II) is considerably decreased irrespective of the electron acceptor(s) used. If vitamin K is the only light-sensitive component, only MTT reduction would be affected, but not that of PMS-DCPIP. The loss of the latter indicates that the flavin region of the respiratory chain is also affected by irradiation.

o-Phenanthorline (10 m*M*) inhibited the reduction of both the dyes in a similar manner as noticed in the irradiated ETP (table II). These observations indicate that flavoprotein in combination with non-heme iron, functions on the substrate side of vitamin K in the malate FAD-pathway of *M. smegmatis.*

Support for the above observation came from electron paramagnetic resonance (EPR) studies. On addition of malate to normal ETP, a signal at $g = 2.00$ was obtained. Irradiated particles alone or in the presence of malate did not show the signal. Many ferredoxin-like proteins have g values between 1.89 and 2.02 (10). Therefore, the EPR signal, by the ETP of *M. smegmatis* may be attributed to a ferredoxin-like protein. Irradiation probably destroyed the binding between flavin and iron in such a way that malate failed to reduce the iron part of the molecule. It probably implies that the environment around the metal is an essential requirement for its reduction by the substrate.

References

1 *Asano, A.; Kaneshiro, T., and Brodie, A.F.:* J. biol. Chem. *240:* 895 (1965).
2 *Bogin, E.; Higashi, T., and Brodie, A.F.:* Proc. natn. Acad. Sci. USA *67:* 1 (1970).
3 *Brodie, A.F. and Ballantine, J.:* J. biol. Chem. *235:* 226 (1960).
4 *Brodie, A.F. and Gutnick, D.L.:* in *King and Klingenberg* Electron and coupled energy transfer in biological systems; vol. 1, part B, p. 599 (Marcel Dekker, New York 1972).
5 *DiMari, S.J.; Snyder, C.D., and Rapoport, H.:* Biochemistry *7:* 2301 (1968).

6 *Gutnick, D.L.; Dunphy, P.J.; Sakamoto, H.; Phillips, P.G., and Brodie, A.F.:* Science *158:* 1469 (1967).
7 *Gutnick, D.L. and Brodie, A.F.:* J. biol. Chem. *240:* 3698 (1965).
8 *Kurup, C.K.R. and Brodie, A.F.:* Biochem. biophys. Res. Commun. *28:* 862 (1967).
9 *Kusunose, E. and Goldman, D.S.:* Biochim. biophys. Acta *73:* 391 (1963).
10 *Palmer, G. and Brintzinger, H.:* in *King and Klingenberg* Electron and coupled energy transfer in biological systems; vol. 1, part B, p. 379 (Marcel Dekker, New York 1972).
11 *Ramakrishnan, T.; Suryanarayana Murthy, P., and Gopinathan, K.P.:* Bact. Rev. *36:* 69 (1972).
12 *Reddy, T.L.P.; Suryanarayana Murthy, P., and Venkitasubramanian, T.A.:* Biochim. biophys. Acta *376:* 210 (1975).
13 *Shetna, Y.I.; Wilson, P.W.; Hansen, R.E., and Beinert, H.:* Proc. natn. Acad. Sci. USA *52:* 1263 (1964).
14 *Snyder, C.D. and Rapoport, H.:* Biochemistry *7:* 2318 (1968).
15 *Suryanarayana Murthy, P.; Bogin, E.; Higashi, T., and Brodie, A.F.:* J. biol. Chem. *244:* 3117 (1969).
16 *Weber, M.M. and Rosso, G.:* Proc. natn. Acad. Sci. USA *50:* 710 (1963).

Dr. *P. Suryanarayana Murthy,* Department of Biochemistry, University College of Medical Sciences, *New Delhi 110 016* (India)

Wld Rev. Nutr. Diet., vol. 31, pp. 216–225 (Karger, Basel 1978)

New Developments in the Study of the Vitamin K-Dependent Carboxylation System

Robert E. Olson

Edward A. Doisy Department of Biochemistry, St. Louis University School of Medicine, St. Louis, Mo.

The discovery of γ-carboxyglutamic acid (GLA) in a tetrapeptide (Leu-Gla-Gla-Val) isolated from bovine prothrombin and representing residues 6–9 by *Stenflow* (25) and similar findings by *Nelsestuen et al.* (20) and *Magnusson et al.* (18) were the first specific clues to the action of the vitamin K. This new amino acid was absent from the corresponding peptide derived from the abnormal inactive prothrombin present in the plasma of cows who had been fed dicoumarol. These findings strengthened the view that vitamin K was involved in a post-translational carboxylation of an inactive precursor peptide. *Magnusson et al.* (18) further observed that in fact all glutamic acids in the first 40 amino acids from the N-terminus (at positions 7, 8, 15, 17, 20, 21, 26, 27, 30 and 33), were γ-carboxylated. These discoveries stimulated a flurry of studies of CO_2 fixation into prothrombin under various conditions. In vitamin K-deficient rats given $(H^{14}CO_3)^-$, *Olson* (21) found little evidence of $(^{14}CO_2)$ incorporation into prothrombin. *Girardot et al.* (12) dosed vitamin K-deficient rats with $(H^{14}CO_3)^-$ and reported that a (^{14}C)-tryptic peptide from plasma prothrombin contained a labeled acidic amino acid which yielded unlabeled glutamate on boiling. Since then many laboratories have taken up the study of the function of vitamin K in peptide-bound glutamate carboxylation.

The first vitamin K-dependent *in vitro* system of post-mitochondrial supernate catalyzing the incorporation of $(H^{14}CO_3)^-$ into the endogenous microsomal precursor protein was described by *Esmon et al.* (7) and *Shah and Suttie* (24). In this *in vitro* system essentially all of the radioactivity was incorporated into γ-carboxyglutamic acid residues in the Fragment 1 portion of prothrombin. The vitamin K-dependent synthesis and modification of precursor prothrombin has also been demonstrated in H-35 hepatoma cells in culture (19).

Three related systems derived from rat liver, which have slightly different properties, have been used to study the vitamin K-dependent carboxylase reaction. These are: (i) post-mitochondrial supernatant suspension (full system)

Table I. Requirements for prothrombin synthesis in rat liver microsomes

Conditions	Prothrombin synthesis, % control[1]
Complete system	100 ± 2
– Vitamin K_1	3 ± 1
– ATP, PC, CPK	50 ± 2
– O_2 (N_2 + glucose + glucose oxidase)	5 ± 3
– Cytosolic proteins + NADH (2 m*M*)	40 ± 10
– Dialysate of cytosol	20 ± 2
– Dialysate of cytosol + NADH (2 m*M*)	89 ± 4
+ Puromycin (100 μg/ml)	95 ± 3
+ Metyrapone (200 μ*M*)	89 ± 3
+ CN^- 0.5 m*M*	90 ± 5
+ Avidin (60–180 μg/ml)	90 ± 5
+ FCCP (2 μ*M*)	95 ± 3

The complete system contained 4 ml of post-mitochondrial supernatant equivalent to 2.0 g liver from a vitamin K-deficient rat, 1.0 ml of an energy-generating system which provided 1 m*M* ATP, 10 m*M* creatine phosphate, 50 μg/ml creatine kinase, and 50 m*M* KCl, 2.5 m*M* $Mg(Ac)_2$, 250 m*M* sucrose, 25 m*M* imidazole buffer pH 7.2 and 20 μg phylloquinone in 20 μl ethanol/ml. Incubation was carried out for 15 min at 37°C in air.

[1] % conversion of precursor to prothrombin in the complete system was 56.7 ± 1.2% (SEM).

which contains microsomes, variable amounts of other non-mitochondrial particles, and cystosolic proteins; (ii) washed microsomes suspended in a buffer fortified with various coenzymes and factors, and (iii) microsomes solubilized with detergents. In all three systems the vitamin K-dependent carboxylation of peptide-bound glutamate residues has been demonstrated. Significant differences in the vitamin K requirements, the effect of vitamin K homologues, prothrombin yield, apparent γ-carboxyglutamate synthesis, ATP requirement and warfarin sensitivity have been observed.

The requirements of the full system are shown in table I. The results are similar to those reported by *Shah and Suttie* (24). The cytosolic proteins are required for maximum yields of prothrombin. The presence of vitamin K reductase and proteins concerned with 'completion' of prothrombin in the cytosol may be responsible for this effect. The system was insensitive to puromycin, metyrapone (an inhibitor of P 450), cyanide, avidin, and FCCP (trifluoromethyl carbonyl cyanide phenylhydrazone, an inhibitor of oxidative phosphorylation).

The dose-response curve for phylloquinone in the presence and absence of warfarin (100 mg/ml) is shown in figure 1. The vehicle for this vitamin (ethanol *vs* tween) made no difference in the response. With phylloquinone, the dose-re-

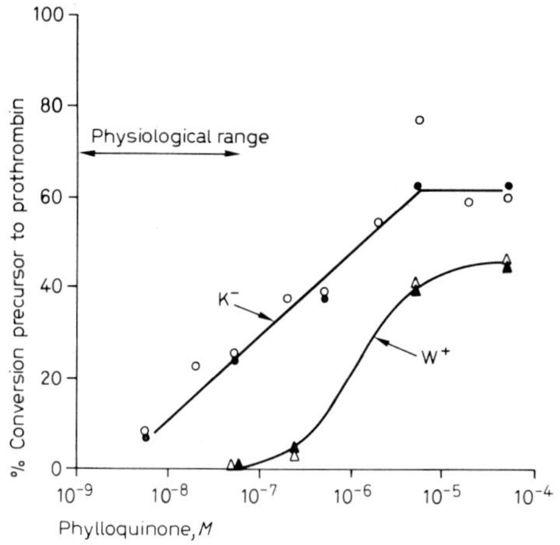

Fig. 1. Effect of dose of phylloquinone upon prothrombin formation in liver microsomes plus cytosol from vitamin K-deficient rats. Phylloquinone was given in ether ethanol OW or tween. The lower curve shows the effect of warfarin (100 μg/ml) at various phylloquinone concentrations.

sponse curve was semi-logarithmic over a wide range (10^{-4} to $10^{-8}M$) which is more typical of whole animals (14) than enzyme-substrate reactions. This reflects the complexity of the carboxylase system and the diversity of vitamin K metabolizing systems in post-mitochondrial suspensions of liver. With warfarin present, little inhibition occurred at pharmacological vitamin K doses ($10^{-5}M$) but at physiological vitamin K doses (10^{-6}–$10^{-8}M$) marked inhibition of conversion was observed. The shape of the dose-response curve shifted from a semi-logarithmic one to a sigmoid one more typical of ligand-protein interactions.

A study of homologues in the full system showed that menaquinone-4, like phylloquinone, showed a broad log dose-response curve encompassing the range between $4 \times 10^{-9}M$ to $4 \times 10^{-6}M$ (14, 16). On the other hand, menaquinone-3 showed a somewhat lower response to high concentrations and menaquinone-2 showed a very different dose-response curve resembling that occurring with phylloquinone in the presence of warfarin. Menaquinone-1 at $4 \times 10^{-5}M$ was only 30% as effective as phylloquinone. Menadione and 2,3-dimethyl, 1,4-naphthoquinone were inactive. When the homologues are studied at different temperatures, it was found that the apparent energy of activation for the vitamin K-dependent conversion varied with the length of the isoprenoid side chain. It was surprising that at 0°C menaquinone-2 had 30% of the activity it manifested at 37°C. The results of a study of vitamins K_1, menaquinone-2, menaquinone-3

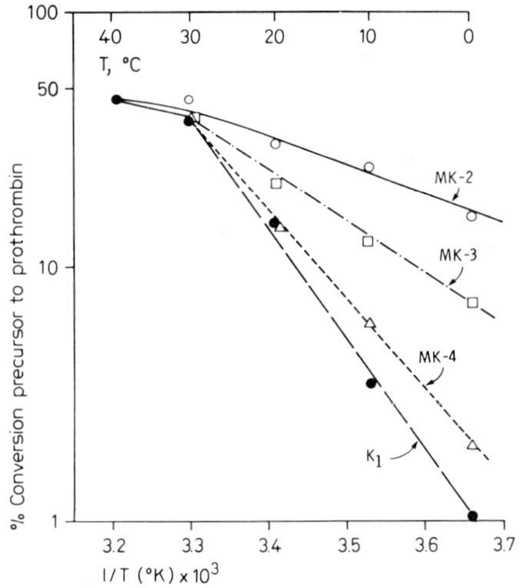

Fig. 2. Effect of temperature upon prothrombin formation in liver microsomes plus cytosol from vitamin K-deficient rats. The conversion rate is plotted against the reciprocal of the absolute temperature according to Arrhenius. The incubations were carried out for 15 min.

and menaquinone-4 are presented in figure 2 as Arrhenius plots. With increasing side chain lengths, there were progressively increasing activation enthalpies. The values for these activation enthalpies varied from 5 kCal/mole for menaquinone-2 to 20 kCal/mole for phylloquinone. Because of the lack of a clear break in the melting curve for menaquinone-2, it is assumed that this homologue does not interact with the bilayer, but may interact with a peripheral portion of the membrane containing the vitamin K-dependent carboxylase. Longer chain homologues show typical break points corresponding to the melting point of the membrane.

Half maximal activity of the reaction was obtained with a $_{p}O_2$ about 10 mm Hg. This value was considerably higher than that of cytochrome oxidase which is of the order 0.5 mm Hg (3), about the same order as that of cytochrome P_{450}-dependent cholesterol 7-α-hydroxylase (1), and lower than that of phylloquinone 2,3-epoxidase (28). Since both reduction and oxidation of vitamin K are required for the carboxylation reaction, it is possible that the oxygen requiring step is a direct oxidation of the reduced quinone or its derivative.

With regard to the bicarbonate requirement, estimates have ranged from 2 m*M* (22) to 20 m*M* (5). We discovered that with an endogenous level of about 4 m*M* bicarbonate in post-mitochondrial supernatant, no additions of CO_2 or bicarbonate were necessary to obtain full activity (28). When cytosol was dialyzed against a CO_2-free buffer, and small amounts of bicarbonate were added, the bicarbonate level required to give half-maximal activity was found to be 0.2 m*M*. Such a low apparent k_m value for 'CO_2' generally indicates that bicarbonate is the active species in this reaction rather than CO_2. Since biotin-deficiency does not reduce plasma prothrombin levels, avidin does not inhibit the reaction (28) and a partially solubilized system does not require ATP (22), it is not likely that this vitamin K-dependent carboxylation is biotin-dependent.

We have (17) investigated the active species of 'CO_2' in the microsomal system by the low temperature method of *Filmer and Cooper* (8). This was possible only because menaquinone-2 is quite active at 10°C in the microsomal system. The reactions were carried out with washed microsomes in the presence of cycloheximide, avidin and acetazolamide to inhibit respectively protein synthesis, biotin-dependent reactions, and carbonic anhydrase. ($^{14}CO_2$) or ($H^{14}CO_3$)– were generated preferentially and the rate of uptake of isotope from each species into γ-carboxyglutamate residues in microsomal protein was measured at minute intervals for 5 min. The incorporation of radioactivity from ($^{14}CO_2$) after 1 min was 5–10 times that from ($H^{14}CO_3$)– as shown in figure 3. The presence of 1 m*M* ATP or the inhibitor ADP-NH-P had no effect on the rate of uptake of either species, indicating that the intrinsic CO_2– fixation reaction is not ATP-dependent.

It has been observed by several investigators (9, 16) that menadione and 2,3-dimethyl-1,4-naphthoquinone have no activity in the membrane associated carboxylase system. Likewise, our studies with menadione and NADH as a reductant and even menadiol showed no activity in the soluble system. When 2 m*M* DTT is added to the soluble system with menadione, however, the vitamin K-dependent system is activated to the extent of 50% when compared with phylloquinone. *Gardner* (11) in my laboratory, has recently observed that when menadione is incubated with dithiothreitol, a thio-ether derivative in the 3 position is formed by alkylation. This compound has been isolated by thin layer chromatography and characterized by UV, NMR and mass spectrometry. It appears that a thio-ether side chain of only 4 carbon atoms will suffice to confer biological activity on menadione (fig. 4). *Carter and Warner* (2) observed earlier that the 3-mercaptopropionic acid adduct of menadione was active in cholecystonephrostomized dogs and in a human patient with liver disease.

A search for artificial synthetic substrates for the carboxylation reaction has been successful. *Suttie et al.* (26) reported that the pentapeptide, Phe-Leu-Glu-Glu-Val analogous to residues 5–9 in bovine precursor prothrombin can be carboxylated in the soluble rat microsomal system. Carboxylation activity was higher with the artificial substrate in solubilized vitamin K-deficient rat liver microsomes as compared to normal ones, suggesting that the carboxylase enzyme is induced or activated in the vitamin K-deficient state.

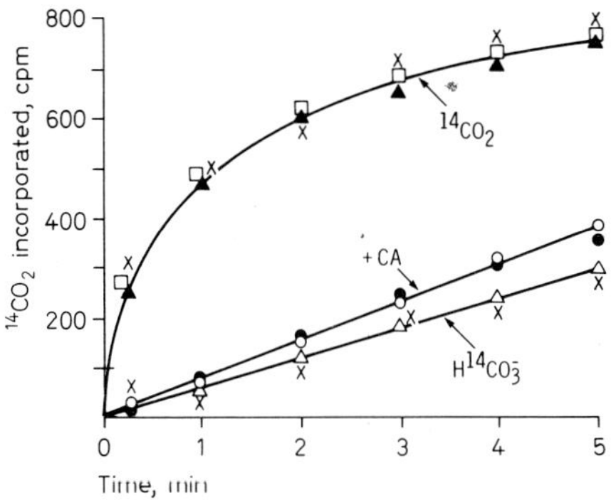

Fig. 3. Menaquinone-2-dependent radioactivity incorporated into γ-carboxyglutamate residues of microsomes when either $(H^{12}CO_3)^-$ + $(^{14}CO_2)$ (▲) or $(H^{14}CO_3)^-$ + $(^{12}CO_2)$ (△) were added initially in the presence of carbonic anhydrase inhibitor Diamox® at 1 m*M* and in the absence of ATP. (X) values were obtained in the presence of 1 m*M* adenylyl-imidodiphosphate and (□) values were obtained in the presence of 1 m*M* ATP. When the carbonic anhydrase inhibitor was omitted from the reaction mixture (+CA) the curves represented by $(^{14}CO_2)$ + $(H^{12}CO_3)^-$ (●) or $(^{12}CO_2)$ + $(H^{14}CO_3)^-$ (○) were obtained.

1.)

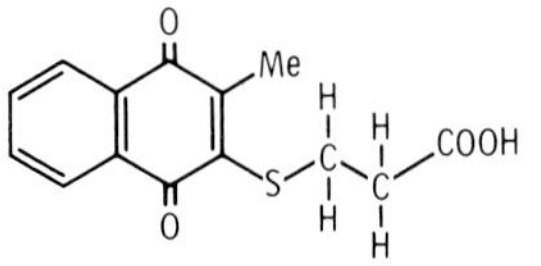

Vitamin K-S: S-(2-methyl-1, 4 napthoquinonyl-3)-β-mercaptopropionic acid

2.)

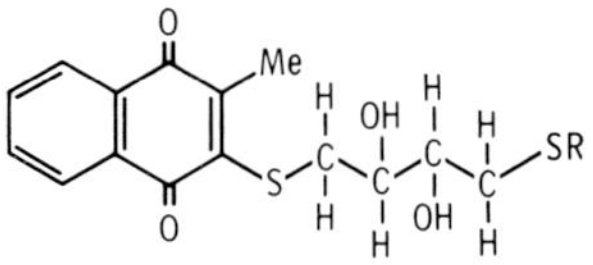

S-(2methyl,-1, 4, napthoquinonyl-3)-dithiothreitol

Fig. 4. Thio-derivatives of vitamin K with biological activity: (1) vitamin K-S and (2) menadione-DTT R = $(DTT)_n$ or/menadione.

We have compared the activity of this pentapeptide, Phe-Leu-Glu-Glu-Val, with the homologous pentapeptide, Phe-Leu-Glu-Glu-Ile which imitates the sequence of prothrombin precursor in the rat (15) and observed that the Ile-peptide was 3 times as active as the Val-peptide in the solubilized rat carboxylation system at concentrations of 3 m*M*. It appears that the vitamin K-dependent carboxylase will recognize short sequences of the physiological substrate.

The biochemical mechanism of the vitamin K-dependent carboxylation of peptide-bound glutamate is still unclear. We have speculated about the possibility of vitamin K serving as a carboxyl carrier in the reaction. A possible mechanism by which vitamin K might serve this function is shown in figure 5. After reduction of vitamin K by NADH to vitamin KH_2, the hydroquinone anion makes a nucleophilic attack on CO_2 to form the hemicarbonate. In the presence of O_2, the hemicarbonate would be reoxidized to the quinone and the CO_2 released for carboxylation of peptide-bound glutamate to yield peptide-bound γ-carboxyglutamate (fig. 5A). This mechanism is analogous to that suggested by *Clark et al.* (6) to explain oxidative phosphorylation. This hypothesis is under active study in several laboratories. The hemicarbonate ethyl ester of menaquinone-2 labeled with (^{14}C) in the carbonate moiety has been synthesized and tested in the microsomal and detergent-solubilized systems in St. Louis without, thus far, demonstrating γ-carboxyglutamate synthesis in either endogenous or synthetic pentapeptide substrates. The problem may be the delivery of the putative intermediate to the active site of the enzyme, particularly since the ethyl ester must be hydrolyzed before the organic carbonate, which is extremely labile, is free to react with the substrate. Although esterases are known to be present in the retinulum, and we have demonstrated generation of free ($^{14}CO_2$) under the conditions of our experiments, the externally added intermediate may be in a different environment to the one generated internally. This mechanism deserves, and will undoubtedly get, much additional study.

Another possibility, which appeared interesting in view of the essentiality of the 2-methyl group of vitamin K for activity involves the formation of the chromenol and subsequently the quinone methine. *Fuson,* in 1935, proposed that quinones of methyl substituents on the ring might react in a tautomeric quinone methine form (10). *Chmielewska and Cieslak* (4) and *Vilkas and Lederer* (27) considered such a tautomerism for vitamin K with chromane formation and proposed a mechanism for the formation of a phosphate involving the double bond of the side chain of vitamin K and the 1,2 addition of a phosphate on a methine quinone. The analogous reaction with CO_2 would result in the function of a cyclic carbonate. Unfortunately, neither vitamin K chromenol or chromanol are active in the carboxylation reaction (11, 13). *Sadowski et al.* (23) were unable to detect the formation of the chromenol in systems studied with D_2O in the reaction medium.

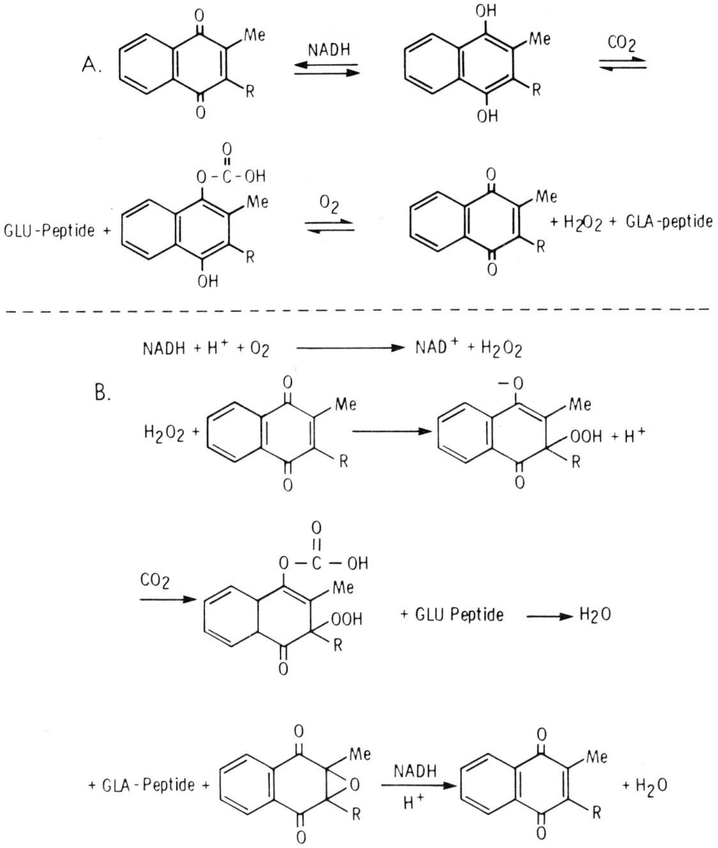

Fig. 5. Vitamin K hydroquinone carbonates as possible intermediates in the vitamin K-dependent carboxylase system.

Another hypothesis is shown in fig. 5B. It postulates that hydrogen peroxide is the driving force in the reaction, generated by a flavin-catalyzed oxidation of NADH. The peroxide anion makes a Michael's addition to the quinone which generates a phenolic anion, which in turn attacks CO_2 to give a hemicarbonate. Upon decarboxylation, vitamin K-2,3-epoxide and water would be formed. This mechanism provides for vitamin K epoxide formation to be linked to transcarboxylation as has been suggested by *Willingham and Matschiner* (28). If this mechanism were true, peroxide should replace the oxygen requirement, and catalase should inhibit the reaction, which so far has not been reported.

Another chemical problem in the reaction mechanism leading to γ-carboxyglutamate synthesis is the need for activation of the γ-proton of peptide bound glutamate in order to produce a carbanion and thus facilitate the introduction of CO_2. In an analogous reaction catalyzed by propionyl-CoA carboxylase, the thioester formed with CoA increases the aldehyde character of the carbonyl, promotes enolization and generates a negative charge on the α-carbon atom. As yet, there is no evidence that CoA esters of the susceptible glutamate residues of preprothrombin are formed, particularly as there is no ATP requirement. Phosphate anhydrides of glutamate are known, but they generally do not promote enolization. Another mechanism for activating the γ-carbon atom would be to bring a nucleophile into the proximity of the appropriate proton. In a lipid medium, hydride ion transfer from NADH to vitamin K might yield an interim species of KH^- which could serve as a nucleophile.

References

1 *Boyd, G.S.; Grimwade, A.M., and Lawson, M.C.:* Studies on rat-liver microsomal cholesterol 7a-hydroxylase. Eur. J. Biochem. *37:* 334 (1973).

2 *Carter, J.R. and Warner, E.D.:* Correction of defects in clotting accelerator activity by administration of methionine and vitamin K and of a new sylfhydryl-substituted methylnaphthquinone, vitamin K-S (11). J. clin. Invest. *37:* 70 (1958).

3 *Chance, B.:* Cellular oxygen requirements. Fed. Proc. Fed. Am. Socs exp. Biol. *16:* 671 (1957).

4 *Chmielewska, I. and Cieslak, J.:* Vitamins and anti-vitamin K. Tautomerism of dicoumarol. Tetra. *16:* 671 (1957).

5 *Chung, G.C.H.; Delaney, R.; Mack, D., and Johnson, B.C.:* Partial purification and characterization of the enzyme which converts precursor liver protein to Factor X. Biochim. biophys Acta *386:* 556 (1975).

6 *Clark, V.M.; Kirby, G.W., and Todd, A.:* Oxidative phosphorylation: a chemical approach using quinol phosphates. Nature *181:* 1650 (1958).

7 *Esmon, C.T.; Sadowski, J.A., and Suttie, J.W.:* A new carboxylation reaction: the vitamin K-dependent incorporation of $H^{14}CO_3$ into prothrombin. J. biol Chem. *250:* 4744 (1975).

8 *Filmer, D.L. and Cooper, T.G.:* Effect of varying temperature of pH upon the predicted rate of 'CO_2' utilization by carboxylases. J. theor. Biol. *29:* 131 (1970).

9 *Friedman, P.A. and Shia, M.:* Some characteristics of a vitamin K-dependent carboxylating system from rat liver microsomes. Biochem. biophys. Res. Commun. *70:* 647 (1976).

10 *Fuson, R.C.:* The principle of vinylogy. Chem. Rev. *16:* 1 (1935).

11 *Gardner, E.J.:* The effect of menadione (MK-0) and its derivatives on the carboxylation of preprothrombin in a detergent-solubilized rat liver microsomal system. Fed. Proc. Fed. Am. Socs exp. Biol. *36:* 307 (1977).

12 *Girardot, J.M.; Delaney, R., and Johnson, B.C.:* Carboxylation, the completion step in prothrombin biosynthesis. Biochem. biophys. Res. Commun. *59:* 1197 (1974).

13 *Girardot, J.M.; Mack, D.O.; Price, J.; Suen, E., and Johnson, B.C.:* On vitamin K-dependent carboxylation reaction. Fed. Proc. Fed. Am. Socs exp. Biol *36:* 307 (1977).
14 *Houser, R.M.; Jones, J.P.; Fausto, A.; Gardner, E.J.; Lee, F.C., and Olson, R.E.:* Vitamin K-dependent carboxylation of preprothrombin in rat liver microsomes. Fed. Proc. Fed. Am. Socs exp. Biol. *35:* 1353 (1976).
15 *Houser, R.M.; Carey, D.J.; Dus, K.M.; Marshall, G.R. and Olson, R.E.:* Partial sequence of rat prothrombin and the activity of two related pentapeptides as substrates for the vitamin K-dependent carboxylase system. FEBS Lett. *75:* 226 (1977).
16 *Jones, J.P.; Fausto, A.; Houser, R.M.; Gardner, E.J., and Olson, R.E.:* Effect of vitamin K homologues on the conversion of preprothrombin to prothrombin in rat liver microsomes. Biochem. biophys. Res. Commun. *72:* 589 (1976).
17 *Jones, J.P.; Gardner, E.J.; Cooper, T.G., and Olson, R.E.:* The species of carbon dioxide utilized in the vitamin K-dependent carboxylation of preprothrombin. Fed. Proc. Fed. Am. Socs exp. Biol. *36:* 307 (1977).
18 *Magnusson, S.; Sottrup-Hansen, L.; Petersen, T.E.; Morris, H.R., and Dell, A.:* Primary structure of the vitamin K-dependent part of prothrombin. FEBS Lett. *44:* 189 (1974).
19 *Munns, T.W.; Johston, M.F.M.; Liszewski M.K., and Olson, R.E.:* Vitamin K-dependent synthesis and modification of precursor prothrombin in cultured liver cells. Proc. natn. Acad. Sci. USA *73:* 2803 (1976).
20 *Nelsestuen, G.L.; Zytkovicz, T.H., and Howard, J.B.:* The mode of action of vitamin K. Identification of γ-carboxyglutamic acid as a component of prothrombin. J. biol. Chem. *249:* 6347 (1974).
21 *Olson, R.E.:* New concepts relating to the mode of action of vitamin K. Vitams Horm. *32:* 483 (1974).
22 *Sadowski, J.A.; Esmon, C.T., and Suttie, J.W.:* Vitamin K-dependent carboxylase. J. biol. Chem. *251:* 2770 (1976).
23 *Sadowski, J.A.; Schnoes, H.K., and Suttie, J.W.:* Vitamin K epoxidase: properties and relationship to prothrombin synthesis. Biochem. J. *16:* 17 (1977).
24 *Shah, D.V. and Suttie, J.W.:* The vitamin K dependent *in vitro* production of prothrombin. Biochem. biophys. Res. Commun. *60:* 1397 (1974).
25 *Stenflo, J.; Fernlund, P.; Egan, W., and Roepstorff, P.:* Vitamin K-dependent modifications of glutamic acid residues in prothrombin. Proc. natn. Acad. Sci. USA *71:* 2730 (1974).
26 *Suttie, J.W.; Hageman, J.M.; Lehrman, S.R., and Rich, D.H.:* Vitamin K-dependent carboxylase. Development of a peptide substrate. J. biol. Chem. *251:* 5827 (1976).
27 *Vilkas, M. and Lederer, E.:* On the possible mechanism of oxidative phosphorylation. Experientia *18:* 546 (1962).
28 *Willingham, A.K. and Matschiner, J.T.:* Changes in phylloquinone and microsomal clotting activity in the rat. Biochem. J. *140:* 435 (1974).

Dr. *R.E. Olson,* Saint Louis University, School of Medicine, Edward A. Doisy Department of Biochemistry, 1402 South Grand Boulevard, *Saint Louis, MO 63104* (USA)

Wld Rev. Nutr. Diet., vol. 31, pp. 226–231 (Karger, Basel 1978)

A Model of Chemical Thermogenesis Regulated by Ubiquinone

T. Ramasarma and S. Sivaramakrishnan
Department of Biochemistry, Indian Institute of Science, Bangalore

Under conditions of exposure to cold, the production of heat to keep the thermal balance becomes paramount and all tissues seem to contribute. The increased thermogenesis *sans* shivering seems to involve increased food consumption, breakdown of caloric sources and combustion to CO_2 via the same metabolic pathways and increase in metabolic rate and oxygen uptake (7). This process normally occurs under conditions of basal metabolism at rest and is referred to as 'basal non-shivering thermogenesis'. When the ambient temperature goes below thermoneutral zone it increases and the heat thus produced is referred to as 'regulatory non-shivering thermogenesis' (11). The whole effect of increased thermogenesis being readily reversible, the mechanism used must be some kind of regulatory modification of existing metabolic capability. There are a variety of ways for generating the extra heat. Uncoupling of oxidative phosphorylation, activation of pumps of Na-K or Ca and futile cycles. These involve an initial increased production of ATP and subsequent hydrolysis by the exergonic reactions (9). In most tissues the rates of mitochondrial oxidations are increased to a small extent and the phosphorylation system unaffected (10). Thermogenic response can occur by oxidations not associated with coupled electron transport such as in microsomal or peroxisomal systems. We address ourselves to the question of the possibility of a general heat-producing mechanism by transfer of electrons via the alternate or shunt pathways (15) for thermogenic response. Evidence is presented for a model wherein mitochondrial ubiquinone acts as a switch (17) at the level of succinate dehydrogenase for channelling energy towards thermogenesis.

Interaction of Ubiquinone and Succinate Dehydrogenase

The natural acceptor of electrons from the succinate dehydrogenase is ubiquinone. In addition to this primary role, ubiquinone in the mitochondrial mem-

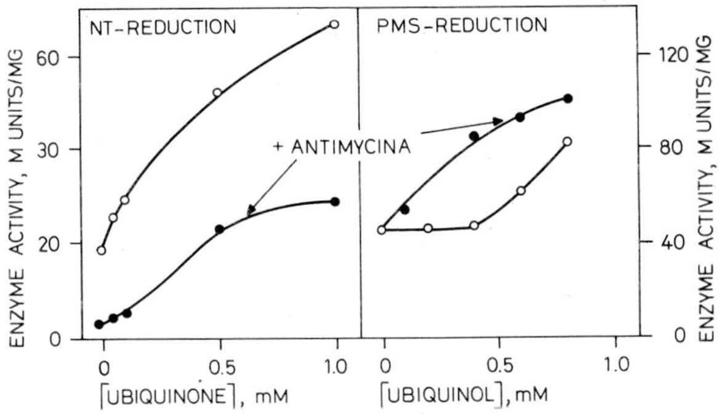

Fig. 1. Activation of succinate dehydrogenase by exogeneous ubiquinone: mitochondria (about 2 mg of protein) from rat liver were preincubated at 37°C for 5 min with varying concentrations of ubiquinone or ubiquinol. Antimycin A (1 μg/mg protein) was incubated in the preincubation medium in the other set of experiments.

brane appears to have a regulatory control on the activity of this enzyme system. In isolated mitochondria, the enzyme from a variety of tissues can be activated by addition of ubiquinone *in vitro.* The activity of the same flavoprotein measured by the reduction of two dyes – phenazine methosulphate (PMS) and neotetrazolium chloride (NT) – are specifically and differently activated by the redox status of ubiquinone. The reduction of PMS is activated by reduced form (12) and that of NT by oxidized form (6). The two activations are specific in the tissues tested: liver, heart, brain, kidney and brown adipose (18).

Significance of Succinate-NT Reduction

A number of properties of NT-reduction are different from that of PMS-reduction. Thus, activation of NT-reduction alone can be obtained on treatment of mitochondria with ubiquinone *in vitro* or the animal *in vivo.* The results in figure 1 show the effect of concentration of ubiquinone or ubiquinol added to liver mitochondria. The PMS-reduction is obtained in the presence of antimycin A, as this protects the added ubiquinol from oxidation. While the PMS-reduction is insensitive to antimycin A, that of NT-reduction is partially sensitive showing thereby that the electron transfer to this dye is dependent on endogenous ubiquinone at an antimycin-sensitive site, but this is bypassed by excess of exogeneous ubiquinone. It is thus possible that NT-reduction represents an alternate way of tapping electrons from the main electron transport sequence at the succinate dehydrogenase level. This should then lead to uptake of oxygen and production of H_2O_2. The two activities – NT-reduction (17) and H_2O_2 production (13) – have some common properties. Both are dependent on succinate as the electron donor and on ubiquinone for the mediation of transfer of electrons. Their site of action is succinate dehydrogenase. Their activities are higher when production or need for ATP is low, such as in state 4 for H_2O_2 production (3) and cold-exposure for NT-reduction (1). Also their activities increased as a 'monotonous function' (4) of added ubiquinone without reaching a saturation limit. It is tempting to speculate that NT-reduction, in fact, may be another measure of that pool of ubiquinone reducible by succinate dehydrogenase and available to interact directly with molecular oxygen for generation of H_2O_2. The regulatory molecules of the quinone must also be differently situated from the main electron transfer component, yet can interact with, and be reducible by, the dehydrogenases. There is evidence that the distribution of ubiquinone in mitochondrial membranes is inhomogeneous (16). Based on these features, it was considered that the activity measured by NT-reduction represents a shunt pathway and energy of electrons passing through this will not be conserved but released as heat (1).

Increase in Hepatic Ubiquinone in Cold Exposure

The liver had been the tissue of choice for experiments with ubiquinone metabolism. Concentration of ubiquinone in the liver progressively increased in rats exposed to low environmental temperature (0–5°C). The overall increase was about 3-fold in acclimated animals (about 30 days) and the increase was mainly accounted for in the particulate fractions, including mitochondrial and microsomal fractions (1). The brown adipose tissue, which is the specialized tissue for thermogenesis in cold-exposed or hibernating or new-born animals, shows a concentration of ubiquinone (about 200 nmol/g) as high as the liver sample from acclimated animals.

Changes in Succinate Oxidation in Thermogenic Conditions

The oxygen uptake by liver slices increased in cold-exposed rats by about 50% (7). This is accompanied by a corresponding change in the succinate oxidase system (1). The activity of succinate dehydrogenase in hepatic mitochondria measured by reduction of either PMS or NT showed increase in both cold-exposed and noradrenaline-treated animals. While the change in PMS-reduction reached a saturation limit by 10 days, that of NT-reduction progressively increased beyond 10 days concomitant with the increase in ubiquinone concentration (1). On the other hand, in the case of noradrenaline treatment both activities reached a maximum at about 2 h and decreased thereafter (fig. 2).

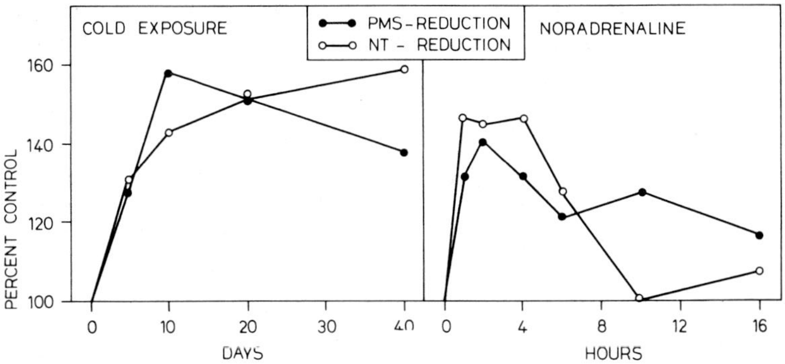

Fig. 2. Hepatic mitochondria were isolated from rats either exposed to cold (0–5°C) or were given noradrenaline (0.2 mg/rat) intraperitoneally for the various periods indicated. The enzymes were assayed as described by *Sivaramakrishnan and Ramasarma* (18). The values are % of control for 4 animals in each group.

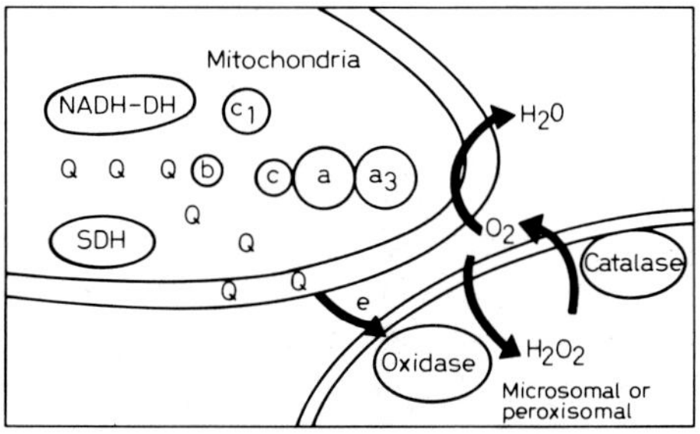

Fig. 3. A model for chemical thermogenesis.

A Model for Chemical Thermogenesis

Alternate pathways of trapping electrons from dehydrogenases yield H_2O_2 as the product. H_2O_2 can also be generated by transferring the reducing equivalents to oxidases in peroxisomes and microsomes. Being cytotoxic, H_2O_2 is normally destroyed rapidly by catalase invariably present in all aerobic cells. It is well known that this is an exergonic reaction and generates heat. In fact such a system is used in an impressive manner by the bombardier beetle for the production of vaporised secretion as a defensive mechanism (5). Their reactor glands possess a mixture of hydroquinone and H_2O_2 which are squeezed into an outer compartment containing peroxidases and catalase in order to trigger the events for production and degradation of H_2O_2 generating sufficient heat for use to vaporize the water. A controlled operation of the same system may provide the basis of intracellular thermogenesis. The model shown in figure 3 proposes that the reducing power in mitochondria is partly transferred to a separate pool of the abundant membrane ubiquinone. This then is oxidized by oxidases present in mitochondria or peroxisomes, or by auto-oxidation producing H_2O_2 which is degraded by catalase. If one mole of O_2 were utilized for each molecule of reduced ubiquinone, oxygen would be recycled. But net increase in oxygen uptake was found in H_2O_2 production in presence of cyanide to abolish cytochrome oxidase activity and also in overall metabolic rate under conditions of increased thermogenesis. This is resolved by the finding that H_2O_2 production requires superoxide dismutase and each set of $(H^+ + e)$ generated one superoxide anion (13). The equations shown below explain the net oxygen uptake of one molecule for a pair of ubiquinol molecules:

$$2\,QH_2 + 4\,O_2 \xrightarrow{\text{Oxidase}} 2Q + 4\,O_2^- + 4\,H^+$$

$$4H^+ + 4\,O_2^- \xrightarrow[\text{Dismutase}]{\text{Superoxide}} 2\,H_2O_2 + 2\,O_2$$

$$2\,H_2O_2 \xrightarrow{\text{Catalase}} 2\,H_2O + O_2$$

$$2\,QH_2 + O_2 \longrightarrow 2\,Q + 2H_2O$$

The reactions leading to formation of H_2O_2 are insensitive to cyanide and antimycin A and will provide oxygen uptake independent of the cytochrome system that accounts for about 30% of the total (11). The energy of electrons passing through this shunt pathway will be released as heat. By suitable modification of available ubiquinone on the membrane and its redox status the extent of energy flow can be regulated with ubiquinone acting as a switch. Ascorbic acid, whose requirement increases in cold exposure is shown to mediate the cyanide-insensitive respiration (2) and may be acting via the above system. This type of alternate electron bypasses leading to cyanide-insensitive respiration and thereby thermogenesis was also observed in plants. The energy expenditure that the plants incur during photorespiration may be justified for generation of localized heat in tissues so that higher metabolic rates be sustained. The inflorescence of a common garden philodendron (14) and the spadix of *Arum maculatum* and *Sanromatum guttalum* (10) exhibit core temperature 10–15°C higher than the ambient. It is more than coincidence that spadix have a high ubiquinone concentration (8). It is, therefore, conjectured that ubiquinol-H_2O_2-catalase system may turn out to be a universal mechanism for all the thermogenic cells.

Acknowledgement

The earlier work in this laboratory was carried out by Drs. *H.N. Aithal* and *L. Susheela.* This forms part of the project on 'Environmental stress and biochemical adaptation' supported by the Office of Naval Research, USA (#N00014-71-C-0348). *S. Sivaramakrishnan* is a Senior Research Fellow of Council of Scientific and Industrial Research, New Delhi.

References

1 *Aithal, H.N. and Ramasarma, T.:* Biochem. J. *123:* 677 (1971).
2 *Arrigoni, R.; Liso, G., and Calabrese:* Science *194:* 332 (1976).
3 *Boveries, A. and Chance, B.:* Biochem. J. *134:* 707 (1973).
4 *Boveries, A.; Cadenas, E., and Stoppani, A.O.M.:* Biochem. J. *156:* 435 (1976).
5 *Eisner, T.:* Chemical ecology; p. 157 (Academic Press, New York 1970).
6 *Gutman, M.; Kearney, E.B., and Singer, T.P.:* Biochem. J. *10:* 2726 (1971).
7 *Hart, J.S.:* Fed. Proc. Fed. Am. Socs exp. Biol. *17:* 1045 (1958).
8 *Hemming, F.W.; Morton, R.A., and Pennock, J.F.:* Proc. R. Soc. B *158:* 291 (1963).
9 *Himms-Hagen, J.:* Ann. Rev. Physiol. *38:* 315 (1976).
10 *Hochachka, P.W.:* Fed. Proc. Fed. Am. Socs exp. Biol. *33:* 2162 (1974).
11 *Jansky, L.:* Biol. Rev. *44:* 85 (1973).
12 *Lester, R.L. and Smith, A.L.:* Biochim. biophys. Acta *47:* 475 (1961).
13 *Loschen, F.; Flohe, L., and Chance, B.:* FEBS Lett. *18:* 261 (1971).
14 *Nagy, K.A.; Odell, D.K., and Seymour, R.S.:* Science *178:* 1195 (1972).
15 *Potter, V.R.:* Fed. Proc. Fed. Am. Socs exp. Biol. *17:* 1060 (1958).
16 *Ramasarma, T. and Lester, R.L.:* J. biol. Chem. *235:* 3309 (1960).
17 *Ramasarma, T. and Susheela, L.:* in *Packer* Biomembranes – architecture, biogenesis, bioenergetic and differentiation; p. 261 (Academic Press, New York 1974).
18 *Sivaramakrishnan, S. and Ramasarma, T.:* Environ. Physiol. Biochem. *5:* 189 (1975).

Dr. *T. Ramasarma,* Department of Biochemistry, Indian Institute of Science, *Bangalore 560012* (India)

Wld Rev. Nutr. Diet., vol. 31, pp. 232–242 (Karger, Basel 1978)

Concluding Remarks

James Allen Olson
Biochemistry and Biophysics Department, Iowa State University, Ames, Iowa

So now, after three and a half days of intense effort, we come to the end of our symposium. This symposium was particularly rich in personal interactions, which are the first tentative steps in the development of new and fruitful professional relationships. In his inaugural address, Professor *Morton* focused on some fascinating modern aspects of visual pigment physiology and some possible molecular transformations in the rhodopsin molecule. The protonated Schiff-base, for example, may well have an exomethylene group, and the initial absorption of light quanta by rhodopsin must involve an energized state prior to the cumbersome time-consuming process of isomerization. We were all shocked to learn of his sudden demise shortly after his return to Liverpool. As one of the great figures in biochemistry of the past half century, his presence and his example will be sorely missed.

After an introduction to isoprenoids by Dr. *Sharman,* we considered the transport of vitamin A. Dr. *Rask* discussed how plasma retinol binding protein (pRBP) is formed in the liver on the rough endoplasmic reticulum, and then secreted. In vitamin A deficiency, the synthesis of RBP is faster and the apo-RBP accumulates in the liver. Professor *Glover* found that free retinol of the liver interchanges rapidly with retinol in holo-RBP ($t_{\frac{1}{2}}$ = 2.7 h), and that the secretion of holo-RBP occurs quickly after retinol is given to a vitamin A-deficient rat. But the pRBP level in the plasma oscillates in two distinct ways: (i) a diurnal cycle, and (ii) a seasonal cycle, which is closely associated with gonadal maturation. Whether pRBP release is predominantly stimulated by estrogen or by some other hormonal factor is not yet clear.

Dr. *Muto* has carefully distinguished: (i) animals with mainly a pRBP-PA complex, which include the human, rabbit, rat, chick, goat, buffalo and frog; (ii) organisms with free pRBP, which include fish, the cow and the shark, and (iii) organisms which, oddly enough, have no pRBP at all, but apparently carry vitamin A in ester form as a lipoprotein. The lamprey, a cyclostome, is the only known member of this latter group. A further study of this unique characteristic and its relation to vitamin A uptake and function by epithelial cells will be most welcome. Mr. *Sreekrishna* showed that goat pRBP binds all-*trans* retinol most tightly, with an association constant 20-fold higher than reported for other species.

Dr. *Pirie* examined pRBP levels in Indian children from Madurai, suffering from xerophthalmia. Whereas initial pRBP levels were around 15 μg/ml, treatment with vitamin A caused them to rise within 4–13 days to a normal level of around 33 μg/ml. When these children were returned to their home environments, however, pRBP levels tended again to slip downward. Thus, emphasis clearly must be placed on educating the mother about proper nutrition during the nutritional rehabilitation. Interestingly, mild cases of corneal xerosis (X2) seem to be cured as effectively by dietary carotenoids as by the administration of a large dose of vitamin A.

Another clinical condition, namely urinary excretion of RBP as a result of cadmium poisoning, was discussed by Professor *Kanai.* During cadmium-induced tubular proteinuria, about 70 mg RBP, 20 mg β_2-microglobulin (11,800 daltons), 70 mg albumin and smaller amounts of other proteins are lost each day in the urine. By plotting the log of albumin excretion *vs* the log of RBP excretion, Professor *Kanai* was able to distinguish readily between normal individuals and cases of either glomerular or tubular proteinuria.

The high specificity of pRBP for all-*trans* retinol was stressed in a fascinating discussion of α-retinol by Dr. *Pitt.* As reported 7 years earlier, α-retinol shows all the hypervitaminotic and membrane effects of retinol while possessing only 2% of the biological activity in the conventional rat growth test. Dr. *Pitt* now attributes the biological inactivity of α-retinol to the inability of pRBP to transport it to peripheral tissue sites. When α-retinol is actually presented to the target tissue, such as in the hamster cheek pouch or in tracheal cell cultures, its activity is similar to that of retinol. Thus, the specificity of plasma retinol binding protein seems to be a major controlling step in the utilization of vitamin A and its derivatives by tissues.

One of the most exciting areas of present vitamin A research is the manner in which vitamin A interacts with target cells. As shown in elegant studies by both Drs. *Rask and Heller,* surface receptors for pRBP exist on target cells. Studying the pigment epithelium of the eye, Dr. *Heller* found that I^{125}-labeled pRBP bound in less than one minute to receptors located on the infolded plasmalemma of the pigment epithelium. Binding occurred only on the outer membrane, and holo-pRBP was more tightly held than apo-pRBP. Retinol apparently is then transferred from pRBP into the membrane, and finally into the cell. Dr. *Rask* presented a similar model based on the use of holo-pRBP covalently bound to a large non-absorbable polysaccharide. By using an immunofluorescent technique for pRBP, Dr. *Rask* found a heavy concentration of pRBP bound to the outer keratinized layers of epithelial tissue, but little or none near the metabolically active basal membrane cells. In all likelihood, the binding of pRBP to all target epithelial cells is similar, but whereas the metabolically active cells take up retinol well and then release apo-pRBP, the less active squamous cells become saturated with unused holo-pRBP. Interestingly, epithelial cells in psoriasis do not contain bound pRBP.

The surface receptor is therfore a second site of control for vitamin A utilization. Some cells have receptors, and consequently are target cells, whereas others do not. In either case, how vitamin A passes through the membrane is still uncertain. Quite possibly a membrane carrier – let's call it a retinol permease – actually strips retinol from the RBP cell receptor complex and facilitates its entrance into cells.

Once within the target cell, the retinol is not free to wander, but rather combines with another specific carrier, termed cellular retinol binding protein (cRBP). Dr. *Chytil* pioneered studies on intracellular binding proteins for retinol and retinoic acid, termed cellular retinol binding protein (cRBP) and cellular retinoic acid binding protein (cRABP). Although approximately of the same size (*ca.* 14,000 daltons), these proteins are relatively specific for their respective ligands. In addition to all-*trans* retinol, cRBP apparently binds some *cis* isomers of retinol, but neither retinal nor retinoic acid. Some tissues have both cRBP and cRABP; namely, the brain, eye, testes, uterus and ovary; some, like the intestinal mucosa, kidney, liver, lung and spleen, have only cRBP, and muscle and heart have neither. The cellular binding proteins are distinct both from pRBP and from the surface receptor. Unlike pRBP, however, the concentrations of cRBP and cRABP are not affected by vitamin A deficiency.

Just why cRABP is present in the testes is at first glance puzzling, inasmuch as retinoic acid, given either orally or injected into testicular tissue, has no spermatogenic effect. To resolve this dilemma, Dr. *Chytil* suggests that *both* cRBP *and* cRAPB are required for spermatogenesis. Since retinol is readily converted enzymically to retinoic acid, the administration of retinol produces a biological effect, whereas retinoic acid itself, which cannot be reduced to retinol, will react only with cRABP.

In a purely diagnostic sense, cRABP may be a useful marker. Tumors of the breast and lung, unlike normal tissues, contain significant concentrations of cRABP. Since the synthetic β-retinoids combine with cRABP, the presence of that carrier in a tumour may indicate a sensitivity to the β-retinoids for anticancer therapy. This interesting observation of Dr. *Chytil* certainly bears attention and careful follow-up.

A surprisingly large cRBP exists in the pigment epithelium and in the cytosol of photoreceptor cells, as shown by Dr. *Heller.* Whereas the association constant of pRBP for retinol is usually around 10^6 *L/M,* that of cRBP is around 10^{12} *L/M,* a much stronger association.

The next metabolic and functional actions of retinol are obviously of great interest. In photoreceptor cells, of course, retinol undergoes oxidation to retinal, which is isomerized in a $FADH_2$-dependent reaction to 11-*cis* retinal, and then associates with one of the retinal binding proteins, the opsins. In epithelial cells, the retinol-cRBP complex probably diffuses into the nucleus, where, in all likelihood, it interacts with the genome, leading ultimately to the formation of a specific set of proteins which are characteristic of a given differentiated state of an epithelial cell. We know essentially nothing of these additional binding proteins; indeed, whether or not they even exist. Before embracing too enthusiastically this model for retinol in differentiation, however, we should soberly realize that no specific gene product for retinol has yet been identified.

Several years ago I referred to vitamin A as an elegant young girl of mysterious and irrestistible charm. She has clearly grown up in recent years, and is now constantly surrounded by a group of protein chaperones, not only to protect her during her travels in the stream of life and to open doors for her passage into cells, but also to direct her rather wilful intracellular activities. Hopefully we might look forward, before too long, to the notice of her marriage, possibly by interaction with the genome to produce specific proteins involved in differentiation, by controlling crucial events in the latter process, or indeed by quite different mechanisms. Predicting a young lady's behavior, however, is always an uncertain task!

Relative to possible modulating effects of vitamin A on differentiation was the fascinating study of the effect of vitamin A on the development of the estrogen-stimulated chick oviduct. Professor *Ganguly* showed that vitamin A-deficient rats responded poorly to estrogen stimulation in terms of cell number, size and acini per lobe. Retinoic acid, although not as satisfactory as retinol, did possess stimulatory activity. In a most interesting *in vitro* study, retinol was found to stimulate by about 50% the uptake of ^{3}H-thymidine into the DNA of oviduct cells. Other experiments with regenerating liver also suggest that vitamin A deficiency markedly depresses cell division and differentiation. Further studies on these interesting models will be watched with attention.

Vitamin A might, of course, act in different ways. Professor *Wolf* described the elegant studies which he and Dr. *Luigi DeLuca* have been conducting over the past 5 or 6 years. Physiologically retinol is activated by ATP to yield retinyl phosphate, which then, upon reaction with GDP-mannose, yields retinyl-phosphomannose. The latter may then transfer mannose to a glycoprotein receptor. In the liver the specific receptor seems to be an α-macroglobulin which is then released into the plasma. Interestingly this α_1-macroglobulin is a proteinase inhibitor, and its absence in vitamin A deficiency may enhance the rapid collagenolytic destruction of the cornea seen in keratomalacia.

Vitamin A might also play a role in membranes, as shown by Dr. *Vakil.* A small but significant amount of vitamin A is associated with most cell membranes. In vitamin A deficiency, more lysolecithin and fewer polyunsaturated fatty acids were present in membranes, the membranes were more fragile, and peroxidative reactions were enhanced. Dr. *Ninjoor* reported that the irradiation of β-carotene or vitamin A gave products which enhanced lysosome fragility. Quite possibly peroxidative reactions are also involved in this case.

In an extensive study on phospholipid metabolism in retinol-fed animals, Dr. *Misra* showed that the pattern of unsaturated fatty acids in phospholipids was altered and that the transfer of phospholipid between microsomes and mitochondria was enhanced, again suggesting a membrane effect of large doses of vitamin A. Dr. *Rama Rao* found that vitamin A-depleted rats had less gangliosides in the brain and catabolized basic brain proteins at a slower rate than normal animals, suggesting a disruption of the process of myelinization in deficient animals. Gluconeogenesis is also reduced in vitamin A deficiency but markedly stimulated by excessive doses of vitamin A. In a careful metabolic analysis of the reaction sequence, Dr. *Singh* found that key enzymes in the pathway, namely PEP carboxykinase, fructose-1,6-diphosphatase and glucose-6-phosphatase, as well as alanine amino-transferase were stimulated in the hypervitaminotic state. Plasma free fatty acids also increased. Although the role of vitamin A in these processes is not well defined, the alterations may well contribute to the clinically described syndrome of either deficiency or toxicity.

Studies on the metabolism of vitamin A itself played a smaller role in this symposium than in previous like conferences. Nonetheless some important and interesting findings were presented. Dr. *Barua,* in studying the formation of 3 dehydroretinol (vitamin A_2) in fish *(S. fossilis),* showed that lutein is converted biologically to dehydrolutein, which then undergoes cleavage, probably, but not necessarily, at the 15,15′ double bond, to yield 3-dehydroretinol and 3-hydroxyretinol. Interestingly, fed β-carotene was not converted to retinol in the liver, but did give rise to retinoic acid in the intestine. Dr. *Sundaresan* summarized his careful studies on the kinetics of vitamin A excretion after dosing rats with labeled vitamin A. Three distinct phases were found: a rapid metabolism phase (to 7 days), a maintenance and liver depletion phase (1–6 weeks) and a final depletion phase. The excretion patterns found were in excellent keeping with known metabolic reactions of vitamin A in the rat. In addition, Dr. *Sundaresan* noted increased activity of retinal oxidase in zinc deficiency and a marked depression (10%) in the retinal concentration in transplanted mucinous adenocarcinomas relative to the parent intestinal mucosa. These interesting observations serve as a useful starting point for defining in greater detail vitamin A interactions in cancer and with zinc.

A major, global nutritional problem in children is vitamin A deficiency, which each year causes blindness in 15–20,000 children in India and 50–80,000 children in the world. Dr. *Srikantia* summarized the outstanding studies which the Hyderabad Laboratory has conducted over the past ten years. Of various possible strategies – nutrition education, distribution of vitamin A capsules, fortification of staples, home gardens, and massive dosing – the latter was selected as the most suitable and immediately effective. An oral dose of 200,000 IU of retinyl palmitate in oil was selected for administration every 6 months to children 1–5 years of age. Symptoms of hypervitaminosis A, which occurred in only a few children, were mild and transient both by clinical and biochemical signs. The efficiency of absorption (66%) and retention (47%) was satisfactory, but tended to be reduced in infections. A prophylactic program has been instituted in nine Indian states, and in the best supervised programs a reduction of 60–75% in the signs of mild deficiency (XIB, etc.) were noted. Although the vitamin A status of treated children has clearly improved, no direct evidence yet exists that the incidence of blindness is decreasing. A study of blindness in treated areas is now being initiated in a hospital in Hyderabad. Mr. *Shivakumar* described the effects of kwashiorkor, gastrointestinal and respiratory infections, and ascariasis on the absorption and storage of vitamin A in children. As expected, both absorption and storage were better at low (1 mg) than at high (60 mg) doses of vitamin A. Infections reduced absorption and storage by 20–30%, but surprisingly protein calorie malnutrition had little adverse effect.

Ultimately, vitamin A nutriture can only be improved by increasing the carotenoid and vitamin A content of the diet. To this end, Mr. *Premachandra* described his studies on crossing the local strain of a tomato, which is high in lycopene and low in β-carotene, with some strains containing high β-carotene and low lycopene. Suitable F_2 generations with roughly equal amounts of β-carotene and lycopene were selected for use in the field. Along a similar line, Dr. *Murthy* described her work on the use of amaranth and carotene-rich leaf protein extracts in improving the vitamin A status of children in Coimbatore, and Dr. *Rajalakshmi* discussed the effect of food usage patterns, food costs and cooking on the ingestion of carotene in Gujarat and Kerala states.

The use of oral contraceptives influences the nutritional status, as shown by Dr. *Bamji.* In women taking estrogen-containing contraceptive drugs, the plasma vitamin A levels increase 30–60% within 10–15 days and then remain elevated. The mechanism seems to be an estrogen-induced increase both of pRBP synthesis and its release from the liver, which is associated with a somewhat more rapid depletion of liver vitamin A reserves. In women with a poor vitamin A status, the drug may exacerbate the condition. The concomitant use of multivitamin pills, including, of course, vitamin A, was therefore recommended.

Inasmuch as the focus in nutrition research and public health tends to be largely on the deficiency state, Dr. *James Olson* suggested that vitamin A status be considered in a broader context than solely in reference to signs of deficiency. Vitamin A status was defined in terms of protection period, i.e., the length of time that a child given a vitamin-free diet would not show any signs of vitamin A deficiency. For a protection period of 100 days, which was selected as the minimal satisfactory period, a 15 kg child needs a liver storage of 20 μg retinol/g weight of liver. Children with liver values of 5 μg retinol/g or below are in imminent risk of clinical vitamin A deficiency. Based on the use of liver autopsy samples, the concept and guidelines developed were tested in Salvador, Brazil, among children dying of various causes. The use of this new approach to vitamin A nutriture might be of considerable value in areas where autopsy samples can be readily obtained.

In his discussion of the metabolism and function of vitamin D, Dr. *Fraser* stressed that suitable physiological mechanisms do not exist for controlling the 25-hydroxycalciferol concentration in the plasma. The natural pathway for vitamin D synthesis is the photochemical conversion of 7-dehydrocholesterol to calciferol in the skin, and then transport in the plasma on a vitamin D binding protein to the liver. Interestingly, deep sea fish who live in constant darkness may have evolved a light-independent enzymatic process of forming vitamin D, inasmuch as considerable quantities exist in the liver, whereas dietary vitamin D is quickly metabolized. Since the rate of photochemical formation of vitamin D is only moderate, the vitamin D binding protein, which is largely in the *apo* form, normally serves as a physiological buffer for the transformation of vitamin D to 25-hydroxycalciferol. Dietary vitamin D, on the other hand, is rapidly converted to 25-hydroxycalciferol, leading to a transiently high concentration in the plasma. Since vitamin D toxicity is due to 25-hydroxycalciferol, serious attention should be given to possible long-term toxic effects of dietary vitamin D.

The function of vitamin E remains rather puzzling. Unquestionably it does serve as an antioxidant, but whether it has other more specific roles is still very much debated. On the other hand, the functional interrelation between vitamin E and selenium, for many years also shrouded in uncertainty, is now becoming much clearer. Among many effects of vitamin E deficiency are kidney abnormalities and liver necrosis. In the kidney of PUFA-fed, vitamin E deficient animals, as discussed by Professor *Moore,* a large number of brown granular bodies appear and the tubules become more susceptible to post-mortem autolysis than are normal kidney tubules. Several other tissues do not show such changes. Liver necrosis in PUFA-fed animals, on the other hand, can be prevented either by selenium or by vitamin E. Dr. *Diplock* focused his attention on this interrelationship. Vitamin E stabilizes membranes as an anti-oxidant, but also shows some specific physiological actions which are not substituted by other antioxidants. Selenium, on the other hand, is an intrinsic part of glutathione peroxidase, which reduces lipid peroxides (or H_2O_2) with a concomitant conversion of reduced glutathione to its oxidized form. Dr. *Diplock* envisioned that vitamin E deficiency causes a change in membrane structure such that phospholipase is able to release PUFA, which, being more accessible to oxygen, are then converted to peroxyradicals. The peroxyradicals may react with any vitamin E present to yield hydroperoxides. In the presence of glutathione and glutathione peroxidase, however, peroxyradicals and hydroperoxides are reduced to hydroxyacids, thereby breaking the chain reaction and protecting the membrane from further degradation. In concordance with this mechanism, Dr. *Fatterpaker* found that lysolecithin increased in mitochondrial membranes from vitamin E deficient animals, probably as a result of increased phospholipase A_2 activity and a fall in the lysolecithin acylating enzyme in the membrane.

Vitamin E tends to associate preferentially with phospholipid containing polyunsaturated fatty acids in model membrane systems. Using the Langmuir trough technique, Professor *Lucy* found, further, that vitamin E reacted poorly with saturated fatty acids and cholesterol, but that a small proportion of unsaturated fatty acids in the lipid mixture strongly promoted association with vitamin E. Of analogues with various chain lengths, α-tocopherol$_{15}$, the natural compound, interacted most strongly with the polyunsaturated fatty acids. Since membranes tend to contain more unsaturated fatty acids on their inner surfaces, vitamin E is probably more highly concentrated there as well. These physicochemical interactions of vitamin E with lipids must certainly contribute significantly to the more complex interactions existing in natural membranes.

The field of vitamin K research is in a most exciting stage, following the observations of *Stenflo* that prothrombin contains a number of γ-carboxy glutamyl residues. Vitamin K is required for the carboxylation of the prothrombin precursor, and all three of the speakers (Dr. *Suttie,* Dr. *Robert Olson* and Dr. *Johnson*) mainly considered the requirements and possible mechanism of this reaction. The carboxylation of prothrombin requires the hydroquinone form of vitamin K, carbon dioxide and molecular oxygen. ATP apparently serves as an allosteric modulator but is not used as a phosphate donor. Biotin is not involved in the reaction and the enzyme system is sensitive to sulfhydryl binding agents. The post-mitochondrial supernatant solution, the microsomal membrane preparation and the solubilized enzyme system have similar properties with some exceptions.

Dr. *Suttie* particularly stressed his recent use of several synthetic pentapeptides, including Phe.Leu.Glu.Glu.Ile, as an acceptor for CO_2 in place of the endogenous prothrombin precursor. Dr. *Johnson* indicated that the β,γ unsaturation in the vitamin K side chain was essential for activity, that a half reduced mixture of quinone and hydroquinone was active in the reaction, and that the methine phosphate of vitamin K was inactive. Tritium from ^3H_2O was not incorporated into the carboxylated product, excluding the β,γ unsaturation of glutamate as a reaction intermediate. Dr. *R. Olson* discussed dose-response relationships, showed that CO_2 and not bicarbonate was the active species at a half-saturation concentration of 0.2 m*M*, and pointed out that menaquinones 2–6 were all equally effective in the reaction, whereas analogues with longer or shorter side chains were less active. The formation of an interesting adduct of menaquinone and dithiothreitol was also discussed.

One possible intermediate for the reaction presented by Dr. *R. Olson* was the O-carboxyl-quinol adduct, although clearly other mechanisms might also be written. Further work on the mechanism of this fascinating reaction will be watched with great interest. In addition, the possible physiological involvement of vitamin K oxide, both as an intermediate in and in the control of the carboxylation reaction, must certainly be considered. And finally, the involvement of vitamin K in other protein carboxylation reactions, both in bone tissues and in the formation of other serum proteins not involved in clotting reactions, suggests that this vitamin might have much broader functions in physiology than previously thought.

In mycobacteria vitamin K is known to be involved in substrate level phosphorylation. Dr. *P.S. Murthy* showed that two systems exist for the reduction of vitamin K by malate, the first via NAD and a flavoprotein and the second via a flavoprotein enzyme alone. The latter enzyme, termed malate vitamin K reductose, generates an EPR signal characteristic of a non-heme iron intermediate during malate oxidation. *M. smegmatis* contains only this latter system, whereas *M. phlei* contains both pathways for vitamin K reduction.

The ring of ubiquinone is synthesized *in vivo* from tyrosine via p-hydroxycinnamic acid, which is followed by methylation and the addition of the isoprenoid side chain. The major control point in the biosynthetic sequence, according to Dr. *Aiyar,* is mevalonate-NADP oxidoreductase of liver microsomes, exactly the same as in cholesterol biosynthesis.

A possible novel role of ubiquinone in thermogenesis was proposed by Dr. *Ramasarma.* Since the production of heat accounts for 30% of the total energy released in the body, heat production is a major and highly controlled aspect of nutrient utilization. The ubiquinone concentration in mitochondria increases significantly in response to cold exposure. Dr. *Ramasarma* suggests that the redox status of ubiquinone may direct the oxidation of succinate towards either heat production or ATP synthesis, depending on the needs of the organism.

In conclusion, we might venture to cite some possibly fruitful areas of future endeavor. Although broad in scope, the symposium really centered on three major topics: carrier proteins for vitamin A, programs and strategies for improving vitamin A nutriture, and the function of vitamin K.

In its overall metabolism vitamin A passes through a series of complexes with lipids and proteins, varying increasingly from the non-specific to the specific. During its digestion to free retinol and its absorption as a lipid micelle in the gut, through its transport as an ester in chylomicra to its storage in a low density lipoprotein in the liver, the association of vitamin A with lipids and proteins tends to be relatively non-specific. The formation of a retinol-RBP complex in the liver and its release into the plasma, is a highly specific and well controlled process, however, and even though complexes between several analogues of retinol and RBP can be formed *in vitro,* all-*trans* retinol is the only vitamin A species normally transported by plasma RBP.

Thereafter retinol always seems to be bound to a protein. In future consideration of any physiological action of vitamin A, therefore, we should always be curious about the nature of its protein carrier. In other words, the complex between vitamin A and a specific protein carrier may well be the active physiological unit, and not vitamin A itself. The absence of a specific protein component, as might occur for example in psoriasis or possibly in retinitis pigmentosa, may well be just as important for vitamin A function as the lack of vitamin A itself.

The actual function of vitamin A in growth and differentiation is not known, and it is premature to assign it any specific role. In general the idea that vitamin A, bound naturally to a specific protein, interacts with the genome and 'turns on' the synthesis of a given group of proteins characteristic of a certain differentiated cell, analogous to the action of 17β-estradiol, is most attractive. But no specific vitamin A-dependent gene product has been noted, and physiologically vitamin A has much less dramatic effects on tissues than does estrogen. Nonetheless this approach is exciting and will certainly be explored by many workers in the field.

A resurgence of interest in the role of vitamin A in membranes may also be expected, mainly in view of the role of rhodopsin, a trans-membrane disc protein, in calcium release and the action of membrane bound bacterio-rhodopsin in directing proton transport in halophilic bacteria. That vitamin A, as a sugar phosphate derivative, serves as a transfer function in the synthesis of specific glycoproteins, must also be carefully considered. These diverse functions are not mutually exclusive, for indeed the overall effects of any of them may be widespread. Nonetheless it would be nice to discover a single molecular action of vitamin A on the basis of which the diverse effects of vitamin A deficiency might be rationalized.

In terms of public health programs for the reduction of vitamin A deficiency, massive dosing has certainly been successfully employed in several countries. But the massive dosing program is labor-intensive, tends to be less effective in reaching its target group on subsequent rounds, and is intrinsically an emergency and fairly costly measure. The problem is to find ways of improving the diet of small children by the use of more wholesome, inexpensive and available foods.

The field of vitamin K research is in a most exciting state, and the enticing leads presented in this symposium on the mechanism of carboxylation of γ-glutamyl residues in the prothrombin precursor have whetted our appetites. Although the mechanism is not immediately evident, one feels that it should soon be clarified. Perhaps we will also then better understand the role of the epoxide of vitamin K in the control of prothrombin synthesis. But perhaps the most interesting aspect is that vitamin K may have a much broader role in metabolism than in the formation of clotting proteins alone.

Some other topics might have been considered in the symposium. For example, attention might well have given to the important carrier functions of dolichylphosphate derivatives, not just in reference to mannosyl retinyl phosphate, but in general. And since vitamin D was included as a topic, a fuller discussion of vitamin D metabolism and function would have been welcome. But these topics might be left for another occasion; indeed, the symposium would probably have been too long and wearying with additional major concerns.

Then, with a final salute to Professor *Cama* and his gracious colleagues at the Indian Institute of Science, we turned and, with bags and tickets in hand, rushed off, either to various parts of India or to the four corners of the world.

Dr. *J.A. Olson,* Biochemistry and Biophysics Department, Iowa State University, *Ames, IA 50011* (USA)

Subject Index